1996
YEAR BOOK OF
VASCULAR SURGERY®

Statement of Purpose

The YEAR BOOK Service

The YEAR BOOK series was devised in 1901 by practicing health professionals who observed that the literature of medicine and related disciplines had become so voluminous that no one individual could read and place in perspective every potential advance in a major specialty. In the final decade of the 20th century, this recognition is more acutely true than it was in 1901.

More than merely a series of books, YEAR BOOK volumes are the tangible results of a unique service designed to accomplish the following:

- to *survey* a wide range of journals of proven value
- to *select* from those journals papers representing significant advances and statements of important clinical principles
- to provide *abstracts* of those articles that are readable, convenient summaries of their key points
- to provide *commentary* about those articles to place them in perspective.

These publications grow out of a unique process that calls on the talents of outstanding authorities in clinical and fundamental disciplines, trained literature specialists, and professional writers, all supported by the resources of Mosby, the world's preeminent publisher for the health professions.

The Literature Base

Mosby and its Editors survey more than 1,000 journals published worldwide, covering the full range of the health professions. On an annual basis, the publisher examines usage patterns and polls its expert authorities to add new journals to the literature base and to delete journals that are no longer useful as potential YEAR BOOK sources.

The Literature Survey

The publisher's team of literature specialists, all of whom are trained and experienced health professionals, examines every original, peer-reviewed article in each journal issue. More than 250,000 articles per year are scanned systematically, including title, text, illustrations, tables, and references. Each scan is compared, article by article, to the search strategies that the publisher has developed in consultation with the 270 outside experts who form the pool of YEAR BOOK editors. A given article may be reviewed by any number of editors, from one to a dozen or more, regardless of the discipline for which the paper was originally published. In turn, each editor who receives the article reviews it to determine whether or not the article should be included in the YEAR BOOK. This decision is based on the article's inherent quality, its probable usefulness to readers of that YEAR BOOK, and the editor's goal to represent a balanced picture of a given field in each volume of the YEAR BOOK. In addition, the editor indicates when to include figures and tables from the article to help the YEAR BOOK reader better understand the information.

Of the quarter million articles scanned each year, only 5% are selected for detailed analysis within the YEAR BOOK series, thereby assuring readers of the high value of every selection.

The Abstract

The publisher's abstracting staff is headed by a physician-writer and includes individuals with training in the life sciences, medicine, and other areas, plus extensive experience in writing for the health professions and related industries. Each selected article is assigned to a specific writer on this abstracting staff. The abstracter, guided in many cases by notations supplied by the expert editor, writes a structured, condensed summary designed so that the reader can rapidly acquire the essential information contained in the article.

The Commentary

The YEAR BOOK editorial boards, sometimes assisted by guest commentators, write comments that place each article in perspective for the reader. This provides the reader with the equivalent of a personal consultation with a leading international authority—an opportunity to better understand the value of the article and to benefit from the authority's thought processes in assessing the article.

Additional Editorial Features

The editorial boards of each YEAR BOOK organize the abstracts and comments to provide a logical and satisfying sequence of information. To enhance the organization, editors also provide introductions to sections or individual chapters, comments linking a number of abstracts, citations to additional literature, and other features.

The published YEAR BOOK contains enhanced bibliographic citations for each selected article, including extended listings of multiple authors and identification of author affiliations. Each YEAR BOOK contains a Table of Contents specific to that year's volume. From year to year, the Table of Contents for a given YEAR BOOK will vary depending on developments within the field.

Every YEAR BOOK contains a list of the journals from which papers have been selected. This list represents a subset of the more than 1,000 journals surveyed by the publisher, and occasionally reflects a particularly pertinent article from a journal that is not surveyed on a routine basis.

Finally, each volume contains a comprehensive subject index and an index to authors of each selected paper.

The 1996 Year Book Series

Year Book of Allergy, Asthma, and Clinical Immunology: Drs. Rosenwasser, Borish, Gelfand, Leung, Nelson, and Szefler

Year Book of Anesthesiology and Pain Management: Drs. Tinker, Abram, Chestnut, Roizen, Rothenberg, and Wood

Year Book of Cardiology®: Drs. Schlant, Collins, Engle, Gersh, Kaplan, and Waldo

Year Book of Chiropractic®: Dr. Lawrence

Year Book of Critical Care Medicine®: Drs. Parrillo, Balk, Calvin, Franklin, and Shapiro

Year Book of Dentistry®: Drs. Meskin, Berry, Kennedy, Leinfelder, Roser, Summitt, and Zakariasen

Year Book of Dermatologic Surgery®: Drs. Swanson, Glogau, and Salasche

Year Book of Dermatology®: Drs. Sober and Fitzpatrick

Year Book of Diagnostic Radiology®: Drs. Federle, Clark, Gross, Latchaw, Madewell, Maynard, and Young

Year Book of Digestive Diseases®: Drs. Greenberger and Moody

Year Book of Drug Therapy®: Drs. Lasagna and Weintraub

Year Book of Emergency Medicine®: Drs. Wagner, Davidson, Dronen, King, Niemann, and Roberts

Year Book of Endocrinology®: Drs. Bagdade, Braverman, Horton, Kannan, Landsberg, Molitch, Morley, Nathan, Odell, Poehlman, Rogol, and Ryan

Year Book of Family Practice®: Drs. Berg, Bowman, Davidson, Dexter, and Scherger

Year Book of Geriatrics and Gerontology®: Drs. Beck, Burton, Rabins, Reuben, Roth, Shapiro, and Whitehouse

Year Book of Hand Surgery®: Drs. Amadio and Hentz

Year Book of Hematology®: Drs. Spivak, Bell, Blume, Ness, Quesenberry, and Wiernik

Year Book of Infectious Diseases®: Drs. Keusch, Barza, Bennish, Klempner, Skolnik, and Snydman

Year Book of Infertility and Reproductive Endocrinology: Drs. Mishell, Lobo, and Sokol

Year Book of Medicine®: Drs. Bone, Cline, Epstein, Greenberger, Malawista, Mandell, O'Rourke, and Utiger

Year Book of Neonatal and Perinatal Medicine®: Drs. Fanaroff and Klaus

Year Book of Nephrology, Hypertension and Mineral Metabolism: Drs. Coe, Curtis, Favus, Henderson, Kashgarian, Luke, and Myers

Year Book of Neurology and Neurosurgery®: Drs. Bradley and Wilkins

Year Book of Neuroradiology: Drs. Osborn, Eskridge, Grossman, Hudgins, and Ross

Year Book of Nuclear Medicine®: Drs. Gottschalk, Blaufox, McAfee, Wackers, and Zubal

Year Book of Obstetrics and Gynecology®: Drs. Mishell, Herbst, and Kirschbaum

Year Book of Occupational and Environmental Medicine®: Drs. Emmett, Frank, Gochfeld, and Hessl

Year Book of Oncology®: Drs. Simone, Bosl, Cohen, Glatstein, Ozols, and Tallman

Year Book of Ophthalmology®: Drs. Cohen, Augsburger, Eagle, Flanagan, Grossman, Laibson, Maguire, Nelson, Rapuano, Sergott, Tasman, Tipperman, and Wilson

Year Book of Orthopedics®: Drs. Sledge, Cofield, Dobyns, Griffin, Poss, Springfield, Swiontkowski, Wiesel, and Wilson

Year Book of Otolaryngology–Head and Neck Surgery®: Drs. Paparella and Holt

Year Book of Pain: Drs. Gebhart, Haddox, Jacox, Janjan, Marcus, Rudy, and Shapiro

Year Book of Pathology and Laboratory Medicine: Drs. Mills, Bruns, Gaffey, and Stoler

Year Book of Pediatrics®: Dr. Stockman

Year Book of Plastic, Reconstructive, and Aesthetic Surgery®: Drs. Miller, Cohen, McKinney, Robson, Ruberg, and Whitaker

Year Book of Podiatric Medicine and Surgery®: Dr. Kominsky

Year Book of Psychiatry and Applied Mental Health®: Drs. Talbott, Ballenger, Breier, Frances, Meltzer, Schowalter, and Tasman

Year Book of Pulmonary Disease®: Drs. Bone and Petty

Year Book of Rheumatology®: Drs. Sergent, LeRoy, Meenan, Panush, and Reichlin

Year Book of Sports Medicine®: Drs. Shephard, Drinkwater, Eichner, Torg, Col. Anderson, and Mr. George

Year Book of Surgery®: Drs. Copeland, Bland, Deitch, Eberlein, Howard, Luce, Seeger, Souba, and Sugarbaker

Year Book of Thoracic and Cardiovascular Surgery®: Drs. Ginsberg, Wechsler, and Williams

Year Book of Ultrasound®: Drs. Merritt, Carroll, and Fleischer

Year Book of Urology®: Drs. DeKernion and Howards

Year Book of Vascular Surgery®: Dr. Porter

1996

The Year Book of VASCULAR SURGERY®

Editor
John M. Porter, M.D.
Professor of Surgery and Head, Division of Vascular Surgery, Oregon Health Sciences University, Portland, Oregon

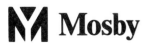 **Mosby**

St. Louis Baltimore Boston Carlsbad Chicago Naples New York Philadelphia Portland
London Madrid Mexico City Singapore Sydney Tokyo Toronto Wiesbaden

Vice President and Publisher, Continuity Publishing: Kenneth H. Killion
Director, Editorial Development: Gretchen C. Murphy
Developmental Editor, Continuity: Kris Horeis, R.N.
Acquisitions Editor: Jennifer Roche
Illustrations and Permissions Coordinator: Lois M. Ruebensam
Manager, Continuity–EDP: Maria Nevinger
Project Manager, Editing: Tamara L. Smith
Senior Project Manager, Production: Max F. Perez
Freelance Staff Supervisor: Barbara M. Kelly
Director, Editorial Services: Edith M. Podrazik, R.N.
Information Specialist: Kathleen Moss, R.N.
Information Specialist: Margery Marble, B.S.N., R.N.
Senior Medical Writer: David A. Cramer, M.D.
Senior Marketing Manager: Eileen M. Lynch
Marketing Specialist: Lynn D. Stevenson

1996 EDITION
Copyright © March 1996 by Mosby–Year Book, Inc.

Printed in the United States of America
Composition by Reed Technology and Information Services, Inc.
Printing/binding by Maple-Vail

Mosby–Year Book, Inc.
11830 Westline Industrial Drive
St. Louis, MO 63146

Editorial Office:
Mosby–Year Book, Inc.
200 North LaSalle Street
Chicago, IL 60601

International Standard Serial Number: 0749-4041
International Standard Book Number: 0-8151-0685-8

Contributing Editors

William Abbott, M.D.
Chief, Vascular Surgery, Massachusetts General Hospital, Boston, Massachusetts

P.R.F. Bell, M.D.
Head, Department of Surgery, University of Leicester, Leicester, England

Thomas O'Donnell, M.D.
Professor and Chair, Department of Surgery, New England Medical Center, Boston, Massachusetts

William Quiñones-Baldrich, M.D.
Associate Professor of Surgery, UCLA Center for Health Sciences, Los Angeles, California

John Ricotta, M.D.
Chairman, Division of Vascular Surgery, Millard Fillard Hospital, Buffalo, New York

Eric S. Weinstein, M.D.
Assistant Professor of Surgery; Chief, Division of Vascular Surgery, University of New Mexico, Albuquerque, New Mexico

Rich Yeager, M.D.
Associate Professor of Surgery, Division of Vascular Surgery, Veterans Administration Medical Center, Portland, Oregon

Table of Contents

Mosby Document Express

Journals Represented

Mosby and its Editors survey more than 1,000 U.S. and foreign medical and allied health journals for its abstract-and-commentary publications. From these journals, the Editors select the articles to be abstracted. Journals represented in this YEAR BOOK are listed below.

Acta Dermato-Venereologica
Acta Neurologica Scandinavica
Acta Radiologica
American Journal of Cardiology
American Journal of Pathology
American Journal of Roentgenology
American Journal of Surgery
American Surgeon
Angiology
Annals of Internal Medicine
Annals of Surgery
Annals of the Royal College of Surgeons of England
Annals of Thoracic Surgery
Annals of Vascular Surgery
Archives of Disease in Childhood
Archives of Internal Medicine
Archives of Otolaryngology–Head and Neck Surgery
Archives of Physical Medicine and Rehabilitation
Archives of Surgery
Arteriosclerosis and Thrombosis
Arthritis and Rheumatism
Artificial Organs
Atherosclerosis
Australasian Radiology
British Journal of Surgery
Cardiovascular and Interventional Radiology
Cardiovascular Surgery
Cerebrovascular Diseases
Circulation
Circulation Research
Clinical Investigator
Clinical Orthopaedics and Related Research
Contemporary Surgery
Critical Care Medicine
European Journal of Surgery
European Journal of Vascular and Endovascular Surgery
European Journal of Vascular Surgery
Journal of Cardiac Surgery
Journal of Cardiovascular Surgery
Journal of Clinical Investigation
Journal of Dermatologic Surgery and Oncology
Journal of General Internal Medicine
Journal of Hypertension
Journal of Internal Medicine
Journal of Interventional Radiology
Journal of Pediatric Surgery
Journal of Rheumatology
Journal of Surgical Research

Journal of the American College of Cardiology
Journal of the American College of Surgeons
Journal of the American Medical Association
Journal of the Royal College of Surgeons of Edinburgh
Journal of Thoracic and Cardiovascular Surgery
Journal of Trauma
Journal of Vascular Surgery
Laboratory Investigation
Lancet
Nature Medicine
New England Journal of Medicine
Radiology
S.A.M.J./S.A.M.T—South African Medical Journal
Stroke
Surgery
Thrombosis and Haemostatis
Ultrasound in Medicine and Biology
World Journal of Surgery

STANDARD ABBREVIATIONS

The following terms are abbreviated in this edition: acquired immunodeficiency syndrome (AIDS), cardiopulmonary resuscitation (CPR), central nervous system (CNS), cerebrospinal fluid (CSF), computed tomography (CT), deoxyribonucleic acid (DNA), electrocardiography (ECG), health maintenance organization (HMO), human immunodeficiency virus (HIV), intensive care unit (ICU), intramuscular (IM), intravenous (IV), magnetic resonance (MR) imaging (MRI), and ribonucleic acid (RNA).

NOTE

The YEAR BOOK OF VASCULAR SURGERY is a literature survey service providing abstracts of articles published in the professional literature. Every effort is made to assure the accuracy of the information presented in these pages. Neither the editors nor the publisher of the YEAR BOOK OF VASCULAR SURGERY can be responsible for errors in the original materials. The editors' comments are their own opinions. Mention of specific products within this publication does not constitute endorsement.

Introduction

With this, the 1996 YEAR BOOK OF VASCULAR SURGERY, I complete my fourth year of editorship. I really do not know how many more years I will be able to stand. As I survey the past year in vascular surgery, I conclude that the major event has been the ongoing revolution in health care delivery. Many cities in the United States, including my own, now have considerably over 50% HMO penetration. Physicians are facing daily restrictions in degrees of freedom, with the whole system being run by gatekeepers, from whom special permission is required for almost everything. Surgical fees continue their precipitous decline while expenses increase. All of us are forced to spend far more time with medical practice administration than we would like. Hopefully, just as with a dog straining at a peach pit, this too shall soon pass.

In reviewing the material contained in this edition of the YEAR BOOK, I conclude that this has not been a year of monumental advances in vascular surgery, but important developments continue to occur. Epidemiologically, the great decrease in both myocardial infarction and stroke mortality represents one of the most important developments in our professional lifetime. The mortality decline appears to be leveling out somewhat, but the current level is drastically reduced. Interestingly, there is no widely accepted explanation for this decrease.

Most of the new information in the lipid area has been negative in the past year. Decreasing lipids with lovastatin or omega-3 fatty acids has not improved the rate of post–coronary angioplasty restenosis. Reducing cholesterol below what is considered to be the normal range appears to convey no benefit.

Perhaps one of the areas of greatest interest in the past year has been study of the fibrous cap overlying atherosclerotic plaques. There is a general belief that the dangerous atheroma is the one with a thin fibrous cap prone to rupture. Evidence indicates that the fibrous cap undergoes inflammation before rupture, and inflammatory cells likely play a role in producing the actual rupture. Fibrous cap rupture with extrusion of atheromatous contents appears to be a frequent cause of abrupt arterial thrombosis, especially in the coronary circulation. One of the most innovative of the many investigations of the past year—attempting to detect fibrous caps at risk for rupture—consisted of sophisticated attenuation slope mapping using ultrasound techniques. The techniques appear promising but are beyond my ability to understand.

The field of coagulation in general, and coagulation-altering drugs in particular, remains a strong focus. There is now a general realization that 25% to 40% of all vascular surgery patients have one or more defined hypercoagulable disorders. The optimal treatment for these disorders, however, is still a matter of intense controversy. In the past year, the clinical syndrome of factor V resistance to activated protein C has been attributed to a point mutation, and many think this will prove to be the most frequently observed hypercoagulable condition in our population. Lipo-protein (a) and homocysteine have both been confirmed as important risk factors for atherosclerosis.

In the drug field in the past year, hirudin has been studied extensively. Although hirudin is a powerful antithrombin, it clearly has a narrow therapeutic window and has a nasty habit of producing intracranial bleed-ing when used in conjunction with thrombolytic agents. Early studies indicate the potential usefulness of a family of antibodies directed against the IIb/IIIa integrin receptors on the platelet surface.

Considerable attention is still being devoted to the phenomenon of shear stress. There is now abundant evidence that both arteries and vein grafts progressively dilate to normalize shear stress, probably through the mecha-nism of receptor-mediated endothelial elaboration of nitric oxide.

The field of imaging continues to attract attention from the vascular surgeons. Ultrafast CT is now beginning to be used clinically. It has been shown definitively in the past year that MRI can be used for quantitative noninvasive flow measurements, and I suspect this technique will have clinical utility in the future. Intravascular ultrasound is providing precise diagnostic information concerning aortic dissection, and many believe intravascular ultrasound is now the diagnostic procedure of choice for this condition. There has been increased appreciation in the past year of the importance of atheromatous disease in the aortic arch and the propensity of this disease to cause both cerebral and peripheral embolization. Ultra-sound, especially transesophageal echocardiography, has proved quite ac-curate in detection of this arch atherosclerosis. Several important studies have examined the ability of the nonenhanced CT scan to predict early rupture of infrarenal abdominal aortic aneurysms. A peculiar nonen-hanced aortic crescent has been found in a significant number of aneu-rysms in the early stages of rupture, before any extraluminal fluid can be noted. On balance, there is little new on causation of abdominal aortic aneurysms. Investigators continue to examine elastase and collagenase, but nothing exciting seems to be happening.

In the leg-bypass field, alternate veins give acceptable clinical perfor-mance, but 20% to 30% require revision within 12 months. If alternate veins are used in the lower extremities, frequent graft surveillance is mandatory.

Perhaps one of the most interesting areas in the past year has been the ongoing saga of the development of a clinically useful endovascular graft for aneurysm repair. The first company to test these grafts in the United States, Endovascular Technologies, had to suspend its clinical trial because of the problem of hooks breaking on the stents. As of this writing, the trial remains suspended. There have been 2 case reports during the past year of delayed rupture of abdominal aneurysms after the apparently successful implantation of endovascular grafts. This is especially worrisome, and reports such as this will be followed very closely. Dr. Parodi, an early innovator of the endovascular graft, is now expressing concern about the future of this device, and he believes major technical improvements will be mandatory before significant clinical utilization will be possible.

A few new features have been included in this edition of YEAR BOOK. I have provided more cross-references to assist the reader in pursuing individual topics. For the first time, I have also commented on invited commentaries from others. I hope you will find this dialogue interesting, and perhaps occasionally amusing. Also for the first time, I have begun to award a special recognition for duplicate publications, failure to appreciate the tenets of clinical research, or sheer silliness. I have termed this award the Camel Dung Award, abbreviated CDA. I hope those who are recognized as recipients of this prestigious award will respond appropriately. Please remember, dear reader: On balance, the most important thing is life is to have fun. Criticisms expressed herein are of specific papers and points of view, certainly not of individuals. Please be kind enough to take it that way, as that is certainly the intent.

As always, I express appreciation for the excellent support I have received from those around me. In my office, Ms. Heather Morin has performed 95% of the enormous amount of secretarial work required of this project, while at the same time taking a full course load in college. I extend to her my profound thanks. The professionals at Mosby, including Jennifer Roche, Kris Horeis, and Emily Veit, have also provided excellent support.

I hope you will find the book of some value as well as, hopefully, fun. Please write me a letter, if so inclined, and tell me your response. I can take it.

John M. Porter, M.D.

1 Basic Considerations

Atherosclerosis

Alcohol Consumption and Carotid Atherosclerosis: Evidence of Dose-Dependent Atherogenic and Antiatherogenic Effects—Results From the Bruneck Study
Kiechl S, Willeit J, Egger G, Oberhollenzer M, Aichner F (Innsbruck Univ Hosp, Austria; Hosp of Bruneck, Italy)
Stroke 25:1593–1598, 1994   145-96-1–1

Background.—Epidemiologic evidence to date supports a U-shaped association between alcohol intake and the risk of ischemic stroke in white populations. Comparatively little is known about the long-term effects of drinking on cardiovascular disease in general and on atherosclerosis in particular.

Methods.—Carotid atherosclerotic disease was quantified by B-mode ultrasonography in a randomly selected group of 460 men entered in 1990 in the Bruneck Ischemic Heart Disease and Stroke Prevention Study.

Results.—A U-shaped age-adjusted relationship between alcohol consumption and carotid artery disease was observed. Light drinkers had a lower risk of atherosclerotic disease (odds ratio, 0.44) than did either nondrinkers (1.00) or heavy drinkers (2.78). Neither smoking nor the inclusion in the reference group of individuals who formerly drank heavily explained this finding. Approximately one fourth of the risk related to heavy drinking was accounted for by risk factors associated with drinking. The benefit associated with a low intake of alcohol appeared to be independent of conventional risk factors.

Conclusion.—Alcohol may have both atherogenic and antiatherogenic effects that influence the risk of cerebrovascular disease.

▶ If one accepts the validity of carotid intimal-medial thickening as being indicative of the atherosclerotic status of the individual, one is forced to the conclusion that moderate alcohol consumption (perhaps up to 50 g/day) decreases the risk of atherosclerosis. Conversely, high alcohol consumption exacerbates the risk, a well-described U-shaped association. Interestingly, only about 25% of the risk of high alcohol consumption can be accounted for by the nonalcohol risk profile of the heavy drinker, primarily cigarette smoking. There does appear to be a direct atherosclerosis-enhancing effect of high alcohol consumption. Evidence such as this must, sadly, temper my previously expressed enthusiasm for alcohol (1).

Reference

1. 1993 Year Book of Vascular Surgery, p 34.

Sex Differences in the Management and Long-Term Outcome of Acute Myocardial Infarction: A Statewide Study
Kostis JB, for the MIDAS Study Group (UMDNJ–Robert Wood Johnson Med School, New Brunswick, NJ)
Circulation 90:1715–1730, 1994   145-96-1–2

Objective.—Women reportedly are less likely than men to undergo invasive procedures to diagnose and treat coronary artery disease. Whether this difference correlates with differential mortality in patients with acute myocardial infarction was evaluated.

Methods.—All discharge records from New Jersey hospitals for patients with acute infarction in the years 1986 and 1987 were reviewed. The total cohort numbered 42,595 patients. The accuracy of the data was assessed by auditing 726 randomly selected patient records.

Findings.—Women were older than men; remained longer in the hospital; and were more likely to have anemia, diabetes, hypertension, and left ventricular dysfunction. Women were less likely than men to be admitted to a hospital that performs invasive procedures. Men more often had past myocardial infarction, arrhythmias, chronic obstructive lung disease, and chronic liver disease. After adjustment for all these differences, women underwent cardiac catheterization less often than men, and the performance of catheterization correlated with reduced mortality. After adjustment for age, race, comorbid conditions, complications, and type of insurance coverage, women as old as 70 years of age had a higher 3-year mortality than men. The difference in mortality was somewhat less when cardiac catheterization and revascularization were taken into account.

Conclusion.—Women with acute myocardial infarction, especially those less than 70 years of age, are less likely than men to have invasive procedures and, as a result, may have a less favorable long-term outcome. The improved outlook for patients who have such procedures may, in part, reflect the selection of relatively low-risk patients.

▶ The witch hunt continues to detect an ever-widening number of areas in health care where sex bias may be invoked as an explanation for fewer procedures being performed in women. These authors conclude that, compared with men, women with acute myocardial infarction are less likely to undergo invasive cardiac procedures and to have a higher 3-year adjusted death rate up to age 70 years. As the authors wisely point out, it is currently unknown whether this represents underuse in women or overuse of such procedures in men. Caution is urged in accepting the results of this study without question, as it was retrospective. There was no quantitation of coronary anatomy, left ventricular function, risk factors, or many other important aspects of patient management. In addition, the study refers to practice patterns more than 5 years in the past.

It appears you are guaranteed publication of almost any paper if you can interject the potential that your paper has discovered yet another example of sex bias, a situation that is guaranteed to offend the politically correct.

Serum Antioxidants and Myocardial Infarction: Are Low Levels of Carotenoids and α-Tocopherol Risk Factors for Myocardial Infarction?
Street DA, Comstock GW, Salkeld RM, Schüep W, Klag MJ (Johns Hopkins Univ School of Hygiene and Public Health, Baltimore, Md; F Hoffmann–La Roche Ltd, Basel, Switzerland)
Circulation 90:1154–1161, 1994   145-96-1–3

Background.—There is evidence from in vitro, animal, and epidemiologic studies that oxidation of lipoproteins may play a key role in atherosclerotic disease, and that antioxidants may protect against this process. In particular, α-tocopherol and β-carotene are able to trap free radicals by interrupting lipid peroxidation, a process that is capable of modifying low-density lipoprotein.

Methods.—A total of 25,802 individuals who were donating blood for a serum bank were studied. The cases included 123 individuals who later had a first myocardial infarction. Two groups of sex- and age-matched controls were defined, with one representing subjects admitted to the hospital and the other representing the total donor group. Serum concentrations of the carotenoids β-carotene, lycopene, lutein, and zeaxanthine were estimated, as well as α-tocopherol and cholesterol levels.

Results.—The risk of myocardial infarction increased significantly as the serum β-carotene level decreased, and less prominently with a decreasing lutein level (table). Only in smokers were low serum carotenoid levels associated with an excessive risk of infarction. Among those with high serum cholesterol levels, higher levels of α-tocopherol appeared to be protective.

Conclusion.—The possibility that β-carotene or other carotenoids may help prevent myocardial infarction is worth pursuing. The Physicians Health Study is evaluating the use of β-carotene supplementation for reducing cardiovascular disease.

▶ Many studies have indicated that lipoprotein oxidation has an important role in causing/facilitating the development of atherosclerosis. Antioxidants may protect against this potentially harmful effect. Specific antioxidants include α-tocopherol, which breaks the chain reaction of lipid peroxidation at high oxygen concentrations, and β-carotene, which accomplishes its beneficial effects at low oxygen concentrations. This retrospective study reports an increasing risk for myocardial infarction associated with decreasing levels of β-carotene, with there being only a suggestive relationship to α-toco-

Percent Difference in Mean Serum Nutrient Levels Between Case and
Combined Control Groups

Serum Nutrient	Cases	Mean (SD) Control Subjects	% Difference	P
β-Carotene, μg/dL	17.2 (12.2)	20.6 (14.4)	−16.5	.03
Lycopene, μg/dL	39.0 (18.6)	40.2 (18.8)	−3.0	.53
Lutein, μg/dL	12.8 (6.2)	13.9 (6.1)	−7.9	.12
Zeaxanthin, μg/dL	3.5 (1.9)	3.6 (1.9)	−2.8	.44
α-Tocopherol, mg/L	12.0 (3.9)	11.4 (3.8)	+5.3	.13
α-Tocopherol: cholesterol ratio × 100	4.9 (1.4)	5.1 (1.4)	−3.9	.20

Note: One individual, a case patient, is missing a cholesterol value.
(Courtesy of Street DA, Comstock GW, Salkeld RM, et al: Serum antioxidants and myocardial infarction: Are low levels of carotenoids and α-tocopherol risk factors for myocardial infarction? *Circulation* 90:1154–1161, 1994. Reproduced with permission. *Circulation*. Copyright 1994 American Heart Association.)

pherol. Numerous ongoing studies continue to examine the potential beneficial effects of a variety of carotenoids in preventing myocardial infarction. Although the lack of effect of α-tocopherol is disappointing, the significant effect of β-carotene is extraordinarily interesting. We will surely hear more about this free radical trapper in the future.

Effect of Lovastatin on Early Carotid Atherosclerosis and Cardiovascular Events

Furberg CD, for the Asymptomatic Carotid Artery Progression Study (ACAPS) Research Group (Bowman Gray School of Medicine, Winston-Salem, NC)
Circulation 90:1679–1687, 1994 145-96-1–4

Background.—The HMG coenzyme A (HMG CoA) inhibitors, or statins, are a new class of lipid-lowering agents that promise more widespread use. They effectively reduce levels of low-density-lipoprotein (LDL) cholesterol and also are better tolerated than older drugs.

Methods.—A total of 919 asymptomatic men and women 40–79 years of age who had B-mode ultrasound evidence of early carotid atherosclerotic disease were entered in a randomized double-blind trial of lovastatin. All participants had LDL-cholesterol levels between the 60th and 90th percentiles. The subjects received lovastatin in a daily dose of 20 or 40 mg or placebo, as well as warfarin (1 mg daily) or placebo. All participants received 81 mg of aspirin daily. The chief variable was the change in the mean maximal intimal-medial thickness (IMT) of the carotid artery wall over 3 years.

Results.—Levels of LDL cholesterol decreased by 28% after 6 months of lovastatin treatment but were mainly unchanged in placebo recipients. Subjects not receiving warfarin had lower mean maximum IMT values after 1 year of receiving lovastatin. Major cardiovascular events (fatal

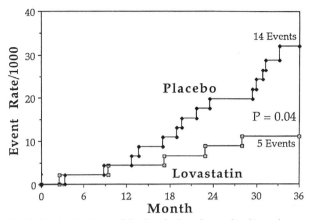

Fig 1–1.—Graph showing incidence of fatal/nonfatal cardiovascular disease by treatment group. (Courtesy of Furberg CD, for the Asymptomatic Carotid Artery Progression Study (ACAPS) Research Group: Effect of lovastatin on early carotid atherosclerosis and cardiovascular events. *Circulation* 90:1679–1687, 1994. Reproduced with permission. *Circulation.* Copyright 1994 American Heart Association.)

coronary heart disease, nonfatal infarction, and stroke) occurred in 5 lovastatin-treated patients and 14 placebo recipients (Fig 1–1). Eight placebo recipients and only 1 patient given lovastatin died.

Conclusion.—Carotid atherosclerotic disease is reversed in patients with moderately increased LDL-cholesterol levels who receive lovastatin, and the risk of major cardiovascular events and death appears to decrease at the same time.

▶ Although the trends in this study are highly favorable, one must note the actual amount of change in intimal-medial thickness actually measured. Thickness in the lovastatin group decreased by 0.009 mm per year, whereas that in the placebo group increased by 0.006 mm per year. Although this is statistically significant, I do have reservations about both the biological significance and the reproducibility of this tiny measurement obtained with ultrasound in patients. It is noted that the LDL cholesterol was reduced by 28% in 6 months and that there were significantly fewer major cardiovascular events in the lovastatin group compared with the placebo group. These authors propose that their data lend support to the suggestion that the cutoff point for initiation of patient treatment be 130 mg/dL of LDL cholesterol. Certainly, the members of the diet-heart group continue to be aggressive in their recommendations for lipid-lowering regimens.

Lack of Effect of Lovastatin on Restenosis After Coronary Angioplasty

Weintraub WS, Boccuzzi SJ, Klein JL, Kosinski AS, King SB III, Ivanhoe R, Cedarholm JC, Stillabower ME, Talley JD, DeMaio SJ, O'Neill WW, Frazier JE II, Cohen-Bernstein CL, Robbins DC, Brown CL III, Alexander RW, and The Lovastatin Restenosis Trial Study Group (Emory Univ, Atlanta, Ga)
N Engl J Med 331:1331–1337, 1994   145-96-1–5

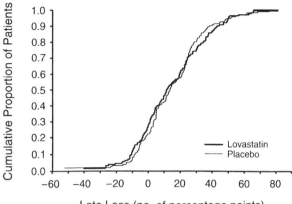

Late Loss (no. of percentage points)

Fig 1–2.—Cumulative distribution curve for the change in the degree of stenosis at the index lesion from the value measured immediately after angioplasty to the value obtained on angiographic restudy (late loss), according to treatment group. Late loss is calculated as the difference in the 2 values, each of which expresses the degree of stenosis as a percentage of the diameter of the vessel. (Reprinted by permission of *The New England Journal of Medicine.* Weintraub WS, Boccuzzi SJ, Klein JL, et al: Lack of effect of lovastatin on restenosis after coronary angioplasty. *New Engl J Med* 331:1331–1337, 1994. Copyright 1994, Massachusetts Medical Society.)

Background.—Both experimental and clinical findings suggest that reducing serum lipids may decrease the risk of coronary restenosis after angioplasty. To demonstrate whether aggressive measures to lower plasma lipid levels will delay or prevent restenosis, the Lovastatin Restenosis Trial, a prospective, randomized, double-blind trial, was conducted.

Methods.—Patients scheduled to undergo coronary angioplasty were randomized 7–10 days before the procedure to receive either 40 mg of lovastatin twice daily or placebo for 6 months. Of 354 patients who successfully underwent angioplasty, 321 had angiography 6 months later to quantify restenosis of the index lesion.

Results.—The lovastatin-treated and placebo patients were similar demographically and clinically at the outset and had comparable angiographic findings. The average stenosis of the index coronary vessel was 64% for the lovastatin group and 63% for the placebo group. Serum low-density-lipoprotein (LDL) cholesterol was decreased by 42% in actively treated patients, but the extent of stenosis at follow-up angiography was nearly identical in the 2 groups (Fig 1–2). There was a trend toward more myocardial infarcts in lovastatin-treated patients.

Conclusion.—Treatment with a high dose of lovastatin for 6 months does not delay recurrent coronary stenosis after angioplasty, despite a substantial reduction in LDL cholesterol.

▶ The purpose of the lovastatin restenosis trial was to determine whether aggressive lipid-lowering therapy with lovastatin for 6 months would decrease the frequency of restenosis after coronary angioplasty. Unfortunately, it did not, despite substantial reductions in LDL cholesterol. One is left to conclude that lipids may not have a primary role in restenosis after coronary angioplasty, and probably not after peripheral angioplasty either. Other agents that have failed to prevent restenosis after angioplasty include ω-3 fatty acids (see comment after Abstract 145-96-1-9) as well as the somatostatin analogue angiopeptin. The addition of lovastatin to the failure bin indicates that, for the time being, restenosis will continue to be a major limitation of the clinical usefulness of angioplasty.

Influence of Serum Cholesterol and Cholesterol Subfractions on Restenosis After Successful Coronary Angioplasty: A Quantitative Angiographic Analysis of 3336 Lesions
Violaris AG, Melkert R, Serruys PW (Thoraxcenter, Erasmus Univ, Rotterdam, The Netherlands)
Circulation 90:2267–2279, 1994   145-96-1–6

Background.—Evidence suggests that hyperlipidemia may correlate with an increased risk for restenosis after successful coronary angioplasty, but these studies have been retrospective and have involved small numbers of patients. Quantitative angiographic follow-up has been inadequate. Quantitative angiography, done at a predetermined interval, was used to examine the association between serum cholesterol levels and restenosis.

Methods.—The participants were 2,753 individuals in 4 major restenosis trials in whom a total of 3,336 lesions were followed up. Cineangiographic films were processed centrally, using an automated interpolated edge-detection method. The total serum cholesterol level was estimated at study entry and after 6 months, and hypercholesterolemia was defined as a value exceeding 7.8 mmol/L. Restenosis was defined (1) as luminal narrowing greater than 50%; and (2) dynamically, on the basis of changes in minimal luminal dimensions after angioplasty.

Results.—Hypercholesterolemia was present on entry in 160 patients with 191 lesions (5.7%). The rates of restenosis were 32% in those patients and 34% in those without hypercholesterolemia. No substantial differences were seen, regardless of the manner in which restenosis was defined; this remained the case when the population was divided into deciles according to total serum cholesterol level. The risk for restenosis could not be related to levels of high- or low-density-lipoprotein cholesterol or to the ratio of these variables.

Conclusion.—Reducing the total serum cholesterol levels does not appreciably decrease the risk for the development of restenosis after coronary angioplasty.

▶ See the comment after Abstract 145-96-1-5. On the flip side of the previous study, these investigators noted the incidence of restenosis in patients with and without hypercholesterolemia after coronary angioplasty. The study population was actually enrolled from 4 major restenosis trials. The results showed no association between cholesterol and restenosis by any of a variety of analytic approaches. These authors conclude that mea-

sures aimed at reducing total cholesterol are unlikely to influence postangioplasty restenosis, an effect also noted in Abstract 145-96-1–5. On balance, the evidence appears persuasive that reducing LDL cholesterol is not
going to have a favorable effect on the outcome of angioplasty.

**Effect on Coronary Atherosclerosis of Decrease in Plasma Cholesterol
Concentrations in Normocholesterolaemic Patients**
Sacks FM, for the Harvard Atherosclerosis Reversibility Project (HARP)
Group (Harvard School of Public Health, Boston)
Lancet 344:1182–1186, 1994   145-96-1-7

Background.—It has been established that lowering the plasma level of
low-density-lipoprotein (LDL) cholesterol benefits some patients with
coronary heart disease whose baseline levels are high, but it is not clear
whether normocholesterolemic patients also will benefit. This possibility
was examined in participants in the Harvard Atherosclerosis Reversibility
Project, an angiographic trial of cholesterol reduction.

Methods.—Seventy-nine nonsmoking patients with coronary heart disease whose total plasma levels of cholesterol ranged from 4.7 to 6.5
mmol/L entered the trial. The 70 men and 9 women had an average age of
58 years. All patients received diet therapy. In addition, 40 were randomly
assigned to receive pravastatin, nicotinic acid, cholestyramine, and gemfibrozil in a stepwise manner until the total cholesterol was lowered to 4.1
mmol/L and the LDL/high-density-lipoprotein (HDL) cholesterol ratio
was 2 or less. The remaining 39 subjects received placebo. Coronary
angiography was repeated after 2.5 years.

Results.—Coronary atherosclerosis did not differ significantly between
the actively treated and placebo subjects at follow-up evaluation. The
mean minimal diameter of the coronary artery decreased significantly in
both groups. There also was no group difference in the percentage of
stenosis. The plasma levels of total cholesterol, LDL cholesterol, triglycerides, and apolipoprotein B all were significantly lower in the actively
treated patients, and the levels of HDL cholesterol were higher.

Conclusion.—Intensive drug treatment over 2.5 years lowers the plasma
level of lipids in normocholesterolemic patients with coronary heart disease, but it does not improve the angiographic status of the coronary
arteries.

▶ These investigators have attempted to extend the envelope. If lipid
lowering in hyperlipidemic patients has a favorable influence on coronary
atherosclerosis, what would be the result of lipid lowering in normocholesterolemic patients? In this nicely conducted, prospective, randomized trial,
one group had their mean cholesterol level reduced by 20% by taking
medications, whereas the other group received placebo. Detailed coronary
angiograms obtained at baseline and 2.5 years after treatment showed
absolutely no difference. There was no detectable angiographic benefit of
reduction of cholesterol in patients who were considered to be normocho-

lesterolemic at the onset. This interesting information appears to be at odds with the message of Abstract 145-96-1–4, which indicates the extension of lipid-lowering therapy to patients with even lower lipid levels. Clearly, the lipid establishment continues to be actively at work attempting to define new uses for their limited skills.

Lack of Association Between Cholesterol and Coronary Heart Disease Mortality and Morbidity and All-Cause Mortality in Persons Older Than 70 Years

Krumholz HM, Seeman TE, Merrill SS, Mendes de Leon CF, Vaccarino V, Silverman DI, Tsukahara R, Ostfeld AM, Berkman LF (Yale Univ, New Haven, Conn; Univ of Connecticut, Farmington)
JAMA 272:1335–1340, 1994   145-96-1–8

Introduction.—It is often recommended that elderly patients with increased serum cholesterol levels be treated to prevent coronary heart disease (CHD). Although the association between CHD and hypercholesterolemia is strongly documented in young and middle-aged adults, there have been conflicting reports of the association in elderly patients. Therefore, the association between total serum cholesterol level, high-density-lipoprotein cholesterol (HDL-C) level, and the ratio of total cholesterol to HDL-C, and survival and hospitalization for heart disease was studied in elderly patients.

Methods.—Data on cardiac history, total serum cholesterol, and HDL-C were collected from a heterogeneous sample of men and women older than 70 years of age, as part of a larger, community-based, longitudinal study. The population was then stratified into those individuals having total serum cholesterol values less than 5.20 mmol/L, between 5.20 and 6.20 mmol/L, and greater than 6.20 mmol/L. They were also separately stratified by tertiles of HDL-C and by tertiles of the ratio of total serum cholesterol to HDL-C. All-cause mortality and CHD mortality rates and incidences of hospitalization for unstable angina or myocardial infarction were compared for the stratified groups.

Results.—Complete data and blood samples were collected for 997 patients with a mean age of 78 years for men and 79 years for women. Total serum cholesterol levels were not significantly associated with survival in either men or women (Figs 1–3 and 1–4). The odds ratios for the group with the highest total cholesterol levels compared with the group with the lowest total cholesterol levels were 0.59 for myocardial infarction or unstable angina, 0.60 for CHD mortality, and 0.99 for all-cause mortality. Similarly, there were no significant differences between the groups in the highest and the lowest tertiles of HDL-C levels or the ratio of total cholesterol to HDL-C for any of the outcome measures.

Discussion.—Hypercholesterolemia does not appear to be a significant independent risk factor for all-cause mortality, CHD mortality, or hospitalization for acute cardiac ischemia in the elderly population.

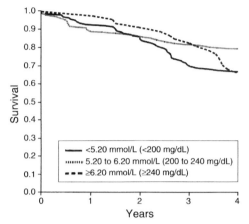

Fig 1–3.—Kaplan–Meier survival curves for men, stratified by total serum cholesterol level. (Reprinted by permission of *The New England Journal of Medicine*. Courtesy of Krumholz HM, Seeman TE, Merrill SS, et al: Lack of association between cholesterol and coronary heart disease mortality and morbidity and all-cause mortality in persons older than 70 years. *JAMA* 272:1335–1340, 1994. Copyright 1994, Massachusetts Medical Society.)

▶ A generally healthy group of elderly individuals (mean age, 79 years) underwent a single serum cholesterol and HDL-C measurement (nonfasting). Lipid abnormalities were not associated with mortality or myocardial infarction during the 4-year follow-up. Considering the study design, patient population, and relatively short duration of follow-up, these results were not surprising. The study population, although elderly, was at relatively low risk for coronary mortality and morbidity, with only 15% having a history of myocardial infarction and only 12% being current smokers. I do not

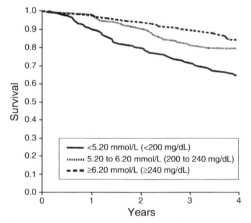

Fig 1–4.—Kaplan–Meier survival curves for women, stratified by total serum cholesterol level. (Reprinted by permission of *The New England Journal of Medicine*. Courtesy of Krumholz HM, Seeman TE, Merrill SS, et al: Lack of association between cholesterol and coronary heart disease mortality and morbidity and all-cause mortality in persons older than 70 years. *JAMA* 272:1335–1340, 1994. Copyright 1994, Massachusetts Medical Society.)

believe we can or should extrapolate these results to our symptomatic vascular surgery patients. There is abundant evidence (mainly in middle-aged individuals) that an elevated serum cholesterol level is associated with cardiovascular disease. This interesting study suggests, however, that routine cholesterol screening is not necessarily indicated in elderly individuals who are otherwise doing well.—R.A. Yeager, M.D.

▶ Although considerable evidence indicates that hypercholesterolemia increases the risk of coronary heart disease in young and middle-aged individuals, there is no such evidence indicating increased risk in individuals older than 70 years of age. Because a significant number of our vascular surgery patients are in this older age cohort, this information is of considerable potential importance.

Do Fish Oils Prevent Restenosis After Coronary Angioplasty?
Leaf A, Jorgensen MB, Jacobs AK, Cote G, Schoenfeld DA, Scheer J, Weiner BH, Slack JD, Kellett MA, Raizner AE, Weber PC, Mahrer PR, Rossouw JE (Massachusetts General Hosp, Charlestown, Mass; Kaiser Permanente, Los Angeles, Calif; Boston Univ Med Ctr, et al)
Circulation 90:2248–2257, 1994   145-96-1–9

Background.—There is considerable evidence from epidemiologic studies that deaths from coronary heart disease decrease as the dietary intake of ω-3 polyunsaturated fatty acids derived from fish oils increases. The resemblance of postangioplasty stenosis to early atherosclerosis suggests that fish oil consumption might prevent restenosis after percutaneous transluminal coronary angioplasty (PTCA).

Methods.—Four hundred seventy patients who successfully underwent angioplasty of one or more coronary vessels were randomly assigned to receive a dietary supplement of ω-3 fatty acids or a corn oil preparation for 6 months. The active supplement provided 4.1 g of eicosapentaenoic acid and 2.8 g of docosahexaenoic acid daily. The groups were well-matched for coronary risk factors. Restenosis was diagnosed when coronary angiography at 6 months demonstrated a 30% or greater increase in narrowing at the previous stenotic site, or loss of at least half of the initial gain with less than half of the luminal diameter remaining. All subjects received 200 mg of α-tocopherol.

Results.—Patients complied well with use of the fish oil supplement. The rate of restenosis was 52% when the fish oil supplement was given and 46% in placebo recipients. There were no apparent ill effects resulting from the ingestion of fish oil.

Conclusion.—This, the largest such trial completed to date, failed to demonstrate that daily use of a sizable fish oil supplement prevents recurrent coronary stenosis after PTCA.

▶ The absence of a beneficial effect of fish oils in reducing restenosis after coronary angioplasty is similar to that reported in Abstracts 145-96-1–5 and

145-96-1–6. We are simply unable to implicate lipid-based atherosclerotic events as having a major role in postangioplasty restenosis. These studies appear to persuasively nail down the lid on the proposition that reducing cholesterol has a favorable effect in this setting.

Cigarette Smoking and Stroke in a Cohort of U.S. Male Physicians
Robbins AS, Manson JE, Lee I-M, Satterfield S, Hennekens CH (Brigham and Women's Hosp, Boston; Harvard Med School, Boston; Harvard School of Public Health, Boston)
Ann Intern Med 120:458–462, 1994   145-96-1–10

Purpose.—Cigarette smoking is a known risk factor for stroke, although there are conflicting data about the strength of this association. Some studies have compared risk of stroke in current smokers with that in never-smokers, and others with that in current nonsmokers. Data from the Physician's Health Study were analyzed to determine the association between cigarette smoking and stroke among men.

Methods.—The Physician's Health Study is a randomized trial of aspirin and β-carotene in 22,071 male physicians. At enrollment, none of the men (age, 40–84 years) self-reported myocardial infarction, stroke, or transient ischemic attack. Based on self-report, 11% were current smokers, 39.3% former smokers, and 49.5% never-smokers. Incidence rates of total, ischemic, and hemorrhagic stroke in these 3 groups were assessed during an average follow-up of 9.7 years.

Results.—After adjustment for age and treatment group, the relative risk for total nonfatal stroke (312 cases) was 1.20 for former smokers, 2.02 for those who currently smoked less than 20 cigarettes/day, and 2.52 for those who currently smoked more than 20 cigarettes/day. The risk of total fatal stroke (28 cases) was not increased in smokers. The findings were essentially the same in proportional-hazards models with simultaneous control for other risk factors, including alcohol consumption.

Conclusions.—Men who are current smokers are at significantly increased risk for stroke. No such association is noted for those who are former smokers. Assuming that the relationship is a causal one, approximately 6% of the stroke incidence in this study population is attributable to smoking. In the general population, with its higher levels of current smoking, approximately 15% of stroke incidence would be attributable to smoking.

▶ This prospective cohort study suffers from the soft end point of self-reporting. A total of 22,000 participants in the Physicians' Health Study were examined to determine the incidence of stroke and to relate this to the cigarette smoking status of the individual. Within the limitations of the study, the results show that current, but not former, smoking increased stroke risk. The authors' conclusion that smoking appears to have an adverse effect on stroke incidence, morbidity, and mortality is hardly surprising. Nonetheless, it does raise at least one more small objective piece of evidence against smoking. Surprisingly, the chief executive officers of the largest tobacco companies in America continue to maintain publicly that they are aware of no persuasive evidence that cigarette smoking has an adverse effect on the cardiovascular system, or even that smoking is addictive. Several have expressed doubts that heart attacks may cause death.

Accumulation of Activated Mast Cells in the Shoulder Region of Human Coronary Atheroma, the Predilection Site of Atheromatous Rupture
Kaartinen M, Penttilä A, Kovanen PT (Univ of Helsinki, Finland)
Circulation 90:1669–1678, 1994   145-96-1–11

Background.—When a coronary atheroma ruptures at the shoulder region, an event ascribed to degradation of extracellular matrix in this vulnerable region, the process might be triggered by mast cells, which are present in coronary atheromas and contain neutral proteases.

Methods.—Specimens of normal and atherosclerotic coronary artery intima from 32 autopsied individuals 13–67 years of age were stained with monoclonal antibodies against tryptase and chymase, the major mast-cell proteases, so as to count these cells in different regions of the intima and atheroma (Fig 1–5).

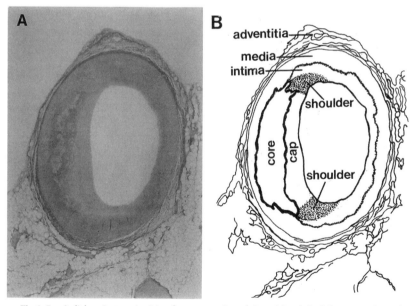

Fig 1–5.—A, light microscopic view of a cross section of the origin of the left anterior descending coronary artery. **B,** schematic representation (*shadow picture*) showing the locations of the regions in which the various cell types were counted separately. (Original magnification, ×20; Elastica–van Gieson.) (Courtesy of Kaartinen M, Penttilä A, Kovanen PT: Accumulation of activated mast cells in the shoulder region of human coronary atheroma, the predilection site of atheromatous rupture. *Circulation* 90:1669–1678, 1994. Reproduced with permission. *Circulation.* Copyright 1994 American Heart Association.)

Results.—On average, 40% of the tryptase-containing mast cells also contained chymase. Only 0.1% of all nucleated cells in the normal coronary intima were mast cells, but a ninefold increase in fatty streaks was evident. Mast cells were increased fivefold in the cap and core of atheromas and tenfold in the shoulder region. Ultrastructural study revealed degranulation of mast cells in the shoulder region, where 85% of the cells were activated. In contrast, only 18% of mast cells in the normal intima were activated.

Conclusion.—The substantial increase in activated mast cells in the shoulder region of coronary atheromas supports a role for these cells in destabilizing atheromas, and thereby triggering acute coronary events.

▶ See References 1 and 2. Increasing evidence indicates that acute thrombotic atherosclerotic events are frequently precipitated by plaque rupture. In fact, it seems that in the coronary circulation, rupture and thrombosis of plaques that are only moderately stenotic at the outset may be more important in the production of myocardial infarction than highly stenotic plaques. Thus, detection of plaques that are at risk for rupture may have profound implications for patient treatment. Accumulation of inflammatory cells in the shoulder region of the plaque is a repetitious finding in this newly emerging science. Perhaps the mast cell does have a central role in matrix degeneration leading to atheroma cap rupture. At present, considerable effort is being directed toward in vivo imaging of plaques at risk for rupture in humans. Stay tuned. I am sure there will be considerably more to follow in this exciting area.

References

1. 1994 YEAR BOOK OF VASCULAR SURGERY, p 32.
2. 1995 YEAR BOOK OF VASCULAR SURGERY, p 4.

Aorta

Analysis of Elastin Cross-Linking and the Connective Tissue Matrix of Abdominal Aortic Aneurysms
Gandhi RH, Irizarry E, Cantor JO, Keller S, Nackman GB, Halpern VJ, Newman KM, Tilson MD (Columbia Univ, New York)
Surgery 115:617–620, 1994   145-96-1–12

Background.—Previous studies of how the connective tissue matrix of abdominal aortic aneurysms (AAAs) is constituted have given mixed results. Data on the glycosaminoglycan content are not available.

Methods.—Matrix components including the cross-link content of residual elastin were examined in specimens of the intrarenal abdominal aorta from 10 patients having surgery for AAA. Control samples were taken from 3 patients with atherosclerotic disease and 4 patients who were organ donors.

	Comparison of Constituents of Urea-Insoluble Connective Tissue Matrix of Control and AAA		
Constituent	NAD	AAA	P Value
Elastin (µg/mg)	196.00 ± 23.00	20.00 ± 8.00	<0.05
Desmosine + isodesmosine (µg/mg)	1.00 ± 0.20	0.10 ± 0.02	<0.05
Desmosine + isodesmosine/valine	6.50 ± 0.16	6.47 ± 0.97	0.97
Collagen (µg/mg)	429.00 ± 21.00	428.00 ± 20.00	0.99
Glycosaminoglycan (µg/mg)	33.50 ± 3.40	17.10 ± 2.00	<0.05
Total protein (µg/mg)	820.00 ± 40.00	700.00 ± 20.00	<0.05

Abbreviation: NAD, no aneurysm disease.
(Courtesy of Gandhi RH, Irizarry E, Cantor JO, et al: *Surgery* 115:617–620, 1994.)

Results.—The elastin content of the connective tissue matrix was markedly reduced in AAA specimens (table). The cross-link content, representing desmosine plus isodesmosine, also was reduced in AAA as a ratio to insoluble matrix dry weight, but the ratio of cross-link content to valine in purified elastin was normal. The protein content of insoluble aneurysmal matrix was significantly reduced, but the collagen content was normal. Significantly less glycosaminoglycan was found in AAA than in control specimens.

Conclusion.—Fundamental biochemical changes appear to be present in the connective tissue matrix of AAAs, but the elastin is not deficient in cross-linked components.

▶ Another detailed study is presented from Dr. Tilson and his associates in New York. They found a reduced amount of elastin in aortic aneurysms from patients and a suggestion of protein and glycosaminoglycan reduction. The problem I have with this and similar studies (see Abstracts 145-96-1–13 and 145-96-1–14) is that the tissue is taken from a necrotic aneurysm. The aneurysms on which I operate tend to be filled with thrombus with apparent necrosis extending well into the wall and only a thin sac left in many places. I have always believed this is the wrong tissue to be studying, because all you are analyzing in this setting is the biochemistry of necrosis. The proper tissue to study is very small 3- to 4-cm aneurysms without necrosis, perhaps obtained from autopsy specimens, if possible. Until then, I will have significant reservations. I suspect the debris theory explains why so many investigators in this area obtain such different results.

Failure of Elastin or Collagen as Possible Critical Connective Tissue Alterations Underlying Aneurysmal Dilatation
Dobrin PB, Mrkvicka R (Loyola Univ, Maywood, Ill; Hines VA Hosp, Ill)
Cardiovasc Surg 2:484–488, 1994   145-96-1–13

Background.—Past studies suggest that, when elastin in the arterial wall is degraded, the vessel tends to dilate, elongate, and become less distensible. In contrast, degradation of collagen leads to a more distensible vessel and promotes rupture. Neither type of change has been seen to produce the gross enlargement typical of human aneurysms.

Methods.—The question of which type of connective tissue is involved in aneurysm formation was addressed by monitoring the dimensions of human common, external, and internal iliac arteries during progressive enzymatic degradation. Six intact vessels were examined along with 2 aneurysmal common iliac arteries. The mounted vessels were subjected incrementally to pressures as high as 200 mm Hg, and pressure-diameter curves were recorded for up to 18 hours as the vessels were exposed to elastase or collagenase.

Results.—Degradation of elastin led to 6% to 10% arterial dilation at 100 mm Hg and decreased distensibility. The pressure load was shifted to the collagen that remained. Degrading collagen led to 10% to 23% dilation at 100 mm Hg (Fig 1–6), increased distensibility of the vessels, and rupture of the aneurysmal arteries.

Conclusions.—Collagen appears to be the critical element of the arterial wall that, when defective, leads to aneurysm formation and rupture. In vessels from individuals having a family history of aneurysms, collagen structure may be defective or endogenous collagenolytic activity increased.

▶ Dr. Dobrin produces another in his series of observations indicating that the important element in aneurysm formation is the failure of collagen. One may legitimately ask the relevance of normal arteries being exposed to toxic concentrations of elastase and collagenase in the laboratory. This highly artificial model has indeed produced information that is of interest but has debatable relevance to the formation of human aneurysms. Nonetheless, as always, Dr. Dobrin's observations must be regarded as important. The progressive load shift from elastin to collagen during experimental aneurysm formation is an interesting observation.

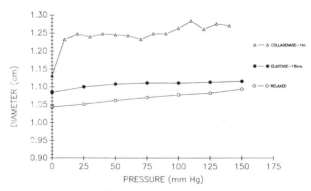

Fig 1–6.—Pressure-diameter curves for a nonaneurysmal external iliac artery. Data are shown for the relaxed vessel (*open circle*), after treatment with elastase (*filled circle*, 18 hours) and after treatment with collagenase (*triangle*, 1 hour). (Courtesy of Dobrin PB, Mrkvicka R: Failure of elastin or collagen as possible critical connective tissue alterations underlying aneurysmal dilatation. *Cardiovasc Surg* 2:484–488, 1994. Reproduced with permission. *Cardiovascular Surgery.* Copyright 1994 American Heart Association.)

The Elastase Infusion Model of Experimental Aortic Aneurysms: Synchrony of Induction of Endogenous Proteinases With Matrix Destruction and Inflammatory Cell Response
Halpern VJ, Nackman GB, Gandhi RH, Irizarry E, Scholes JV, Ramey WG, Tilson MD (St Luke's/Roosevelt Hosp Ctr Columbia Univ, NY; New York Univ School of Medicine, NY)
J Vasc Surg 20:51–60, 1994   145-96-1–14

Introduction.—When the rat aorta is isolated and perfused with a saline solution containing pancreatic elastase, an abdominal aortic aneurysm (AAA) results. The phenomenon is a latent one, suggesting that steps beyond the initial injury are required for an aneurysm to form. The latency period for aneurysmal aortic dilation in this model was correlated with the appearance of endogenous proteinases and the interval until infiltration of inflammatory cells.

Methods.—Forty aortas of Wistar rats were perfused with either saline solution containing pancreatic elastase or normal saline solution. The aortas were measured and harvested by laparotomy on days 1, 2, 3, and 6. Alterations in matrix proteins were evaluated by histochemical studies and the appearance of endogenous proteinases by substrate gel enzymography. Immunohistochemical studies were also performed with the use of monoclonal antibodies to T cells, i.e., CD-4, CD-5, and CD-8; monocytes/macrophages, i.e., ED-2; B cells, i.e., LC-A; immunoglobulin G; and immunoglobulin M.

Results.—After day 2, there was no detectable exogenous elastase. However, the aorta did not dilate to aneurysmal proportions until sometime between days 3 and 6. During this interval, several endogenous matrix proteinases became detectable in aortic tissue preparations. On immunohistochemical studies, various subsets of inflammatory cells were found to progressively infiltrate the aorta.

Conclusion.—The latency in aneurysm formation appears to correspond with a complex sequence of biochemical and cellular events. An interesting "early window" into the early phases of aneurysm formation is provided.

▶ Herein we learn that elastase will produce an aneurysm in rats after an interesting biological delay accompanied by significant inflammatory reaction. The inflammatory reaction has been a consistent message from Dr. Tilson's laboratory; its significance is unknown, as is almost everything else about aneurysm causation. This group hypothesizes that elastase initiates a complex inflammatory reaction, resulting in the elaboration of proteases that ultimately attack collagen, the destruction of which, all agree, is essential for aneurysm formation. On balance, I have had about all the elastase-collagenase inflammatory cell theories of aneurysm formation that I can profit from. I do not believe we are going to go any further using either highly artificial elastase-collagenase animal models or necrotic mature human aneurysms.

We are simply going to have to switch to early analysis of human aneurysm tissue to make significant further progress. See also the comment after Abstract 145-96-1–13.

The Impact of Gelatin-Resorcinol Glue on Aortic Tissue: A Histomorphologic Evaluation
Ennker J, Ennker IC, Schoon D, Schoon HA, Dörge S, Meissler M, Rimpler M, Hetzer R (German Heart Inst Berlin, Germany; Univ of Leipzig, Hannover, Germany; Hannover Med School, Germany)
J Vasc Surg 20:34–43, 1994   145-96-1–15

Introduction.—A new tissue adhesive, gelatin-resorcinol-formaldehyde glue, was developed in the 1960s and was soon used to treat aortic dissections in France. It thereby earned the sobriquet "French glue." Concern over mutagenic and carcinogenic effects led to the development of a gelatin-dialdehyde glue in which formaldehyde is replaced by 2 less toxic aldehydes, glutaraldehyde and glyoxal.

Methods.—The infrarenal aorta of domestic pigs was glued around an implanted prosthesis using gelatin-dialdehyde glue; the histomorphologic findings were examined 1 and 4 weeks after the procedure.

Results.—Histologic observations suggested that both collagenous and smooth-muscle fibers disintegrate and that the proteoglycan interstitial substance of the aortic wall changes. Healing appeared to be equally adequate with both the formaldehyde-free glue and the initial product. All the implants remained securely affixed 4 weeks after surgery. The seal of fiber and vascular granulation tissue appeared to be nearly completely organized and luminal and was covered by endothelialized granulation tissue, which itself had vascularized to varying degrees.

Conclusion.—Gelatin-dialdehyde glue appears to be suitable for use in repairing acute aortic dissections.

▶ I have no idea whether this new tissue adhesive (GRF) will have any significant clinical value. It has been used since the late 1970s in France for the treatment of aortic dissection and has been commonly referred to as "French glue." Interestingly, the original product was developed in the United States at the NIH's Battelle Memorial Institute. Although the new version of GRF, called GR-DIAL, may be superior to the original version, the clinical value of this compound is extraordinarily uncertain. The new compound has a higher adhesiveness than fibrin glue, does not require refrigeration, and apparently is fully absorbed in the body. The authors suggest that the new GR-DIAL be recommended for clinical trials of acute aortic dissection, and apparently such trials are under way in Europe. On balance, the biological glues have played little role to date in vascular surgery.

Measurement of Regional Elastic Properties of the Human Aorta: A New Application of Transesophageal Echocardiography With Automated Border Detection and Calibrated Subclavian Pulse Tracings

Lang RM, Cholley BP, Korcarz C, Marcus RH, Shroff SG (Univ of Chicago Hosps)

Circulation 90:1875–1882, 1994   145-96-1–16

Background.—In vivo data on regional aortic elastic properties are difficult to obtain. Information on instantaneous aortic pressure, wall thickness, and the cross-sectional area or diameter currently can be acquired only through the use of invasive techniques. Transesophageal echocardiography is a new, noninvasive technique for measurement of the regional aortic elastic properties.

Methods.—Twenty-five patients undergoing transesophageal echocardiography were studied. An automated border detection algorithm was applied to the short-axis transesophageal 2-dimensional echocardiograms of the proximal descending thoracic aorta to acquire measurements of instantaneous aortic cross-sectional area (Fig 1–7). These and combined

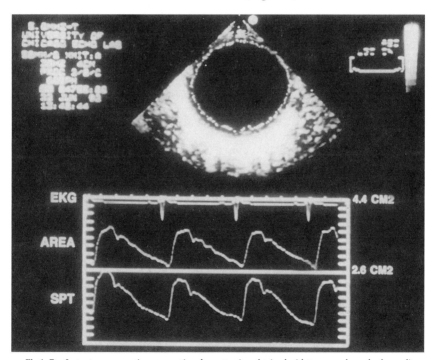

Fig 1–7.—Instantaneous aortic cross-sectional area tracing obtained with transesophageal echocardiography with an automated border detection (short-axis view). The aortic waveform was recorded simultaneously with an electrocardiogram (*EKG*) and a subclavian pulse tracing (*SPT*). (Courtesy of Lang RM, Cholley BP, Korcarz C, et al: Measurement of regional elastic properties of the human aorta: A new application of transesophageal echocardiography with automated border detection and calibrated subclavian pulse tracings. *Circulation* 90:1875–1882, 1994. Reproduced with permission. *Circulation.* Copyright 1994 American Heart Association.)

2-dimensional targeted M-mode end-diastolic wall thickness measurements were used to obtain instantaneous measurements of aortic wall thickness. Simultaneously recorded calibrated subclavian pulse tracings were used to estimate instantaneous aortic pressures, and aortic area-pressure loops were generated with the use of digitized data. The mechanical properties of the regional aorta were quantified in terms of compliance per unit length (C is the slope of the area-pressure regression), aortic midwall radius (R_m), and incremental elastic modulus of the aortic wall (E_{inc}). The values for R_m and E_{inc} were compared at a common level of aortic midwall stress to determine the independent effects of age.

Results.—The mean values in the 25 patients were 0.01 cm^2/mm Hg for C, 1.14 cm for R_m, and 7.059 × 10^6 dynes/cm^2 for E_{inc}. Aortic compliance per unit length was correlated with age in an inverse, linear fashion. The relationship between the incremental elastic modulus and age was nonlinear, increasing markedly after age 60 years. The correlation between midwall radius and age was weaker. The findings were similar to those of previously reported studies in which invasive techniques were used.

Conclusions.—The transesophageal echocardiography technique provides a noninvasive means of measuring the regional elastic properties of the human aorta and will help improve the clinical evaluation of these properties in patients with various disease states.

▶ We have here a solution in search of a problem. Without question, the use of transesophageal echocardiography with automated border detection and calibrated pulse tracings does allow an accurate characterization of regional aortic elastic properties, which the authors theorize may be useful in a variety of disease states. I agree with them right up to the point of clinical value. Generally, I find myself in agreement with the Faber College motto "Knowledge is Good" ("Animal House"). Nonetheless, I am currently unable to identify the problems for which this technique provides a solution.

Coagulation

Lp(a) Lipoprotein Is an Independent, Discriminating Risk Factor for Premature Peripheral Atherosclerosis Among White Men
Valentine RJ, Grayburn PA, Vega GL, Grundy SM (Veterans Affairs Med Ctr, Dallas; Univ of Texas, Dallas)
Arch Intern Med 154:801–806, 1994   145-96-1–17

Background.—An increased plasma level of Lp(a) lipoprotein has been associated with premature atherosclerosis in the coronary circulation and, possibly, at other sites; however, previous patient populations have not been closely screened for premature coronary artery disease (CAD).

Methods.—Fifty-five consecutive white men in whom peripheral vascular disease (PVD) began before 46 years of age were evaluated prospectively to determine whether Lp(a) lipoprotein is a risk factor. Thirty-eight of them had CAD in addition to PVD. Twenty-six age-matched men with premature CAD and 32 control men also were assessed.

Results.—Patients with CAD had higher plasma apolipoprotein B-100 levels than controls. The mean plasma Lp(a) lipoprotein level was higher in patients with PVD alone than in controls and also was increased in the entire group of men with PVD. Premature PVD correlated significantly with a plasma Lp(a) lipoprotein level greater than 30 mg/dL and also with an apolipoprotein B level exceeding 95 mg/dL.

Conclusion.—The plasma Lp(a) lipoprotein concentration is an independent risk factor for premature PVD in white men.

▶ This well-performed study documents the relationship between increased levels of Lp(a) lipoprotein and premature atherosclerosis and its complications. Unfortunately, isoforms of Lp(a) lipoprotein were not measured. There were no women in the study, and there was an uneven distribution of smoking, hypertension, and diabetes among the different groups. However, these variables were adjusted through statistical methods, and Lp(a) lipoprotein remained the single most important atherogenic risk factor in this defined patient population. The underlying mechanism for this association may be related to the plasminogen system. Two theories have been proposed: one in which the homologous structure of Lp(a) lipoprotein competitively inhibits the binding of plasminogen to endothelial cells, resulting in an inhibitory influence on the fibrinolytic system, leading to further intimal damage from the effects of local thrombus formation; and a second theory favoring the attraction of cholesterol to areas where Lp(a) lipoprotein has been attached to the endothelial cells because of its homology to the plasminogen molecule. Both mechanisms may lead to increased plaque formation, a process that has been identified in the early development of atherosclerosis. For the clinician, this is an important correlation, as patients with premature atherosclerosis who are identified with increased Lp(a) lipoprotein should be candidates for aggressive control of their lipid profile.—W. Quiñones-Baldrich, M.D.

▶ Dr. Quiñones-Baldrich is being very kind. It is difficult to draw any conclusions from this very small study. I believe Lp(a) lipoprotein is probably important, but I cannot prove it from this study.

A Prospective Investigation of Elevated Lipoprotein (a) Detected by Electrophoresis and Cardiovascular Disease in Women: The Framingham Heart Study

Bostom AG, Gagnon DR, Cupples A, Wilson PWF, Jenner JL, Ordovas JM, Schaefer EJ, Castelli WP (Boston Univ; Tufts Univ, Boston, Mass)
Circulation 90:1688–1695, 1994   145-96-1–18

Background.—Lipoprotein (a) [Lp(a)] is an antigenic determinant sometimes found in the low-density lipoprotein fraction. An electrophoretic band with pre–β mobility, termed "sinking pre–β," now has been confirmed as representing Lp(a). Five of 7 recent prospective studies have suggested that increased levels of Lp(a) are an independent predictor of coronary heart disease in men, but no prospective data are available for women.

Methods.—Sinking pre–β-lipoprotein was sought by paper electrophoresis in 3,103 women participating in the Framingham Heart Study. These women did not have cardiovascular disease when studied from 1968 through 1975. The 434 women who had a sinking pre-β band, representing 14% of the study population, were followed for a median of approximately 12 years.

Results.—Multivariate analysis yielded relative risk estimates of 2.4 for myocardial infarction, 1.9 for intermittent claudication, and 1.9 for cerebrovascular disease in subjects having a sinking pre–β-lipoprotein band. The relative risk of any coronary heart disease was 1.6, and that of total cardiovascular disease was 1.44. The finding of a sinking pre-β band was 51% sensitive and 95% specific for a plasma Lp(a) level exceeding 30 mg/dL—the threshold value associated with an increased risk of cardiovascular disease in men.

Conclusion.—The presence of a sinking pre–β-lipoprotein band is a valid marker for increased plasma Lp(a) in women currently free of cardiovascular disease. This finding is predictive of future atherothrombotic events, particularly myocardial infarction.

▶ Through the summer of 1994, at least 7 prospective studies of Lp(a) and CHD in men had been reported. Five found a significant association, whereas 2 did not. This interesting study, which incidentally used a sinking pre–β-lipoprotein on electrophoresis, which is not the same as Lp(a) but apparently is a valid surrogate marker, found that the presence of this marker was a strong independent predictor of myocardial infarction, claudication, and cerebrovascular disease in 3,100 patients taken from the Framingham Heart Study. Without question, Lp(a) is a valid marker for symptomatic atherosclerotic vascular disease. Whether the actual mechanism is primary through the induction of atherosclerosis or thrombosis is currently unknown, although perhaps thrombosis precedes atherosclerosis in many patients.

Lipoprotein(a) Levels and Risk of Coronary Heart Disease in Men
Schaefer EJ, Lamon-Fava S, Jenner JL, McNamara JR, Ordovas JM, Davis CE, Abolafia JM, Lippel K, Levy RI (Tufts Univ, Boston; Univ of North Carolina, Chapel Hill; National Heart, Lung, and Blood Inst, Bethesda, Md)
JAMA 271:999–1003, 1994   145-96-1–19

Objective.—The relationship, if any, between an increased serum level of lipoprotein(a) [Lp(a)] and coronary heart disease was examined in a prospective case-control study of men enrolled in the Lipid Research Clinics Coronary Primary Prevention Trial.

Study Population.—The 3,806 men in the trial were aged 35–59 years and were mostly white. All had a plasma cholesterol level of 265 mg/dL or greater at the outset, a low-density-lipoprotein (LDL) cholesterol level of 190 mg/dL or greater, and a triglyceride level of less than 3.39 mmol/L. The participants were randomly assigned to receive cholestyramine or a placebo. The plasma levels of Lp(a) were measured before randomization in 233 subjects who later had coronary heart disease (CHD) and in 390 matched controls who remained free of CHD.

Findings.—Men who had CHD had significantly higher levels of LDL cholesterol and triglycerides and lower levels of high-density-lipoprotein (HDL) cholesterol than the matched controls, and they more often smoked. Plasma levels of Lp(a) were 21% higher in those who had CHD, a significant finding. The association remained significant after adjustment for age, body mass index, smoking, blood pressure, and levels of LDL and HDL cholesterol. The distribution of Lp(a) in cases of CHD was shifted slightly toward higher levels than in controls.

Conclusion.—The plasma level of Lp(a) may be a significant pathogenetic and prognostic factor in atherosclerotic disease in hypercholesterolemic white men.

▶ This important study describes a group of patients recruited from the Lipid Research Clinics Coronary Primary Prevention Trial. All patients were men (age, 35–59 years) who had increased cholesterol levels. Lipoprotein(a) levels were measured in plasma samples obtained before randomization. Carefully selected controls were recruited. The results indicated that the Lp(a) levels averaged 21% higher in case-patients than in controls, even after careful control of body mass index, cigarette smoking, blood pressure, LDL cholesterol level, and HDL cholesterol level. The data are interpreted, probably accurately, as showing that Lp(a) is a strong independent risk factor for coronary heart disease in hypercholesterolemic white men. On balance, the evidence continues to accumulate that Lp(a) is either a significant risk factor or at least a marker for advanced symptomatic atherosclerotic disease in multiple areas.

Warfarin Versus Aspirin for Prevention of Thromboembolism in Atrial Fibrillation: Stroke Prevention in Atrial Fibrillation II Study
McBride R, for the Stroke Prevention in Atrial Fibrillation Investigators (Statistics and Epidemiology Research Corp, Seattle)
Lancet 343:687–691, 1994   145-96-1–20

Introduction.—Although warfarin is an established preventive treatment for stroke in patients with atrial fibrillation, its value relative to aspirin has not been defined. The Stroke Prevention in Atrial Fibrillation II study (SPAF-II) compared the effectiveness of these 2 treatments.

Study Design.—Warfarin and aspirin were compared for the prevention of stroke and embolism in 2 parallel randomized trials involving 715 patients younger than 75 years and 385 patients older than 75.

Results.—In the younger group of patients, warfarin decreased the absolute rate of primary events by 0.7% per year, so that the primary event rate was 1.3% per year. The rate with aspirin was 1.9% per year. The rate of primary events in low-risk younger patients receiving aspirin was 0.5% per year. Among the older patients, warfarin decreased the rate of primary events by 1.2% per year, so that the rate was 3.6%. With aspirin, the event rate was 4.8% per year (Fig 1–8).

Conclusions.—The SPAF-II study was designed to compare the reduction in ischemic stroke with warfarin treatment with that of aspirin treatment in patients with atrial fibrillation. Only a modest benefit of warfarin over aspirin was achieved. Patients younger than 75 years with few risk factors are at low risk for thromboembolism when treated with aspirin. Younger patients with risk factors may require warfarin. In older patients, the rate of stroke was high no matter which agent was used, and the search for better preventive modalities for this group continues.

▶ Many of our elderly patients with arteriopathy have chronic atrial fibrillation. Although vascular surgeons generally do not determine the primary medication for treatment of heart disease, we should be familiar with the

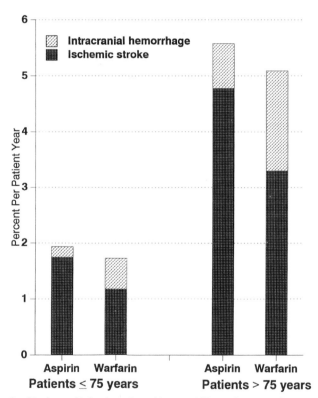

Fig 1–8.—Combined rate of ischemic stroke and intracranial hemorrhage according to antithrombotic therapy and age group. (Courtesy of McBride R, for the Stroke Prevention in Atrial Fibrillation Investigators: Warfarin versus aspirin for prevention of thromboembolism in atrial fibrillation: Stroke Prevention in Atrial Fibrillation II Study. *Lancet* 343:687–691, 1994. Copyright by *The Lancet* Ltd.)

literature. Abundant evidence indicates that patients with nonrheumatic atrial fibrillation are best treated with some sort of anticoagulant, but heretofore it has been unclear whether simple aspirin was as effective as warfarin, with its much more significant complications. The SPAF II Trial (Stroke Prevention in Atrial Fibrillation–II) reported herein conclusively shows that aspirin is just as effective as warfarin in patients without the risk factors of hypertension, previous embolism, or congestive heart failure. For patients with these risk factors, warfarin is incrementally better, although this slight improvement is purchased at the expense of increased complications (1, 2).

References

1. 1993 YEAR BOOK OF VASCULAR SURGERY, p 19.
2. 1994 YEAR BOOK OF VASCULAR SURGERY, p 13.

Use of a Monoclonal Antibody Directed Against the Platelet Glycoprotein IIb/IIIa Receptor in High-Risk Coronary Angioplasty
Califf RM, for The EPIC Investigators (Duke Univ, Durham, NC)
N Engl J Med 330:956–961, 1994   145-96-1–21

Background.—Platelets are believed to play a role in the ischemic complications of coronary angioplasty, such as abrupt closure of the treated coronary vessel during or soon after the procedure. The platelet glycoprotein IIb/IIIa receptor binds circulating adhesive macromolecules, particularly fibrinogen and von Willebrand's factor, which can cross-link receptors on adjacent platelets. This receptor is the final common pathway for platelet aggregation, and a mouse monoclonal antibody, 7E3, against this receptor can inhibit platelet aggregation. Whether the chimeric monoclonal-antibody Fab fragment (c7E3 Fab) may be beneficial in coronary angioplasty or atherectomy was investigated.

Study Design.—In a prospective, randomized, double-blind trial, 2,099 patients in 56 centers were enrolled in the Evaluation of 7E3 for the Prevention of Ischemic Complications study group. The patients were assigned to 1 of 3 treatment groups: a bolus and an infusion of placebo, a bolus of c7E3 Fab and an infusion of placebo, or a bolus and an infusion of c7E3 Fab. The patients were scheduled to undergo coronary angioplasty or directional atherectomy in high-risk clinical situations such as severe unstable angina, evolving acute myocardial infarction, or high-risk coronary morphologic characteristics. The primary end point of the trial included any of the following events in the first 30 days after randomization: death, a nonfatal myocardial infarction, an unplanned surgical revascularization, an unplanned repeat percutaneous procedure, an unplanned implantation of a coronary stent, or the insertion of an intra-aortic balloon pump for refractory ischemia.

Outcome.—Compared with the placebo only group, the c7E3 Fab groups exhibited a graded effect, from a 10% reduction in the rate of the primary end point with a c7E3 Fab bolus alone to a 35% reduction with a c7E3 Fab bolus and infusion. With the c7E3 Fab bolus and infusion, the reduction in the number of events occurred primarily in the rate of non-fatal myocardial infarction and unplanned revascularization procedures, but this beneficial effect was achieved with a significant increase in bleeding complications and blood transfusions. The doubling of the transfusion rate in these patients occurred primarily as a result of bleeding at the femoral puncture site. The treatment effect and major episodes of bleeding in patients given c7E3 Fab bolus and infusion were inversely related to weight.

Conclusions.—A substantial and sustained blockade of the platelet glycoprotein IIb/IIIa receptor is beneficial in patients undergoing high-risk percutaneous revascularization procedures. The use of a monoclonal antibody directed against this receptor reduces ischemic complications of coronary angioplasty and atherectomy but at the risk of increased bleeding. Future studies should be directed toward averting bleeding and transfusions and the determination of effective doses.

▶ The integrin glycoprotein receptor IIb/IIIa on the platelet surface has a critical role in platelet aggregation, binding both fibrinogen and von Willebrand's factor. The mouse monoclonal antibody, 7E3, was produced in 1985 against this platelet receptor, and its antithrombotic effects were demonstrated (1). The use of a bolus followed by an infusion of c7E3 Fab antibody resulted in a significant reduction of primary end points in this prospective randomized study. As I have stated before in these publications, I do believe that we are approaching an era when the shotgun approach to anticoagulation, consisting of aspirin, warfarin, and heparin, will be badly outdated. In the future, we are going to have monoclonal antibody preparations, genetically engineered compounds such as hirudin, and numerous exotic agents to neutralize highly specific areas in the coagulation cascade. The demonstration of efficacy of the agent reported herein is important. The next phase of investigation must surely use an active control, namely, aspirin itself. Until we see the comparison with the active control, this material is hard to put in perspective. Worrisomely, the amount of transfusion requiring bleeding was almost double in the experimental as in the placebo group.

Reference

1. Coller BS: *J Clin Invest* 76:101–108, 1985.

Randomised Trial of Coronary Intervention With Antibody Against Platelet IIb/IIIa Integrin for Reduction of Clinical Restenosis: Results at Six Months
Topol EJ, Califf RM, Weisman HF, Ellis SG, Tcheng JE, Worley S, Ivanhoe R, George BS, Fintel D, Weston M, Sigmon K, Anderson KM, Lee KL, Willerson JT, on behalf of the EPIC Investigators (Cleveland Clinic Found, Ohio)
Lancet 343:881–886, 1994   145-96-1–22

Purpose.—One third of patients will experience restenosis in the first 6 months after coronary angioplasty. There currently is no known treatment to reduce the frequency of this complication. The monoclonal antibody Fab fragment c7E3 is directed against the platelet glycoprotein IIb/IIIa integrin, which is the receptor that mediates the final common pathway of platelet aggregation. The ability of c7E3 to reduce the frequency of clinical restenosis was assessed in a randomized trial.

Methods.—The study patients all had unstable angina, recent or evolving myocardial infarction, or high-risk morphological findings on angiography. They were randomized to receive a c7E3 bolus followed by a 12-hour c7E3 infusion (708 patients); a c7E3 bolus followed by a placebo infusion (695 patients); or a placebo bolus and placebo infusion (696 patients). The patients were followed in double-blind fashion for at least 6 months. The groups were compared in regard to their need for repeat angioplasty or surgical coronary revascularization and the occurrence of ischemic events.

Results.—The 30-day rate of major ischemic events—i.e., death, myocardial infarction, or urgent revascularization—was 13% in the placebo bolus/placebo infusion group vs. 8% in the c7E3 bolus/c7E3 infusion group. The difference of 4.5% represented a 35% reduction for the latter group. By 6 months, there was an 8% absolute difference in the occurrence of a major ischemic event or elective revascularization, for a 23% reduction in risk for the c7E3 bolus/c7E3 infusion group (Fig 1–9). Most of the long-term benefit stemmed from the reduced need for bypass or repeat angioplasty in patients with an initially successful procedure. The c7E3 bolus/c7E3 infusion group had a 26% lower need for repeat target vessel revascularization than the placebo group (Fig 1–10). The outcomes of the

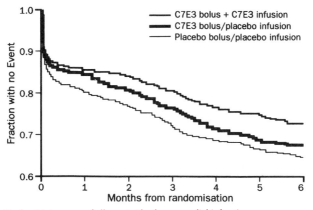

Fig 1–9.—Kaplan-Meier curve of all events (death, myocardial infarction, coronary revascularization) for all patients enrolled. There was a significant reduction of events for the c7E3 bolus/c7E3 infusion group compared with the active bolus only or placebo treatments ($P = 0.001$). A substantial proportion of events occurred after 1 month. (Courtesy of Topol EJ, Califf RM, Weisman HF, et al: Randomised trial of coronary intervention with antibody against platelet IIb/IIIa integrin for reduction of clinical restenosis: Results at six months. *Lancet* 343:881–886, 1994. Copyright by *The Lancet* Ltd.)

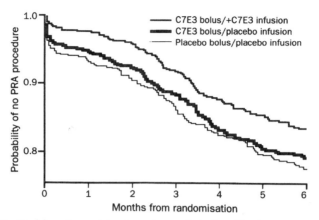

Fig 1–10.—Need for subsequent target vessel revascularization, either by coronary angioplasty or coronary artery bypass surgery. Repeat revascularization was significantly reduced in the bolus and infusion group ($P = 0.007$). (Courtesy of Topol EJ, Califf RM, Weisman HF, et al: Randomised trial of coronary intervention with antibody against platelet IIb/IIIa integrin for reduction of clinical restenosis: Results at six months. *Lancet* 343:881–886, 1994. Copyright by *The Lancet* Ltd.)

c7E3 bolus/placebo infusion group were intermediate but not significantly better than those of the placebo bolus/placebo infusion group.

Conclusions.—For patients undergoing coronary angioplasty, treatment with a c7E3 bolus followed by a c7E3 infusion reduces the frequency of abrupt closure and adverse outcomes in the acute phase and decreases the need for later coronary revascularization procedures. More study is needed before c7E3 can be used in groups other than high-risk angioplasty patients because this treatment carries some risk of bleeding complications.

▶ See the preceding comment on Abstract 145-96-1–21. This study had a generally similar end point and found a similar significant reduction of primary outcome events in the experimental group. I still do not understand why an active control with aspirin was not used, but it was not. Because monoclonal antibody to IIb/IIIa is a much more potent platelet inhibitor than aspirin, we are left to speculate that platelet-derived growth factor or some similar substance emanating from activated platelets must have a measurably adverse effect on outcome in acutely manipulated coronary arteries. On balance, I find the ongoing IIb/IIIa antibody saga fascinating.

Thrombotic Risk of Women With Hereditary Antithrombin III-Protein C- and Protein S-Deficiency Taking Oral Contraceptive Medication
Pabinger I, Schneider B, and the GTH Study Group on Natural Inhibitors (Univ of Vienna; Univ Hosp, Frankfurt, Germany; Univ Hosp Vienna; et al)
Thromb Haemost 71:548–552, 1994   145-96-1–23

Purpose.—There have been no data on the additional thrombotic risk associated with oral contraceptive (OC) use by women with a heterozygous natural clotting inhibitor deficiency. Randomized prospective studies of this issue are not feasible. In a retrospective, controlled cohort study, the relative risk of thrombosis was compared in women with established hereditary clotting inhibitor deficiencies with or without exposure to an OC.

Methods.—This study was conducted at 8 European coagulation laboratories and thrombosis units. Two groups of 48 women who were heterozygous for hereditary type I deficiency of antithrombin III (AT III), protein C, or protein S were studied. One group of women had taken an OC at least once in their life, and the other group had never taken an OC. The deficiency state was diagnosed at the participating centers. The patient or a physician completed a questionnaire that provided data on the onset and duration of OC use and the date and site of any thrombotic events. In patients taking OCs, the observation period began with the start of OC use and continued until a thromboembolic event had occurred or until OC use was discontinued. For control patients, observation began at an age matched to that of the patient taking OCs and continued until a thromboembolic event occurred or as long as the corresponding patient taking OCs was receiving treatment.

Results.—Among women with AT III deficiency, use of an OC was associated with a significantly increased probability of thrombosis. No significant OC-associated differences in thrombosis were noted for women with protein C or S deficiency. In the OC group, the incidence of thrombosis per patient year was 28% for AT III–deficient women, 12% for protein C–deficient women, and 7% for protein S–deficient women. The corresponding values in the control group were 3%, 7%, and 9% (table).

Conclusions.—In women with hereditary AT III deficiency, OC use is associated with an increased risk of venous thromboembolism. These women should strictly avoid OC use, and their female relatives must undergo AT III measurement before starting OC use. Oral contraceptive use does not appear to increase the risk of thrombosis in women with

Incidence of Thrombosis Per Patient Year in Deficient Female Patients
With and Without the Use of OCs

	AT III-deficiency	PC-deficiency	PS-deficiency
OC-patients			
Total observation time (years)	36.3	67.2	92.3
Incidence per patient year	27.5%	11.95%	6.5%
Patients not on OC (controls)			
Total observation time (years)	29.1	57.2	59.0
Incidence per patient year	3.4%	6.9%	8.6%

Abbreviations: ATIII, antithrombin III; *OC,* oral contraceptive; *PC,* protein C; *PS,* protein S.
(Courtesy of Pabinger I, Schneider B, and the GTH Study Group on Natural Inhibitors: *Thromb Haemost* 71:548–552, 1994.)

protein S deficiency. No significant increase in thrombosis is noted among protein C–deficient women who use an OC, but an increased risk cannot be excluded.

▶ The data contained in this article are soft, derived from retrospective control cohort studies done in multiple centers. The authors interpreted the results as showing that females deficient in AT III should not take birth control pills, as this increases the incidence of thrombosis per patient year from 3.4% to 27.5%. Interestingly, thrombosis associated with protein C and protein S deficiency appeared to be unaffected by birth control medication.

Vascular surgeons are occasionally asked their opinion about the advisability of using birth control medication in patients with a history of thrombosis. I have always believed the available literature does not produce any convincing evidence that birth control medication per se leads to thrombosis. However, the data presented convince me that women with AT III deficiency should not take birth control medication. Until better information comes along, I am going to accept this as sufficient to affect my clinical practice.

Safety Observations From the Pilot Phase of the Randomized r-Hirudin for Improvement of Thrombolysis (HIT-III) Study: A Study of the Arbeitsgemeinschaft Leitender Kardiologischer Krankenhausärzte (ALKK)
Neuhaus K-L, v Essen R, Tebbe U, Jessel A, Heinrichs H, Mäurer W, Döring W, Harmjanz D, Kötter V, Kalhammer E, Simon H, Horacek T (Städtische Kliniken Kassel, Germany)
Circulation 90:1638–1642, 1994   145-96-1-24

Background.—Adjunctive measures used with thrombolysis in patients with acute myocardial infarction include the use of aspirin as a platelet inhibitor and administration of heparin to inhibit thrombin. The latter effect may be enhanced by using hirudin.

Methods.—A recombinant hirudin, HBW 023, was compared with IV heparin in a randomized, double-blind phase III trial, the r-Hirudin for Improvement of Thrombolysis study. The goal was to randomize 7,000 patients seen within 6 hours of the onset of symptoms of acute infarction to receive either IV heparin in a bolus of 70 IU/kg, followed by an infusion of 15 IU/kg/hr; or hirudin in a bolus dose of .4 mg/kg, followed by .15 mg/kg/hr. Infusions lasted 48–72 hours and were adjusted to maintain the activated partial thromboplastin time at 2–3.5 times baseline. All patients received an initial dose of 250 mg of aspirin. Front-loaded alteplase was used as a thrombolytic agent.

Results.—The trial was ended after enrollment of 302 patients, when 5 of 148 hirudin-treated patients (3.4%) had intracranial bleeding develop. None of the 154 patients given heparin bled intracranially. The respective rates of stroke of all types were 3.4% for the hirudin group and 1.3% for the heparin group. Five patients who were given hirudin and 3 of those in the heparin group had major bleeding at other sites; ventricular rupture occurred in 3 patients and 1 patient, respectively. Of 19 hospital deaths, 13 occurred in the hirudin group.

Conclusion.—The risk of intracranial bleeding may be increased in patients with acute myocardial infarction who receive both hirudin and aspirin in conjunction with alteplase.

▶ Unfortunately, the specific antithrombin hirudin used in this study in combination with thrombolysis produced an unacceptable incidence of intracranial bleeding, leading to premature cessation of the study. Sadly, almost identical problems and premature study terminations occurred in the Global Use of Strategies to Open Occluded Arteries II and the Thrombolysis in Myocardial Ischemia IV trials as well. One is forced to conclude that recombinant hirudin has a very narrow therapeutic range when used in combination with thrombolytic drugs. Although I have noted in previous comments that the multitude of new anticoagulant drugs may be more powerful and more focused than those currently available, perhaps I should add that they may also be more dangerous. Unquestionably, this new family of anticoagulants should be used with extreme care, as clearly shown in this article.

Recombinant Hirudin for Unstable Angina Pectoris: A Multicenter, Randomized Angiographic Trial
Topol EJ, Fuster V, Harrington RA, Califf RM, Kleiman NS, Kereiakes DJ, Cohen M, Chapekis A, Gold HK, Tannenbaum MA, Rao AK, Debowey D, Schwartz D, Henis M, Chesebro J (Cleveland Clinic Found, Ohio; Duke Univ, Durham, NC; Massachusetts General Hosp, Boston; et al)
Circulation 89:1557–1566, 1994   145-96-1–25

Introduction.—The pathophysiologic role of coronary artery thrombosis in unstable angina and non–Q-wave myocardial infarction has been well demonstrated. Attempts at treatment using heparin and thrombolytic agents have met with limited success. Recombinant hirudin is a direct thrombin inhibitor that might be better than heparin in preventing accumulation of coronary artery thrombus. The use of recombinant hirudin for patients with unstable angina pectoris was assessed in a multicenter, randomized trial.

Methods.—There were 166 patients with ischemic pain at rest, ECG abnormalities, and baseline angiogram showing a 60% or greater stenosis of a culprit coronary artery or saphenous vein graft with visual evidence of thrombus. The patients were randomized to receive either 1 of 2 different doses of heparin—with a target-activated partial thromboplastin time (aPTT) of 65–90 seconds or 90–110 seconds—or 1 of 4 doses of hirudin— 0.05, 0.10, 0.20, or 0.30 mg·kg^{-1}·h^{-1} infusion—in a dose-escalating protocol. One hundred sixteen patients received hirudin, and 50 received heparin. Repeat coronary angiograms obtained 72–120 hours after treatment were compared with the baseline studies by quantitative analysis.

The results were assessed in terms of the primary end point of a change in the average cross-sectional area of the culprit lesion, and by the secondary end points of changes in the dimensions of the culprit lesion and Thrombolysis in Myocardial Ischemia flow grade.

Results.—Recombinant hirudin increased aPTT in a dose-dependent manner, with an apparent plateau at the 0.2-mg/kg dose. The aPTT was within the 40 second range for 71% of patients in the hirudin groups vs. 16% of those in the heparin groups. The hirudin-treated patients tended to show greater improvement than the heparin-treated patients in terms of average and minimal cross-sectional areas, minimal luminal diameter, and percent diameter stenosis.

Conclusions.—Recombinant hirudin is a promising treatment for the inhibition of coronary artery thrombus in patients with unstable angina pectoris. Large-scale comparative trials of recombinant heparin and hirudin are needed.

▶ Hirudin, as used in this study, was marginally but significantly more effective than heparin in a prospective randomized study. Everyone agrees that there is a need for a more effective antithrombotic therapy in patients with unstable angina. Perhaps hirudin will prove to be such an agent. No excess bleeding was noted in this study.

Randomized Trial of Intravenous Heparin Versus Recombinant Hirudin for Acute Coronary Syndromes
(The Global Use of Strategies to Open Occluded Coronary Arteries (GUSTO) IIa Investigators) (Cleveland Clinic Found, Ohio)
Circulation 90:1631–1637, 1994   145-96-1–26

Background.—Intravenous heparin has many drawbacks when used as an anticoagulant in patients with acute coronary syndromes. It requires antithrombin III as a co-factor, has no affinity with clot-bound thrombin, and is bound or rendered inactive by a number of plasma proteins as well as platelet factor 4. Improved angiographic and clinical outcomes have been reported with the use of recombinant hirudin, a direct thrombin inhibitor.

Methods.—Patients in 12 countries who went to 1 of 275 participating hospitals within 12 hours of the onset of ischemic chest discomfort and who had abnormal ECG findings were randomized into the study. Heparin was infused for 3–5 days at a rate of 1,000–1,300 units/hr, after an initial bolus of 5,000 units. The infusion rate was adjusted to maintain an activated partial thromboplastin time (aPTT) of 60–90 seconds. Hirudin was given in a bolus of .6 mg/kg, followed by infusion at a fixed rate of .2 mg/kg/hr.

Results.—The goal was to recruit 12,000 patients for the trial, but it was stopped after 2,564 were enrolled because of an excess of intracerebral bleeding. Hemorrhagic stroke developed in 1.3% of patients treated with hirudin. The incidence was significantly increased in patients given thrombolytic treatment (1.8% vs. .3%). The risk was greatest (3.2%) for patients given streptokinase and hirudin. Patients with intracerebral bleeding had significantly increased aPTT values after 12 hours of treatment compared with event-free patients (110 seconds vs. 87 seconds).

Conclusion.—Patients who were given hirudin in conjunction with thrombolytic treatment were at increased risk of intracerebral bleeding. The trial has been resumed using lower doses of both hirudin and heparin.

▶ See also the comment after Abstract 145-96-1–24. Again, an excess of intracranial bleeding associated with the combination of thrombolytic therapy and hirudin was noted compared with a combination of thrombolytic therapy and heparin. On the basis of the results described in this article a new trial using lower doses of hirudin has begun. As noted in the comment after Abstract 145-96-1–24, there undoubtedly is a very narrow therapeutic window for hirudin when used in combination with thrombolytic therapy.

Safety and Anticoagulation Effect of a Low-Dose Combination of Warfarin and Aspirin in Clinically Stable Coronary Artery Disease
Langer A, for the Coumadin Aspirin Reinfarction (CARS) Pilot Study Group (St Michael's Hosp, Toronto)
Am J Cardiol 74:657–661, 1994   145-96-1–27

Objective.—Whether combining low-dose aspirin with warfarin is more effective than aspirin alone in preventing recurrent myocardial infarction, stroke, and cardiovascular death was determined in patients participating in the Coumadin Aspirin Reinfarction Study.

Methods.—A pilot series of 114 patients with stable coronary artery disease entered the study. The average age of the participants was 64 years; 85% were men. A 3-mg dose of warfarin and 80 mg of aspirin were given daily for 8 weeks. The international normalized ratio (INR) was measured within 72 hours of starting treatment and then at weekly intervals.

Results.—The dose of warfarin was reduced to 1 mg daily (+80 mg of aspirin) in 19 of 110 patients whose INRs were assessable. Four other patients withdrew because their INR was consistently 4.5 or higher. The average steady-state INR was 1.48 in patients taking the assigned doses of warfarin and aspirin and 1.21 in those whose warfarin dose was reduced. Interpatient variability (the mean of standard deviations at steady state) was 0.49, and intrapatient variability was 0.13. Age did not influence the distribution of INRs (table). One fifth of the patients had microscopic hematuria, but it occurred independently of the INR. Three patients were withdrawn because of persistent hematuria or epistaxis.

Conclusion.—A fixed combination of warfarin and aspirin in low doses led to a stable and predictable increase in the INR in many patients with clinically stable coronary artery disease.

▶ In the past, I was advised by our very good institutional coagulation service that the combination of aspirin and warfarin was inherently danger-

International Normalized Ratio (INR) Analysis by Age Group					
Analysis	50–59 Years		60–69 Years		70–80 Years
Group (mg)	No. of Patients	INR	No. of Patients	INR	No. of Patients	INR
3 + 80	20	1.43 ± 0.11	38	1.52 ± 0.47	19	1.54 ± 0.35
1 + 80	3	1.12 ± 0.11	12	1.24 ± 0.25	4	1.09 ± 0.05

Note: Steady-state INR (mean ± standard deviation).
(Courtesy of Langer A, for the Coumadin Aspirin Reinfarction Pilot Study Group: *Am J Cardiol* 74:657–661, 1994. Reprinted with permission from the *American Journal of Cardiology.*)

ous and should be avoided. In recent years, this proposition has been reexamined both locally and nationally, as evidenced by this publication. Herein is reported a preliminary study from an ongoing clinical trial in which 114 patients received 3 mg of warfarin daily plus 80 mg of aspirin. Four of 110 patients had to discontinue medication because of increased INR and 3 patients because of bleeding events, primarily hematuria and epistaxis. The authors accurately observe that an overwhelming majority of patients appear to be safely treated with the combination if an early INR is obtained to detect hypersensitive individuals. Whether this combination will be more effective than other anticoagulant therapy in the prevention of reinfarction remains to be determined.

Inhibition of Growth of Thrombus on Fresh Mural Thrombus: Targeting Optimal Therapy

Meyer BJ, Badimon JJ, Mailhac A, Fernández-Ortiz A, Chesebro JH, Fuster V, Badimon L (Massachusetts Gen Hosp, Boston; Mt Sinai School of Medicine, New York)
Circulation 90:2432–2438, 1994   145-96-1–28

Background.—When mural thrombus remains on a severely damaged arterial wall, the risk of thrombosis is considerable. It was hypothesized that directly inhibiting thrombin might prevent the growth of fresh thrombus more effectively than indirectly suppressing thrombin, inhibiting cyclooxygenase, or both measures.

Methods.—Fresh mural thrombus was produced by perfusing the aortic tunica media of Yorkshire pigs—used as a model of severe damage to the arterial wall—ex vivo with fresh porcine blood for 5 minutes at a high shear rate. The amounts of platelets and fibrinogen deposited in 5 minutes were quantified. Thrombus growth was measured by perfusing blood from pigs with indium-111–labeled platelets and ^{125}I-labeled fibrinogen over preformed mural thrombus. Treatments included recombinant hirudin; aspirin, a cyclooxygenase inhibitor; heparin in both moderate (100 IU/kg/hr) and high (250 IU) doses; and low-dose heparin combined with aspirin. All treatments were given intravenously.

Results.—Thrombus growth was only mildly countered by aspirin. The effects of heparin were dose-dependent: deposition of both platelets and

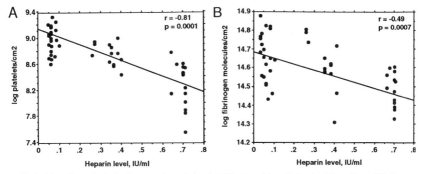

Fig 1–11.—Plots of relation between heparin levels (IU/mL) and log of platelet (**A**) and log of fibrinogen (**B**) depositions during growth of thrombus onto a mural thrombus in pigs treated with different heparin doses. The significant inverse relations are shown. (Courtesy of Meyer BJ, Badimon JJ, Mailhac A, et al: Inhibition of growth of thrombus on fresh mural thrombus: Targeting optimal therapy. *Circulation* 90:2432–2438, 1994. Reproduced with permission. *Circulation.* Copyright 1994 American Heart Association.)

fibrinogen correlated inversely with the mean plasma heparin concentration (Fig 1–11). Recombinant hirudin markedly inhibited thrombus growth, to an extent that significantly exceeded the effect achieved with even the higher dose of heparin.

Conclusions.—Thrombin seems to be the means by which fresh thrombus activates platelets, and specifically inhibiting thrombin markedly inhibits the growth of fresh mural thrombus.

▶ This is an interesting model in which to study experimental thrombus accretion. Specific thrombin inhibition with hirudin markedly inhibited platelet and fibrin deposition on a fresh mural thrombus, whereas aspirin and heparin had little effect. This is strong indirect evidence favoring hirudin in difficult situations, where retardation of thrombus accretion is essential. As noted in prior comments, however, hirudin unfortunately has a real chance of producing intracranial bleeding. Caution is clearly indicated.

Hypercoagulable States in Patients With Leg Ischaemia
Ray SA, Rowley MR, Loh A, Talbot SA, Bevan DH, Taylor RS, Dormandy JA
(St George's Hosp, London)
Br J Surg 81:811–814, 1994   145-96-1–29

Background.—Hypercoagulable states are found in up to 10% of patients with a history of unexplained venous thrombosis. Increasing evidence points to a similar incidence of hypercoagulation abnormalities in patients with arterial thrombosis. The prevalence and nature of hypercoagulable states were investigated in a large group of patients who had undergone peripheral arterial reconstruction.

Method.—Thrombophilia screening was done in 124 patients with a history of lower-limb surgical revascularization, 45 patients with claudication, and 27 controls. Screening involved measurement of hematocrit, platelet count, liver function, and levels of serum cholesterol and triglycerides. Protein C, protein S, and antithrombin III assays were performed twice on the same sample. Any level that was less than the laboratory normal range of 70 to 130 units/dL was considered abnormal.

Results.—Of patients who had undergone revascularization, 40% had a hypercoagulation abnormality, which was shown by low levels of protein C, protein S, and antithrombin III, or by the presence of the lupus anticoagulant. In contrast, 27% of patients with claudication and 11% of controls had abnormalities. Moreover, patients who had experienced reocclusion after revascularization were significantly more likely to have a hypercoagulation abnormality than were those who had not, even if 6 months had elapsed between time of the occlusion and the study. The most frequently detected abnormality was lupus anticoagulant; like low protein C levels, it was seen only in patients with peripheral vascular disease (table).

Conclusion.—To determine whether hypercoagulation abnormalities are an independent risk factor for early occlusion after revascularization of the leg, thrombophilia screening is now being done on all patients pre- and post surgery.

▶ These authors found that about 40% of patients who undergo lower extremity revascularization have a defined hypercoagulable state, predominantly a low protein C level. Although we have found almost the same number here in Oregon, we infrequently find a low protein C level; instead, our major offender is anticardiolipin antibody (1). Presently, we screen all patients admitted to the Vascular Surgical Service for coagulation abnormality. This probably is not cost-effective, and perhaps this screening should be limited to individuals with a prior history of failed bypass. When we discover a coagulation abnormality in someone who has a current bypass or a history of a failed bypass, we routinely use warfarin anticoagulation. We currently

Prevalence of Abnormal Thrombophilia Screen

	Patent (n=49)	Revascularization Recent occlusion (n=31)	Old occlusion (n=44)	Claudication (n=45)	Controls (n=27)
Low antithrombin III level	1 (2)	0 (0)	0 (0)	0 (0)	0 (0)
Low protein C level	2 (4)	9 (29)	7 (16)	2 (4)	0 (0)
Low protein S level	4 (8)	7 (23)	6 (14)	4 (9)	3 (11)
Lupus anticoagulant	9 (18)	3 (10)	16 (36)	6 (13)	0 (0)
Multiple abnormalities	2* (4)	2† (6)	7‡ (16)	0 (0)	0 (0)
Any abnormality	13 (27)	17 (55)	20 (45)	12 (27)	3 (11)

Note: Values in parentheses are percentages.

* One patient had low antithrombin III and low protein C and S levels, and 1 had a low protein S level and lupus anticoagulant.

† One patient had low protein C and S levels, 1 had a low protein S level and lupus anticoagulant.

‡ Four patients had lupus anticoagulant and a low protein C level, 1 had lupus anticoagulant and a low protein S level, and 2 had lupus anticoagulant and low protein C and S levels.

(Courtesy of Ray SA, Rowley MR, Loh A, et al: Hypercoagulable states in patients with leg ischaemia. *Br J Surg* 81:811–814, 1994. Copyright 1994, Blackwell Science, Ltd.)

have a higher percentage of our patients who have undergone leg revascularization receiving warfarin than we have ever had in the past, and we seem to be adding more every day. From our perspective, vascular surgery and hypercoagulable states are becoming increasingly intertwined. The material on Lp(a) lipoprotein presented earlier (see the comments after Abstracts 145-96-1–17 to 145-96-1–19) is undoubtedly part of the same patient population. See also the comment after Abstract 145-96-1–33.

Reference

1. Taylor LM, et al: *Ann Surg* 220:544–551, 1994.

Endothelial Expression of Thrombomodulin is Reversibly Regulated by Fluid Shear Stress
Malek AM, Jackman R, Rosenberg RD, Izumo S (Harvard Med School–Massachusetts Inst of Technology, Boston; Beth Israel Hosp, Boston)
Circ Res 74:852–860, 1994   145-96-1–30

Background.—The vascular endothelium participates critically in regulating thrombosis and fibrinolysis. Part of this role is mediated by thrombomodulin (TM), a surface receptor that binds thrombin and activates the protein C anticoagulant pathway. The expression of TM is controlled by various cytokines, but the role of biomechanical stimuli is uncertain.

Methods.—The effects of fluid shear stress on the expression of TM messenger RNA (mRNA) and protein were examined in vitro in bovine aortic endothelial (BAE) cells and bovine smooth muscle cells.

Results.—When BAE cells were exposed to moderate shear stress at 15 dynes/cm^2, or elevated stress at 36 dynes/cm^2, levels of TM mRNA increased transiently and then decreased to 16% of baseline 9 hours after the onset of blood flow. Shear stress at 4 dynes/cm^2 had no effect, and no effect was noted when bovine smooth muscle cells were exposed to moderate shear stress. Only BAE cells altered their shape and became aligned in the direction of blood flow. The TM protein decreased to 33% after 36 hours of exposure of BAE cells to moderate shear stress. Levels of TM mRNA returned to baseline within 6 hours after the end of shear stress. Steady laminar shear stress, turbulent flow, and pulsatile flow all had similar effects on the expression of TM. The expression of tissue-type plasminogen activator in BAE cells increased threefold with moderate shear stress and 22-fold with elevated stress.

Conclusion.—Thrombomodulin may protect against thrombosis in areas of circulatory stasis or low blood flow. In turn, blood flow appears to regulate the expression of TM in vascular endothelial cells.

▶ This fascinating study presents convincing evidence that the endothelial cell is profoundly affected by shear stress, producing an excess of TM at low shear stress (stasis) and a high level of tissue plasminogen activator at high shear stress (high flow). This appears to be another clear example that shear stress has a major role in determining the phenotypic expression of the adjacent cell, in this case, endothelium. The observation that shear stress affects both TM and tissue plasminogen activator mRNA expression by endothelial cells may be of pivotal importance in our understanding of the increasingly complex blood-endothelium interface.

Association of Idiopathic Venous Thromboembolism With Single Point-Mutation at Arg^{506} of Factor V
Voorberg J, Roelse J, Koopman R, Büller H, Berends F, ten Cate JW, Mertens K, van Mourik JA (Central Lab of The Netherlands Red Cross Blood Transfusion Service, Amsterdam; Academic Med Centre, Amsterdam)
Lancet 343:1535–1536, 1994   145-96-1–31

Background.—Venous thromboembolism has been linked with molecular defects in a number of hemostatic components. As many as 30% of patients who are disposed to thromboembolism for reasons that are not obvious have a poor anticoagulant response to activated protein C (APC); this, in turn, is associated with a plasma factor that seems to be identical to coagulation factor V.

Methods.—Point mutations in the APC-sensitive region of factor V were sought in 27 consecutive patients with recurrent idiopathic thromboembolism.

Results.—Ten patients had a single base-pair mutation that resulted in a substitution of Arg^{506} to Gln. This mutation was linked to a significant degree with in vitro resistance to APC.

Conclusion.—Some cases of "idiopathic" thromboembolism may result from a mutation that renders APC unable to inactivate the procoagulant factor V.

▶ Our local coagulation experts tell us that factor V resistance to APC may be the most frequently observed cause of hypercoagulability in the entire population. This important study cleverly identifies a single base-pair mutation resulting in a substitution of Arg to Gln in patients with factor V resistance to APC. They speculate, and I suspect correctly, that this mutation may form the molecular basis for thrombotic events associated with resistance to APC. Stay tuned. There surely will be more to follow in this fascinating area.

Aprotinin Significantly Decreases Bleeding and Transfusion Requirements in Patients Receiving Aspirin and Undergoing Cardiac Operations
Murkin JM, Lux J, Shannon NA, Guiraudon GM, Menkis AH, McKenzie FN,

Novick RJ (Univ of Western Ontario, London, Ont, Canada; Miles Canada Inc, Etobiocoke, Ont, Canada)
J Thorac Cardiovasc Surg 107:554–561, 1994   145-96-1–32

Background.—Aprotinin is known to reduce bleeding in patients undergoing cardiac surgery. A double-blind, placebo-controlled, randomized trial was done to establish whether aprotinin decreases bleeding and to determine the need for blood transfusions in patients receiving aspirin.

Methods.—Patients undergoing first-time coronary bypass or valvular surgery who had received at least 1 week of aspirin therapy and had discontinued its use 48 hours or less before surgery were randomized to receive intraoperative aprotinin (up to 7 million kallikrein inactivator units) or placebo. All patients were given heparin to maintain the activated clotting time (ACT) at greater than 450 seconds during surgery.

Results.—Fifty-four evaluable patients completed the study over 14 months. The aprotinin-treated group had significantly less blood loss and fewer transfusion requirements. Forty-one percent of aprotinin-treated patients received no blood products at all throughout the hospital stay. Twelve percent of placebo recipients required no exogenous blood. Among patients receiving packed red blood cells, aprotinin treatment resulted in significantly fewer units transfused, even in conjunction with the use of internal mammary artery grafts. Aprotinin did markedly prolong intraoperative ACT. Time for sternal closure and total operative duration were significantly shorter in the aprotinin group.

Discussion.—Aprotinin use may eliminate the need to delay cardiac surgery in patients receiving aspirin. In contrast to prior studies, no greater tendency for myocardial infarction was noted. Larger trials are indicated to confirm this finding as well as the trend toward shorter intensive care and hospital lengths of stay.

▶ Aprotinin, which is the current name for the ancient serine protease inhibitor trasylol, is widely used in cardiac surgery as a nonspecific agent to diminish bleeding. It apparently works both by antifibrinolytic and platelet preservation mechanisms. This study again attests to the efficacy of this agent in patients receiving aspirin who are undergoing heart surgery. I wonder whether this agent has been used in any vascular surgery population. It would seem to be a reasonable thing to try in selected cases, such as ruptured aneurysm, in which hemostasis frequently is so difficult.

Antiphospholipid Antibodies in Vascular Surgery Patients: A Cross-Sectional Study
Taylor LM Jr, Chitwood RW, Dalman RL, Sexton G, Goodnight SH, Porter JM (Oregon Health Sciences Univ, Portland)
Ann Surg 220:544–551, 1994   145-96-1–33

Background.—The presence of autoantibodies against phospholipids (aPL) has been associated with vascular thrombosis in the cerebral and coronary circulations as well as at peripheral arterial and venous sites. However, there are no data on the frequency of aPL in patients with peripheral arterial disease.

Methods.—An enzyme-linked immunosorbent assay was used to detect aPL in 234 consecutive patients with peripheral arterial disease who were admitted for vascular surgical procedures. All patients were receiving aspirin.

Results.—Sixty patients (26%) had aPL. Those with positive titers were nearly twice as likely as antibody-negative patients to have had vascular surgery on the lower extremity (table). Among patients who previously had undergone surgery, those with aPL were more than 5 times as likely to have had graft occlusion. In these patients, occlusion took place much earlier. Women were over-represented among aPL-positive patients with occluded grafts.

Conclusions.—Approximately 1 in 4 patients with marked symptoms of peripheral arterial disease have serum aPL. These patients—particularly women—are at increased risk for premature graft failure after vascular surgery is done on the lower extremity.

▶ In this rather large cross-sectional study, 26% of all patients admitted to our Vascular Surgical Service were found to have aPL antibodies. Others had other anticoagulation abnormalities, as noted in the comment after Abstract 145-96-1–29. Patients with aPL antibody had a distinctly different vascular history from those without, including many more failed grafts and a shorter duration of prior graft patency. As shown in Abstract 145-96-1–29, increasing evidence indicates that a remarkable proportion of patients admitted to a vascular surgery service will have a distinct hypercoagulable disorder if it is searched for diligently. This information will be important when selecting optimal treatment for these patients.

Positive Associations With Presence of Antiphospholipid Antibodies Confirmed by Logistic Regression Analysis

Factor	Odds Ratio	95% Confidence Interval	p Value
Previously lower extremity vascular procedure	1.8	1.0–3.3	0.047
Occlusive failure of previous lower extremity procedure	5.6	1.9–16.8	0.003
Female sex and previous lower extremity procedure	4.0	1.4–11.3	0.018

(Courtesy of Taylor LM Jr, Chitwood RW, Dalman RL, et al: *Ann Surg* 220:544–551, 1994.)

Anti-Cardiolipin Antibodies and Risk of Myocardial Infarction in a Prospective Cohort of Middle-Aged Men

Vaarala O, Mänttäri M, Manninen V, Tenkanen L, Puurunen M, Aho K, Palosuo T (Univ of Helsinki)
Circulation 91:23–27, 1995   145-96-1–34

Background.—Mixed results have been reported from studies relating titers of antiphospholipid antibodies to myocardial infarction in subjects lacking overt evidence of autoimmune disease. These studies have focused on patients with established coronary heart disease and survivors of myocardial infarction.

Objective.—A prospective study was done in male employees participating in the Helsinki Heart Study, a coronary primary prevention trial, to determine whether the presence of anticardiolipin (aCL) antibodies increases the risk of myocardial infarction.

Methods.—Serum samples were taken from middle-aged men who were dyslipidemic and whose baseline level of non–high-density-lipoprotein cholesterol was 5.2 mmol/L or greater. For 5 years, the subjects participated in a double-blind trial of gemfibrozil. Active treatment was associated with a 34% reduction in coronary heart disease. Sera were tested by an enzyme-linked immunosorbent assay for IgG antibody to cardiolipin. A group of 133 patients who had myocardial infarction or who died suddenly were matched for treatment condition and site of residence with the same number of controls.

Results.—Patients had significantly higher aCL antibody titers than matched controls. In those whose titers were in the highest quartile, the relative risk of myocardial infarction compared with the rest of the population was 2. The elevated risk was independent of age, smoking, systolic blood pressure, and low- and high-density-lipoprotein levels. High triglyceride levels augmented the risk associated with aCL antibody (Table 1), as

TABLE 1.—Joint Effect of Anticardiolipin Antibodies and Serum Triglycerides on Coronary Risk in the Helsinki Heart Study Case-Control Population

Elevated aCL Ab*	High TG†	Odds Ratio	95% Confidence Interval
No	No	1	
Yes	No	1.7	0.8 to 3.5
No	Yes	1.2	0.7 to 2.3
Yes	Yes	3.3	1.0 to 10.4

* Highest quartile (≥ 0.47).
† Highest tertile (≥ 2.3 mmol/L).
Odds ratios and 95% confidence intervals based on logistic regression analysis with age, smoking, and systolic blood pressure as co-variates.
Abbreviations: aCL Ab, anticardiolipin antibodies, *TG*, triglycerides.
(Courtesy of Vaarala O, Mänttäri M, Manninen V, et al: Anti-cardiolipin antibodies and risk of myocardial infarction in a prospective cohort of middle-aged men. *Circulation* 91:23–27, 1995. Reproduced with permission. *Circulation.* Copyright 1995 American Heart Association.)

TABLE 2.—Joint Effect of Anticardiolipin Antibodies and Antibody Against Oxidized IDL on Coronary Risk in the Helsinki Heart Study Case-Control Population

Elevated aCL Ab*	Elevated Ox-LDL Ab†	Odds Ratio	95% Confidence Interval
No	No	1	
Yes	No	1.7	0.8 to 4.0
No	Yes	2.3	1.1 to 4.7
Yes	Yes	3.1	1.3 to 7.3

* Highest quartile (≥ 0.47).
† Highest tertile (≥ 0.41).
Odds ratio and 95% confidence intervals based on logistic regression analysis with age, systolic blood pressure, and high-density lipoprotein cholesterol as co-variates.
Abbreviations: aCL Ab, anticardiolipin antibodies, *Ox-LDL Ab,* antibody against oxidized low-density lipoprotein (*LDL*).
(Courtesy of Vaarala O, Mänttäri M, Manninen V, et al: Anti-cardiolipin antibodies and risk of myocardial infarction in a prospective cohort of middle-aged men. *Circulation* 91:23–27, 1995. Reproduced with permission. *Circulation.* Copyright 1995 American Heart Association.)

did the presence of antibody against oxidized low-density lipoprotein (Table 2). A substantial increase in risk was found in smokers with increased aCL titers (Table 3).

Conclusion.—An elevated titer of aCL antibody is an independent risk factor for myocardial infarction or cardiac death in healthy middle-aged men.

▶ In this study, patients with a high level of aCL antibody had a markedly increased relative risk for myocardial infarction compared with the rest of the population. Interestingly, a correlation was noted between the levels of aCL and antibodies to oxidized low-density-lipoprotein cholesterol. These investigators concluded that the presence of a high level of aCL antibody is an independent risk factor for myocardial infarction or cardiac death. What we do not know, of course, is whether anticoagulation therapy has the potential to diminish the cardiogenic risk of antiphospholipid-anticardiolipin antibodies. Hopefully, such information will be available soon.

TABLE 3.—Joint Effect of Anticardiolipin Antibodies and Smoking on Coronary Risk in the Helsinki Heart Study Case-Control Population

Elevated aCL Ab*	Smoking	Odds Ratio	95% Confidence Interval
No	No	1	
Yes	No	1.6	0.7 to 3.9
No	Yes	2.5	1.4 to 4.5
Yes	Yes	5.4	2.3 to 12.6

* Highest tertile (≥ 0.47).
Odds ratios and 95% confidence intervals based on logistic regression analysis with age, systolic blood pressure, and triglycerides as co-variates.
Abbreviations: aCL Ab, anticardiolipin antibodies.
(Courtesy of Vaarala O, Mänttäri M, Manninen V, et al: Anti-cardiolipin antibodies and risk of myocardial infarction in a prospective cohort of middle-aged men. *Circulation* 91:23–27, 1995. Reproduced with permission. *Circulation.* Copyright 1995 American Heart Association.)

Claudication

Augmentation of Blood Flow in Limbs With Occlusive Arterial Disease by Intermittent Calf Compression
van Bemmelen PS, Mattos MA, Faught WE, Mansour MA, Barkmeier LD, Hodgson KJ, Ramsey DE, Sumner DS (Southern Illinois Univ School of Medicine, Springfield)
J Vasc Surg 19:1052–1058, 1994   145-96-1–35

Background.—Surgery on the peripheral vasculature attempts to increase blood flow in ischemic distal vascular beds. There is little evidence that reducing peripheral resistance in a vascular bed is helpful. Another approach may be to increase tissue perfusion by reducing venous pressure so it is below the normal level.

Methods.—The effects of intermittent calf compression on blood flow in the popliteal artery were examined in 41 extremities of symptomatic patients in whom the ankle pressure was reduced and in 11 legs of controls. One third of the patients had diabetes. Duplex ultrasonography was performed with the patient in the sitting and prone positions and was repeated immediately after a pneumatic cuff on the calf was inflated for 2 seconds at pressures of 20–120 mm Hg and then deflated.

Results.—Arterial blood flow increased 2–8 times (average, 4.4 times) on cuff deflation in seated controls, with a duration of 4–14 seconds. Little change was noted when they were prone. In seated patients with arterial obstruction, arterial flow increased an average of 3.2 times the resting flow (Fig 1–12). The peak increase in blood flow did not correlate closely with the ankle-brachial index.

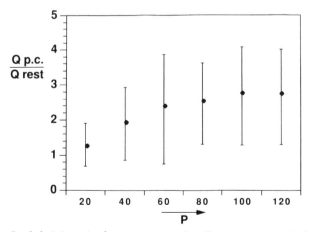

Fig 1–12.—Graph depicting ratio of mean postcompression ($Q_{p.c.}$) to precompression (resting) blood flow (Q_{rest}) vs. cuff pressure (*P* in mm Hg) during compression in 38 legs with decreased ankle pressures. (Courtesy of van Bemmelen PS, Mattos MA, Faught WE, et al: *J Vasc Surg* 19:1052–1058, 1994.)

Conclusions.—The increase in arterial flow associated with intermittent external limb compression reflects both transient vasodilatation and an increased arteriovenous pressure gradient. The effect is not dependent on an increased in-flow pressure and is not lessened by a low resting ankle-brachial pressure index, suggesting that this measure may be a useful nonoperative measure in patients with severe arterial insufficiency.

▶ Voices in the angiologic wilderness have been trying to convince us for years that intermittent pneumatic compression of the end-stage ischemic limb may enhance arterial circulation and result in some patient benefit. I have always thought this to be ridiculous, and I am surprised that Drs. van Bemmelen and Sumner have jumped on this shaky bandwagon. I officially award them the Camel Dung Award because I think this study is silly.

Superiority of Treadmill Walking Exercise Versus Strength Training for Patients With Peripheral Arterial Disease: Implications for the Mechanism of the Training Response
Hiatt WR, Wolfel EE, Meier RH, Regensteiner JG (Univ of Colorado Health Sciences Ctr, Denver)
Circulation 90:1866–1874, 1994   145-96-1–36

Background.—Programmed walking exercise is able to increase peak performance and enhance function in daily life in patients with intermittent claudication. Weak limb muscles may contribute to the difficulty in walking experienced by patients with peripheral arterial disease, but the potential value of other types of exercise has been largely unexplored.

Methods.—Strength training was compared with treadmill walking in 29 patients who had disabling claudication. They were randomized to 12 weeks of supervised walking on a treadmill; resistive strength training of muscle groups in each leg; or a nonexercising control group. Both types of exercise were performed for 3 hours a week. The walking group trained at a level sufficient to produce claudication. Peak exercise performance was determined by graded treadmill testing.

Results.—Peak walking time increased by 74% after 12 weeks of treadmill training and by 36% in those given strength training (Fig 1–13). Peak oxygen consumption improved with treadmill training but did not change in the strength training group. Another 12 weeks of supervised walking led to an additional 49% increase in peak walking time. When walking was added to strength training, performance increased to the level achieved by treadmill training alone.

Conclusion.—Supervised treadmill walking can effectively optimize exercise performance in patients with intermittent claudication.

▶ Dr. Hiatt and his group in Colorado are arguably the primary claudication scientists among the emerging group of vascular internists. In this article, they ask the haunting question of whether leg muscle training in a nonwalking mode will result in the same claudication benefit as walking exercise.

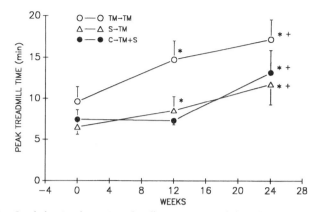

Fig 1–13.—Graph showing changes in peak walking time on a graded treadmill protocol with training. Patients randomized to the treadmill group (*TM*) were treated with a 24-week treadmill training program. Patients initially randomized to strength training (*S*) crossed over to treadmill training in the final 12 weeks. Patients in the control group (*C*) crossed over to a combined treadmill and strength (*TM ± S*) training program in the final 12 weeks. *$P < 0.05$ compared with entry value; *plus sign*, $P < 0.05$ week 24 compared with week 12. (Courtesy of Hiatt WR, Wolfel EE, Meier RH, et al: Superiority of treadmill walking exercise versus strength training for patients with peripheral arterial disease: Implications for the mechanism of the training response. *Circulation* 90:1866–1874, 1994. Reproduced with permission. *Circulation*. Copyright 1994 American Heart Association.)

They concluded, predictably, that muscle training without walking is not nearly as effective as walking training for claudication treatment. They also found, interestingly, that strength training, whether sequential or concomitant, didn't augment response to a walking exercise program. This information is interesting. A nearly identical version of this paper is in press in the *Journal of Vascular Surgery*, and it will probably be published before this YEAR BOOK. You will be able to read the publication of your choice.

An Objective Assessment of Intermittent Claudication by Near-Infrared Spectroscopy
Komiyama T, Shigematsu H, Yasuhara H, Muto T (Univ of Tokyo)
Eur J Vasc Surg 8:294–296, 1994   145-96-1–37

Background.—It has proved difficult to assess the severity of claudication because there is no accurate means of quantifying muscle ischemia during exercise. Peak walking distance does not correlate well with the degree of extremity ischemia.

Methods.—Near-infrared spectroscopy (NIRS) is a new approach to noninvasively monitoring the oxygenation of tissue in vivo. Change in oxygenation in the calf muscle were examined by NIRS in 62 patients describing intermittent claudication at this site during treadmill testing.

Results.—Three distinct patterns of serial change in oxygenated hemoglobin and deoxygenated hemoglobin were observed (Fig 1–14). All pa-

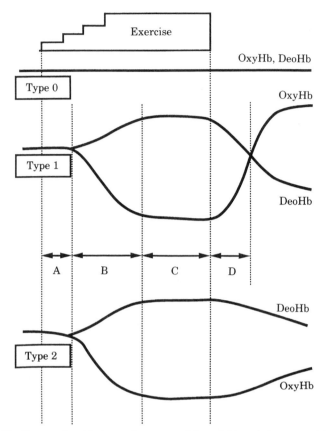

Fig 1–14.—Patterns of serial changes in oxygenated hemoglobin and deoxygenated hemoglobin. *Abbreviations: OxyHb,* oxygenated hemoglobin; *DeoHb,* deoxygenated hemoglobin. (Courtesy of Komiyama T, Shigematsu H, Yasuhara H, et al: *Eur J Vasc Surg* 8:294–296, 1994.)

tients with the type 0 pattern were able to walk for 5 minutes or longer. Severe ischemia was present in 37% of patients with a type 1 pattern and in 82% of those with type 2 changes. The latter patients were significantly compromised in walking, but the mean ankle–brachial pressure index at rest did not differ significantly from that in patients with a type 1 pattern.

Conclusions.—Near-infrared spectroscopy is a useful means of accurately determining the severity of intermittent claudication. It may also be helpful in evaluating the efficacy of medical measures.

► Near infrared spectroscopy measures the muscle oxygenated hemoglobin level by passing a light wave through the skin. Three patterns of dermal hemoglobin oxygenation generally conforming to clinical states of ischemic severity were recognized. These authors speculate that this device can be used to accurately assess the severity of intermittent claudication, and that it may provide objective information regarding the effects of medical treatment. This suggestion warrants further testing.

Electromyographic Signal Frequency Analysis in Evaluating Muscle Fatigue of Patients With Peripheral Arterial Disease

Casale R, Buonocore M, Di Massa A, Setacci C (Univ of Siena, Italy)
Arch Phys Med Rehabil 75:1118–1121, 1994   145-96-1-38

Background.—Patients with peripheral arterial disease (PAD) frequently are classified according to their subjective assessments of pain and fatigue on walking. It may be possible to objectify the process of evaluating these patients by quantifying muscle fatigue—a failure to maintain stable contraction that results in a decrement in performance.

Methods.—Surface electromyography (EMG) was performed in 15 patients with PAD and in 15 healthy subjects matched with the patients for age and sex. The EMG was recorded over the medial gastrocnemius muscle as it was contracted at 60% of maximum effort for 100 seconds. The recordings were analyzed off-line to derive the power spectrum. The median frequency was estimated in the first 30 seconds (T_0) and between 70 and 100 seconds (T_1).

Results.—In both patients with PAD and controls, T_1 values were significantly lower than initial frequencies. Whereas T_0 values did not differ between the patient and control groups, the patients with PAD had significantly lower T_1 values (Fig 1–15).

Conclusion.—Frequency analysis of the surface EMG is a convenient and painless means of objectively assessing muscle performance in patients with PAD.

▶ Just as Abstract 145-96-1-37 attempts to quantitate limb ischemia using near-infrared spectroscopy, this study attempts to quantitate claudication by using surface EMG to study peripheral muscle fatigue. Power spectral analyses were compared at the beginning and end of exercise, and significant differences were found. The values were also significantly different in patients with PAD compared with controls. These authors conclude that surface EMG may provide objective information on claudication. As I noted in the comment on Abstract 145-96-1-37, this is an interesting suggestion that warrants further investigation.

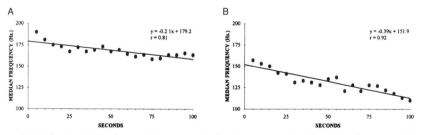

Fig 1–15.—Typical simple regression analysis obtained from a control subject (**A**) and a patient with peripheral arterial disease (**B**). Note that in the control subject, the straight line starts at a higher level and has a less steep gradient. (Courtesy of Casale R, Buonocore M, Di Massa A, et al: *Arch Phys Med Rehabil* 75:1118–1121, 1994.)

Homocystinemia

Premature Carotid Atherosclerosis: Does It Occur in Both Familial Hypercholesterolemia and Homocystinuria? Ultrasound Assessment of Arterial Intima-Media Thickness and Blood Flow Velocity
Rubba P, Mercuri M, Faccenda F, Iannuzzi A, Irace C, Strisciuglio P, Gnasso A, Tang R, Andria G, Bond MG, Mancini M (Univ Federico II, Naples, Italy; Wake Forest Univ, Winston-Salem, NC)
Stroke 25:943–950, 1994   145-96-1–39

Background.—Both familial hypercholesterolemia and homocystinuria caused by a deficiency of cystathionine β-synthase are inherited metabolic disorders that lead to premature cardiovascular disease. Whether different patterns of carotid wall damage and cerebral blood flow are present in these 2 metabolic diseases was investigated.

Methods.—Twelve patients with homocystinuria and 10 with homozygous familial hypercholesterolemia were studied, as were 11 healthy control subjects. The groups had a mean age of 24–26 years. B-mode ultrasonography was used to obtain the intima-media thickness in the common and internal carotid arteries and the carotid bifurcation (Fig 1–16). Cerebral blood flow velocity was estimated using transcranial Doppler scanning of the middle cerebral artery.

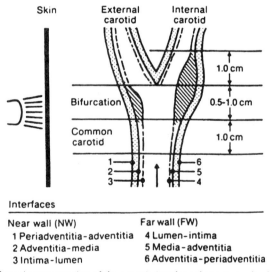

Interfaces

Near wall (NW)	Far wall (FW)
1 Periadventitia-adventitia	4 Lumen-intima
2 Adventitia-media	5 Media-adventitia
3 Intima-lumen	6 Adventitia-periadventitia

Fig 1–16.—Schematic representation of the acoustic interfaces that are visualized by B-mode ultrasound imaging at the level of the common carotid artery, bulb, and internal carotid artery on the arterial wall near and far from the echo transducer. (Courtesy of Rubba P, Mercuri M, Faccenda F, et al: Premature carotid atherosclerosis: Does it occur in both familial hypercholesterolemia and homocystinuria: Ultrasound assessment of arterial intima-media thickness and blood flow velocity. *Stroke* 25:943–950, 1994. Reproduced with permission. *Stroke.* Copyright 1994 American Heart Association.)

Results.—The average maximum intima-media thickness was 1.4 mm in the patients with familial hypercholesterolemia compared with 0.6 mm in each of the other groups (Fig 1–17). The diastolic flow velocity in the middle cerebral artery was significantly lower in the patients with familial hypercholesterolemia than in those with homocystinuria or the controls, but there were no such differences in systolic or mean flow velocity. The patients with familial hypercholesterolemia had significantly increased pulsatility indices, and the pulsatility index of the middle cerebral artery was correlated directly with the mean maximum intima-media thickness of the ipsilateral carotid vessels.

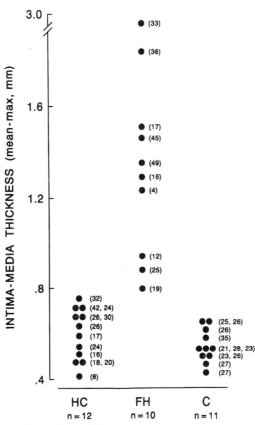

Fig 1–17.—Plot showing carotid wall thickness (mean-max [mean maximum intima-media thickness] estimate of the extent of atherosclerosis) determined with B-mode ultrasound imaging in healthy control subjects (*C*), homocystinuric patients (*HC*), and homozygotes for familial hypercholesterolemia (*FH*). Individual ages of patients and control subjects are indicated in parentheses. (Courtesy of Rubba P, Mercuri M, Faccenda F, et al: Premature carotid atherosclerosis: Does it occur in both familial hyper-cholesterolemia and homocystinuria? Ultrasound assessment of arterial intima-media thickness and blood flow velocity. *Stroke* 25:943–950, 1994. Reproduced with permission. *Stroke.* Copyright 1994 American Heart Association.)

Conclusions.—Carotid plaques are infrequent in patients with homocystinuria but, in those with familial hypercholesterolemia, the carotid vessels typically are diffusely and focally thickened. In addition, endothelial dysfunction of the small resistance arteries secondary to hyperlipidemia may lead to disordered cerebral blood flow in these patients.

▶ These conclusions are interesting. As reported in the 1994 YEAR BOOK (1), Dr. Malinow and associates found that among asymptomatic adults, those who had evidence of carotid wall thickening had a higher plasma homocysteine level than those who did not. These authors are examining the other side of the coin; namely, do individuals with increased homocysteine have arterial wall thickening? They conclude that such people do not, which leads them to speculate that perhaps the mischief caused by an increased homocysteine level is related to thrombosis. One must note, however, that the patients in this study were categorized by homocystinuria, which is, indeed, a rather primitive method. Homocystinemia is much preferred as the method of patient categorization. I am inclined to dismiss this study because of these methodological problems.

Reference

1. 1994 YEAR BOOK OF VASCULAR SURGERY, p 44.

Treatment of Mild Hyperhomocysteinemia in Vascular Disease Patients
Franken DG, Boers GHJ, Blom HJ, Trijbels FJM, Kloppenborg PWC (Univ Hosp Nijmegen, The Netherlands)
Arterioscler Thromb 14:465–470, 1994   145-96-1–40

Introduction.—Mild hyperhomocysteinemia is a known risk factor for premature arteriosclerotic disease. Blood homocysteine levels can be lowered by treatment with vitamin B_6, folic acid, or betaine, all of which are involved in methionine metabolism. However, these treatments have not been reported to normalize increased blood homocysteine concentrations. The screening and treatment of mild hyperhomocysteinemia in patients with vascular disease were reported.

Methods.—Oral methionine loading tests were performed to screen for mild hyperhomocysteinemia in 421 patients who had premature peripheral or cerebral occlusive arterial disease. The screening test was positive in 33% of the patients with peripheral disease and in 20% of those with cerebral disease, in 14% of the men, and in 34% of the premenopausal and 26% of the postmenopausal women. Mild hyperhomocysteinemia was treated with vitamin B_6, 250 mg/day. The methionine loading test was repeated after 6 weeks to evaluate the effects of treatment. If the homocysteine concentration had not normalized, further treatment with vitamin B_6, 250 mg/day; folic acid, 5 mg/day; or betaine, 6 g/day, was given. These treatments were given alone or in any combination.

Results.—Initial treatment with vitamin B₆ normalized the afterload homocysteine concentration in 56% of the patients. This treatment was successful in 71% of the men, 45% of the premenopausal women, and 88% of the postmenopausal women (Fig 1–18). In 95% of the remaining patients, further treatment normalized homocysteine levels.

Conclusions.—Mild hyperhomocysteinemia is common in patients with premature peripheral or cerebral arteriosclerotic disease. In almost all such cases, the homocysteine concentration can be normalized safely and easily by treatment with vitamin B₆, folic acid, and betaine.

▶ These authors make the profound observation that hyperhomocysteine-mia can be reduced to normal by giving a patient vitamin B₆, folic acid, or betaine. Because this has been known for decades, I am amazed that any editor would publish this information. Although the material published in this article is accurate, it was already well known by everyone working in this field. This paper earns at least a junior-grade Camel Dung Award.

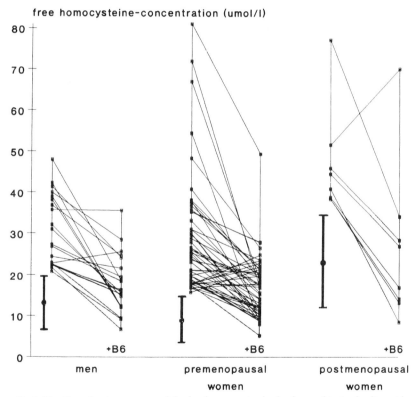

Fig 1–18.—Plots showing response of the free homocysteine levels after methionine loading with a 6-week treatment of vitamin B6, 250 mg daily, in 82 hyperhomocysteinemic vascular disease patients. (Courtesy of Franken DG, Boers GHJ, Blom HJ, et al: Treatment of mild hyperhomocysteinemia in vascular disease patients. *Arterioscler Thromb* 14:465–470, 1994. Reproduced with permission. *Arteriosclerosis Thrombosis* Copyright 1994 American Heart Association.)

Role of Blood Pressure, Uric Acid, and Hemorheological Parameters on Plasma Homocyst(e)ine Concentration

Malinow MR, Levenson J, Giral P, Nieto FJ, Razavian M, Segond P, Simon A (Oregon Regional Primate Research Ctr, Beaverton; Hosp Broussais, Paris; Johns Hopkins Univ, Baltimore, Md; et al)

Atherosclerosis 114:175–183, 1995   145-96-1–41

Background.—An increased plasma concentration of homocyst(e)ine is an independent risk factor for clinical atherosclerotic disease, and basal levels often are increased in patients with arterial occlusive disease.

Methods.—Plasma homocyst(e)ine levels were estimated in 208 men with no history of atherosclerotic disease, and were correlated with various hemodynamic, rheologic, and biochemical values. The study group included 87 individuals with hypertension, 142 subjects with hypercholesterolemia, and 86 smokers.

Results.—Hypertensive men had higher plasma homocyst(e)ine levels than did those who were normotensive. Elevated homocyst(e)ine levels correlated with a number of risk factors, but some associations no longer held after adjusting for other variables. On multivariate analysis, the plasma concentration of homocyst(e)ine correlated with systolic blood pressure, the plasma uric acid level, and the hematocrit, all of which are possible risk factors for atherosclerosis.

▶ These interesting observations come from the individual who really has pioneered the recognition of hyperhomocysteinemia: Dr. M.R. Malinow. He observes that multivariate analysis indicates that systolic blood pressure, plasma uric acid, and hematocrit are independent predictors of the plasma homocysteine concentration. We have previously recognized that renal failure, aging, and deficiency of vitamins B_{12}, B_6, and folic acid are independent predictors. These factors must be carefully considered by epidemiologists before conclusions are reached. We have attempted to minimize the effect of such variables in our own studies of homocysteine by recognizing as positive only those individuals with marked increases in plasma homocysteine.

Association Between Plasma Homocysteine Concentrations and Extracranial Carotid-Artery Stenosis

Selhub J, Jacques PF, Bostom AG, D'Agostino RB, Wilson PWF, Belanger AJ, O'Leary DH, Wolf PA, Schaefer EJ, Rosenberg IH (Tufts Univ, Boston; Boston Univ; Geisinger Med Ctr, Danville, Pa)

N Engl J Med 332:286–291, 1995   145-96-1–42

Background.—Epidemiologic studies suggest that increased plasma homocysteine levels may be a risk factor for atherosclerosis. Moderate hyperhomocysteinemia has been associated with symptomatic peripheral, cerebral, and coronary vascular disease. Fasting homocysteine levels may be one third higher in such patients than in normal individuals.

Objective.—The relationship between carotid artery stenosis, evaluated ultrasonographically, and the plasma homocysteine concentration was examined in a cross-sectional study of 1,041 men and women 67–96 years of age from the Framingham Heart Study. In addition, levels of folate, vitamin B_{12}, and pyridoxal-5'-phosphate (the co-enzyme form of vitamin B_6) were estimated.

Findings.—Peak carotid stenosis of 25% or greater was found in 43% of the men and 34% of the women in the study. The odds ratio for this degree of stenosis in individuals having the highest plasma homocysteine levels (greater than 14.4 µmol/L) compared with those having the lowest levels (9.1 µmol/L or less) was 2.0. This figure was adjusted for age, sex, systolic blood pressure, smoking status, and the plasma level of high-density-lipoprotein cholesterol. Adjusted plasma levels of folate and pyridoxal-5'-phosphate were correlated inversely with carotid stenosis.

Discussion.—In the elderly, a high plasma level of homocysteine is associated with an increased risk of extracranial carotid artery stenosis. The plasma homocysteine level may be brought into the normal range by administering innocuous amounts of folate and vitamins B_6 and B_{12}.

▶ In yet another approach to harvesting of epidemiologic data, these investigators performed a cross-sectional study of 1,041 elderly subjects from the Framingham Heart Study, examining both the extracranial carotid arteries, using ultrasound, and the plasma level of homocysteine. A clear relationship between serum plasma levels of homocysteine and increasing carotid stenosis was noted. Low serum concentrations of folate and vitamin B_6 were also related to an increased risk for carotid disease. These are essential vitamins in the metabolism of homocysteine.

On balance, we have to accept the undisputed association between homocysteine and clinical atherosclerosis, despite what was reported in Abstract 145-96-1-39. What we do not know is whether the increased homocysteine level in one third of the patients with significant atherosclerosis has a cause-and-effect relationship to the atherosclerosis or, rather, is a fellow traveler or marker. I see no way to resolve this other than with a prospective, randomized treatment trial that uses progression of atherosclerosis and clinical atherosclerotic events as end points. Such trials are currently being contemplated by the NIH, but to my knowledge none has yet been funded.

Intimal Hyperplasia

The Expression and Function of G-Proteins in Experimental Intimal Hyperplasia
Davies MG, Ramkumar V, Gettys TW, Hagen P-O (Duke Univ, Durham, NC; Southern Illinois Univ, Springfield; Med Univ of South Carolina, Charleston)
J Clin Invest 94:1680–1689, 1994   145-96-1–43

Background.—Vein bypass grafts develop intimal hyperplasia, with an increased response to norepinephrine; additionally, they develop a contractile response to serotonin. The latter changes suggest significant changes in the smooth muscle cells of the vein grafts compared with their venous progenitors. The G-proteins are membrane-bound signal transduction proteins that couple extracellular receptor signals to various effectors. Changes in responsiveness to norepinephrine and serotonin may be caused by alterations in the expression of G-proteins. The expression and function of G-proteins in experimental intimal hyperplasia of vein bypass grafting were investigated.

Methods.—A reversed jugular vein interposition bypass of the right common carotid artery using the ipsilateral external jugular vein was performed in 30 male rabbits. At 28 days, both the vein graft and the contralateral jugular vein (control) were harvested. Isometric tension studies were performed on rings from 10 veins and vein grafts, and Western blot and messenger RNA (mRNA) analyses were performed in another 20 vessels. The expression and functional coupling of G-proteins (α_1, α_s, α_q, and α_o) were determined.

Results.—Vein grafts demonstrated significant intimal hyperplasia compared with the control vein. Vein grafts demonstrated a fivefold increase in α_q, a 2.7-fold increase in the α_{i2}, and a 3.3-fold increase in α_s expression. In addition, α_{i3} expression was detected only in vein grafts. Furthermore, vein grafts expressed a 3.8-fold increase in β-subunits and increased mRNA for α_s, α_{i3}, and α_{i2}. There was no detectable α_{i1} protein or its mRNA in either the veins or the vein grafts. Contractile responses to norepinephrine were not inhibited by pertussis toxin in the veins, but they were enhanced twofold in vein grafts. In addition, responses to serotonin developed de novo in vein grafts only. Pertussis toxin partially inhibited the contractile responses to both norepinephrine and serotonin in the vein grafts, although there was a 100% adenosine diphosphate ribosylation with pertussis toxin in both the veins and vein grafts.

Implications.—Intimal hyperplasia is associated with increased or novel expression of G-proteins in vivo, which occur simultaneously with the development of pertussis toxin-sensitive contractile responses. Changes in G-proteins at a transcriptional level or at the level of RNA stability may be involved in the response of smooth muscle cells to injury and to intimal hyperplasia formation.

▶ Guanine nucleotide regulatory proteins are intimately involved in signal transduction in many cell functions. These experiments indicate that vein graft adaptation in the arterial system is associated with increased or novel expression of G-proteins, which in turn may be involved in the response of smooth muscle cells to injury. The authors have failed to show a linear response to intimal hyperplasia, and I wonder whether what they are measuring may really be normal vein adaptation to arterial pressure, which may have nothing to do with intimal hyperplasia. Studies relating vein graft behavior to G-protein alterations are welcome, as it is undoubtedly true that these regulatory proteins have a major role in vascular biology. On balance, this is an interesting study.

Intimal Hyperplasia After Vascular Injury Is Inhibited by Antisense cdk 2 Kinase Oligonucleotides
Morishita R, Gibbons GH, Ellison KE, Nakajima M, von der Leyen H, Zhang L, Kaneda Y, Ogihara T, Dzau VJ (Stanford Univ, Calif; Inst for Cellular and Molecular Biology, Osaka, Japan; Osaka Univ Med School, Japan)
J Clin Invest 93:1458–1464, 1994   145-96-1-44

Background.—Cyclin-dependent kinase (cdk) 2 kinase is an enzyme that helps regulate the cell cycle and is activated in the rat carotid artery after injury by balloon inflation. The enzyme may mediate the proliferation of smooth muscle cells. Whether inhibiting the expression of cdk 2 kinase will suppress intimal hyperplasia was examined.

Methods.—A 2-F catheter was used to injure the common carotid artery in rats. The animals received cdk 2 kinase intraluminally in the form of hemagglutinating virus of Japan (HVJ)-liposome complexes. Groups of animals received the active complex, liposome complex without HVJ particles, or antisense phosphorothioate oligodeoxynucleotides (ODN).

Results.—Treatment with antisense ODN markedly reduced the level of messenger RNA for cdk 2 kinase in injured vessels. Administration of antisense ODN 2 weeks after transection decreased neointima formation by 60%. Antisense cell division cycle 2 ODN alone reduced intima formation by 40%, whereas combined antisense treatment almost totally abolished neointima formation. Fluorescence studies of transfected vessels showed that ODN was localized in the media and persisted for up to 2 weeks after transection.

Conclusion.—These findings indicate that the antisense approach is a potentially effective means of preventing recurrent arterial stenosis.

▶ Before reading this paper, I did not know that there was such a thing as cell cycle regulatory genes. These authors report that transfection of vascular wall cells with the antisense version of this substance profoundly inhibits fibrointimal hyperplasia. This is a very basic molecular biological study that points to yet another substance that may be of benefit in the ultimate reduction of the common enemy: intimal hyperplasia.

Inhibition of Integrin Function by a Cyclic RGD-Containing Peptide Prevents Neointima Formation
Matsuno H, Stassen JM, Vermylen J, Deckmyn H (Ctr for Molecular and Vascular Biology, Leuven, Belgium)
Circulation 90:2203–2206, 1994   145-96-1-45

Background.—There is evidence that peptides containing the Arg-Gly-Asp (RGD) sequence, which is found in many adhesive molecules, can prevent the binding of ligands to certain integrin molecules, including glycoprotein IIb/IIa. For this reason, they inhibit platelet aggregation and the migration of smooth muscle cells, processes that are both involved in the formation of neointima.

Methods.—Hamster carotid arteries were injured by a catheter with a roughened tip, and the formation of neointima was monitored by computer-assisted microscopic image analysis. Experimental animals received a cyclic RGD-containing peptide, G4120, delivered IV by an implanted osmotic pump.

Results.—The RGD-containing peptide inhibited neointima formation in a dose-dependent manner. Its suppressive effect was most evident when treatment began before the vessel was injured and was continued throughout the observation period. A lesser effect was achieved when treatment began after injury or when it was begun before injury but then withdrawn.

Conclusions.—Inhibiting integrin function reduces development of a neointima after vascular injury, probably through a dual action inhibiting the secretion of platelet-derived growth factor and, at a later stage, interfering with integrin in smooth muscle cells.

▶ The RGD-containing peptide competitively inhibits the IIb/IIIa integrin receptor on the surface of platelets. Such inhibition in this experimental model reduces the development of neointimal hyperplasia. This appears to be similar to the effect seen using the monoclonal antibody to IIb/IIIa described in Abstract 145-96-1–21.

Halofuginone: A Specific Collagen Type I Inhibitor Reduces Anastomotic Intimal Hyperplasia
Choi ET, Callow AD, Sehgal NL, Brown DM, Ryan US (Washington Univ, St Louis, Mo; Boston Univ)
Arch Surg 130:257–261, 1995   145-96-1–46

Background.—Arterial stenosis is chiefly caused by intimal hyperplasia resulting from both smooth muscle cell proliferation and accumulation of extracellular matrix within the vascular lumen. Fibrillar collagen types I and III have been shown to promote synthetic activity in smooth muscle cells from rabbit artery.

Methods.—Halofuginone hydrobromide, which specifically inhibits the production of type I collagen, was used in an attempt to prevent intimal hyperplasia in rabbits that had the right common carotid artery incised and reapproximated end to end by using interrupted 10-0 Prolene sutures. Randomly selected animals were fed a nontoxic dose of halofuginone, and the arteries were harvested 4 weeks later.

Results.—The administration of halofuginone inhibited smooth muscle cell proliferation in vitro without altering cell viability. Morphometric

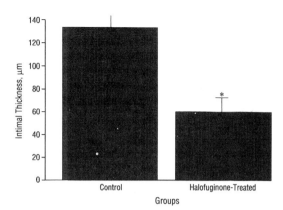

Fig 1–19.—Comparison of maximal intimal thickness at the anastomosis for the control and halofuginone hydrobromide–treated groups. *Asterisk* indicates $P < 0.01$. (Courtesy of Choi ET, Callow AD, Sehgal NL, et al: Halofuginone: A specific collagen type I inhibitor reduces anastomotic intimal hyperplasia. *Arch Surg* 130:257–261, 1995. Copyright 1994/1995, American Medical Association.)

studies demonstrated that active treatment significantly lessened intimal thickness at the anastomotic site (Fig 1–19).

Conclusion.—It may be feasible to limit intimal hyperplasia after arterial anastomosis by blocking collagen production.

▶ Halofuginone, an antifungal agent, inhibits the production of type I collagen. Type I collagen appears to be essential for smooth muscle cell proliferation and conversion to a synthetic phenotype. In this very preliminary animal study, halofuginone appeared to diminish intimal hyperplasia significantly at a vascular anastomotic site. I have absolutely no idea whether this will prove to be a safe or effective agent.

Endovascular Low-Dose Irradiation Inhibits Neointima Formation After Coronary Artery Balloon Injury in Swine
Waksman R, Robinson KA, Crocker IR, Gravanis MB, Cipolla GD, King SB III (Emory Univ, Atlanta, Ga)
Circulation 91:1533–1539, 1995   145-96-1–47

Background.—Restenosis remains a major obstacle to long-term success in patients undergoing percutaneous transluminal coronary angioplasty. Low doses of radiation have effectively inhibited exuberant wound healing in various clinical settings. Because restenosis is a form of wound healing, the efficacy of irradiation was examined in a porcine model of balloon angioplasty injury.

Methods.—Neointimal lesions resembling those seen in restenosed human coronary arteries were made in normal pigs by overinflating an angioplasty balloon. A high-activity iridium-192 source was placed in some of the injured vessels long enough to deliver 350, 700, or 1,400 cGy of gamma radiation, and the vessels were fixed by pressure perfusion after

2 weeks. Other miniswine had their carotid and coronary arteries irradi-ated with 700 or 1,400 cGy and were followed for 6 months.

Results.—Neointima formation was consistently inhibited by irradia-tion, as shown by computer-assisted planimetric measurements. The ratio of intimal area to the length of the medial fracture was correlated inversely with the radiation dose delivered (Fig 1–20). Delaying the delivery of 700 cGy for 2 days after injury further limited neointima formation. The long-term studies confirmed the suppressive effect of irradiation on neoin-tima formation and showed no excessive vascular or perivascular fibrosis.

Conclusions.—It may be feasible to prevent recurrent coronary stenosis after percutaneous angioplasty by exposing the intraluminal surface to gamma radiation.

▶ In this remarkable study, low-dose intracoronary irradiation delivered di-rectly to the site of overstretched balloon dilatation injury of the coronary artery in animals inhibited intimal hyperplasia with, importantly, demonstra-tion of a dose-response relationship. You may remember my prior expression

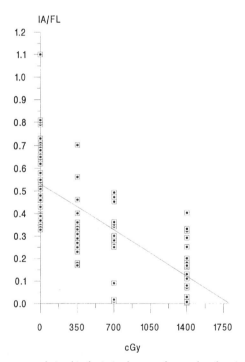

Fig 1–20.—Dose-response relationship for intimal area-to-fracture length ratio (*IA/FL*) as a function of radiation dose in immediately treated groups: slope = −0.0028, P < 0.0001, r = −0.75. The linear model, as opposed to the curvilinear (exponential) model, best described the data. (Courtesy of Waksman R, Robinson KA, Crocker IR, et al: Endovascular low-dose irradiation inhibits neointima formation after coronary artery balloon injury in swine. *Circulation* 91:1533–1539, 1995. Reproduced with permission. *Circulation.* Copyright 1995 American Heart Association.)

of concern regarding this subject (1). I continue to regard this as a worrisome type of treatment to extend to humans, even in a phase I trial. I hope extreme caution will be the order of the day.

Reference

1. 1995 YEAR BOOK OF VASCULAR SURGERY, p 92.

Vasospasm

On the Existence of Functional Beta-Adrenoceptors on Vascular Sympathetic Nerve Endings in the Human Forearm
Chang PC, Grossman E, Kopin IJ, Goldstein DS (Natl Inst of Neurological Disorders and Stroke, Natl Insts of Health, Bethesda, Md)
J Hypertens 12:681–690, 1994   145-96-1–48

Background.—Both in vitro and animal studies have suggested that β-adrenoceptors on sympathetic nerve terminals modulate the release of norepinephrine during sympathetic stimulation. This effect underlies the so-called epinephrine hypothesis of hypertension, according to which a high circulating level of epinephrine in hypertensive patients amplifies sympathetically mediated pressor responses by activating presynaptic β-adrenoceptors and thereby promoting the release of norepinephrine.

Methods.—The presence of presynaptic β-adrenoceptors that modulate the release of norepinephrine in the forearm was examined by infusing isoprenaline intra-arterially to stimulate β-adrenoceptors in 31 healthy individuals. Terbutaline was infused to stimulate β_2-adrenoceptors, propranolol to block β-adrenoceptors, metoprolol to block β_1-adrenoceptors, isoprenaline combined with metoprolol to stimulate β_2-adrenoceptors, epinephrine to stimulate α- and β-adrenoceptors, yohimbine to block α_2-adrenoceptors, and sodium nitroprusside to directly augment forearm blood flow. The spillover of norepinephrine in forearm venous plasma and its rate of appearance in the forearm were determined by infusing tritiated norepinephrine intra-arterially.

Results.—None of the infusions led to systemic hemodynamic changes or altered the arterial plasma concentration of norepinephrine. Metoprolol and propranolol decreased both the norepinephrine spillover and its rate of appearance without changing forearm blood flow. Isoprenaline and nitroprusside increased the spillover of norepinephrine in the forearm, whereas epinephrine decreased it. Terbutaline increased forearm norepinephrine spillover and its rate of appearance more than nitroprusside or isoprenaline did at a given level of forearm blood flow. Isoprenaline infusion had no effects beyond those expected from increased forearm blood flow. The administration of epinephrine increased the spillover and forearm appearance rate of norepinephrine during the intra-arterial infusion of yohimbine.

Conclusion.—These findings affirm that β-adrenoceptors promote the release of norepinephrine from vascular sympathetic nerve endings in normal humans.

▶ This complicated study in humans examines the role of a variety of drugs that stimulate and block α- and β-adrenoceptors. The authors conclude that presynaptic β-adrenoceptors do modulate norepinephrine release. This important study further defines the complex interaction of α_1-, α_2-, β_1-, and β_2-adrenoceptors in human upper extremity circulation.

Molecular Biology

Treatment of Murine Hemangioendotheliomas With the Angiogenesis Inhibitor AGM-1470
O'Reilly MS, Brem H, Folkman J (Children's Hosp, Boston; Harvard Med School, Boston)
J Pediatr Surg 30:325–330, 1995   145-96-1–49

Background.—Although most angiomatous disorders of childhood are self-limited and do not cause serious harm, some cause significant morbidity and may even threaten life. Interferon-α is a weak inhibitor of angiogenesis that reportedly reduces the mortality risk associated with life-threatening hemangiomas. AGM-1470 is a synthetic analogue of fumagillin, a fungus-derived product, that strongly inhibits angiogenesis in vitro and also in vivo.

Objective and Methods.—Syngeneic mice were given implants of cells derived from a spontaneous murine hemangioendothelioma. After tumors had developed in 2–3 days, either AGM-1470 or saline was administered systemically.

Results.—Tumor volumes were substantially smaller in mice given AGM-1470 than in saline-injected animals after 3 weeks (Fig 1–21). The survival of actively treated animals was prolonged, and there was no apparent drug-related toxicity.

Conclusion.—Antiangiogenic agents such as AGM-1470 may prove to be effective and safe when used to treat hemangiomas and related angiomatous disorders.

▶ The potential of angiomatous lesions to regress with drug therapy has attracted considerable attention in recent years. Alpha-interferon appears to be a weak inhibitor of angiogenesis and has been used in some of these patients. Recently, a substance known as AGM-1470, a synthetic analogue of a substance called fumagillin, isolated from fungus, has been shown to be a potent inhibitor of angiogenesis. In this experimental study, the substance appeared to be extremely effective in reducing the volume of a spontaneously occurring mouse hemangioendothelioma. I have no idea whether any of these substances will prove effective in clinical treatment, but I do know that surgery for these lesions is frequently disfiguring and generally unsuccessful.

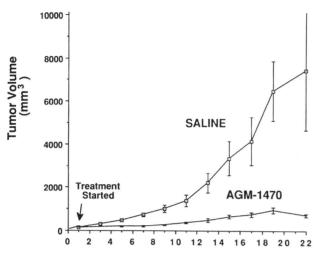

Fig 1–21.—Inhibition of the growth of mouse hemangioendotheliomas by systemic treatment with AGM-1470. (Courtesy of O'Reilly MS, Brem H, Folkman J: *J Pediatr Surg* 30:325–330, 1995.)

Smooth Muscle Cell Expression of Extracellular Matrix Genes After Arterial Injury
Nikkari ST, Järveläinen HT, Wight TN, Ferguson M, Clowes AW (Univ of Washington, Seattle)
Am J Pathol 144:1348–1356, 1994   145-96-1-50

Background.—Extracellular matrix (ECM) accumulates after arterial injury and contributes to intimal thickening. This process is modulated by heparin.

Methods.—The expression of matrix protein was examined by using the Northern blot technique to determine levels of messenger RNA for a number of ECM proteins in a rat model of balloon-induced injury of the carotid artery. The RNA was extracted from normal vessels and from intima-medial preparations 2 days and 1, 2, and 4 weeks after injury. The animals were given either heparin or saline by infusion.

Results.—Transcripts for the heparin sulfate proteoglycans perlecan (Fig 1–22), syndecan, and ryudocan were increased starting a week after injury. Increased expression of the chondroitin sulfate proteoglycan versican, the dermatan sulfate proteoglycan biglycan, type I procollagen, and tropoelastin also was observed. In situ hybridization studies showed that the transcripts for elastin and biglycan were mainly present in intimal smooth muscle cells. They were decreased in samples from heparin-treated animals, in proportion to the decrease in intimal area. Transcripts for perlecan and ryudocan were increased in the intima and media, independently of exposure to heparin.

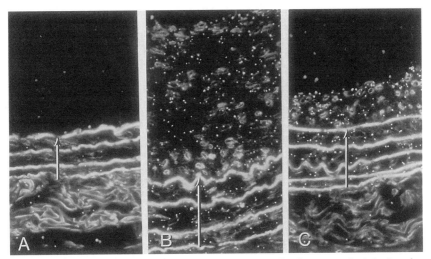

Fig 1–22.—Dark-field photomicrographs showing localization of perlecan transcript induction after rat carotid artery injury by in situ hybridization. A, uninjured carotid. B, 2 weeks after injury with saline treatment. C, 2 weeks after injury with heparin treatment. Induction of transcripts is in both intimal and medial cells in both groups. *Arrows,* span the width of the media and point at the internal elastic lamina. Lumen is at the top. (Magnification, ×800.) (Courtesy of Nikkari ST, Jarvelainen HT, Wight TN, et al: *Am J Pathol* 144:1348–1356, 1994.)

Conclusion.—Extracellular matrix genes are expressed some time after aterial injury. Some of these genes are expressed in the arterial intima only, and others are expressed in both the intima and media.

▶ This exotic publication presents a nice discussion of a whole host of extracellular matrix proteins. The authors conclude that ECM gene expression is a relatively late-occurring event after arterial injury, with some genes expressed only in the intima and others expressed in both the intima and media. On balance, I find this interesting, although I really do not know what it means.

Shear Stress Selectively Upregulates Intercellular Adhesion Molecule-1 Expression in Cultured Human Vascular Endothelial Cells
Nagel T, Resnick N, Atkinson WJ, Dewey CF Jr, Gimbrone MA Jr (Harvard Med School, Boston; Massachusetts Inst of Technology, Cambridge, Mass)
J Clin Invest 94:885–891, 1994   145-96-1–51

Background.—Functional changes in the vascular endothelium result from hemodynamic forces. Some of these changes have been found to reflect alterations in gene expression. In a recent report, investigators described a *cis*-acting transcriptional regulatory element, the shear stress response element (SSRE). The SSRE, which is found in the promoters of several genes, may serve as a common pathway by which biomechanical forces affect gene expression. The effects of shear stress on endothelial expression of adhesion molecules that do and do not express the SSRE were studied.

Methods.—With a cone and plate apparatus, cultured human umbilical vein endothelial cells were subjected to a physiologic range of laminar shear stresses—2.5–46.0 dyne/cm^2—for up to 48 hours. The effects of shear stress on endothelial expression of intercellular adhesion molecule–1 (ICAM-1), which includes the SSRE in its promoter, as well as E-selectin and vascular cell adhesion molecule-1, which do not contain the SSRE, were examined.

Results.—Exposure to shear stress increased surface immunoreactive ICAM-1 in a time-dependent but force-independent manner (Fig 1–23). Expression of ICAM-1 was upregulated in correlation with increased adhesion of the JY lymphocytic cell line. On Northern blotting, increased ICAM-1 transcript was demonstrated after as little as 2 hours of shear stress exposure. At no time was there any upregulation of E-selectin or vascular cell adhesion molecule–1 transcript or cell-surface protein.

Conclusion.—Shear stress causes selective upregulation of adhesion molecule expression by vascular endothelial cells. Along with humoral stimuli, biomechanical forces may play a role in differential endothelial

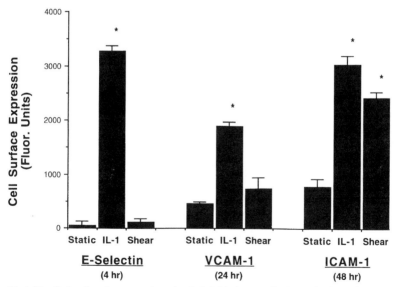

Fig 1–23.—Peak cell-surface expression of endothelial-leukocyte adhesion molecules in human umbilical vein endothelial cells (*HUVEC*) subjected to IL-1β or shear stress. The HUVEC monolayers were maintained under static conditions, exposed to laminar shear stress (10 dyne/cm²), or treated with a maximally effective concentration of IL-1β (10 U/mL) for periods corresponding to the peak cytokine-induced surface expression of E-selectin (4 hours), vascular cell adhesion molecule–1 (*VCAM-1*) (24 hours), or intercellular adhesion molecule–1 (*ICAM-1*) (48 hours), respectively. Cell-surface protein was measured using a fluorescence immunobinding assay. *n* = 3–4 replicate coverslips for each controlled variable; data expressed as mean ± SD, *P < 0.01 stimulus vs. static (Student's *t*-test). (Courtesy of Nagel T, Resnick N, Atkinson WJ, et al: *J Clin Invest* 94:885–891, 1994.)

gene expression. These forces may have pathophysiologic relevance in settings such as inflammation and atherosclerosis.

▶ The article by Malek et al. (Abstract 145-96-1–30) dramatically demonstrated the effect of shear stress on endothelial expression. Abstract 145-95-1–1 examines the effect of shear stress on endothelial expression of 3 adhesion molecules. Intercellular adhesion molecule–1 appeared to be selectively upgraded by shear stress, whereas E-selectin and vascular cell adhesion molecule–1 appeared unaffected. The authors conclude—correctly, I suspect—that biomechanical forces clearly have a role in directing differential endothelial gene expression. If true, shear stress must represent a relevant stimulus in the development of both inflammation and atherosclerosis. I do believe this abstracted paper, along with Abstract 145-96-1–30, contributes important new information.

Mechanical Stretch Increases Proto-Oncogene Expression and Phosphoinositide Turnover in Vascular Smooth Muscle Cells
Lyall F, Deehan MR, Greer IA, Boswell F, Brown WC, McInnes GT (Univ of Glasgow, Royal Infirmary, Scotland; Western Infirmary, Glasgow, Scotland)
J Hypertens 12:1139–1145, 1994   145-96-1–52

Objective.—The effects of hemodynamic loading on biochemical signaling were studied in vitro in a model designed to mechanically stretch cultured vascular smooth muscle cells.

Methods.—Smooth muscle cells from the rat mesenteric artery were cultured on silicone sheets coated with collagen, fibronectin, gelatin, or polylysine, and they were stretched by as much as 20% between Perspex blocks. Expression of messenger RNA (mRNA) for the proto-oncogene c-*fos* was monitored by Northern blotting for 6 hours. Breakdown of phosphoinositide was estimated by measuring the release of tritiated inositol phosphates from prelabeled cells.

Results.—Stretching the cells by 20% led to the rapid induction of c-*fos* mRNA, which peaked within 15 minutes. The level of expression correlated with the degree of cell stretching. A 20% fixed stretch led to a 3.2-fold increase in total inositol phosphates at 20 minutes.

Conclusion.—That mechanically stretching vascular smooth muscle cells leads to early signaling events that are associated with cell growth supports a role for stretching in the development of vascular hypertrophy.

▶ In this study, mechanical stretch in tissue culture is shown to increase proto-oncogene expression as well as phosphoinositide turnover in vascular smooth muscle cells. This is another biomechanical stimulus that appears to be capable of altering a cell's phenotypic expression. Although it is different from shear stress, it is related.

Enhanced Revascularisation After Angiogenic Stimulation in a Rabbit Model of Bilateral Limb Ischaemia

Pu L-Q, Gadowski GR, Graham AM, Ricci MA, Brassard R, Sniderman AD, Symes JF (Mcgill Univ, Montreal; Univ of Vermont, Burlington)
Eur J Vasc Endovasc Surg 9:189–196, 1995   145-96-1–53

Background.—Previous observations have suggested that endothelial cell growth factor (ECGF) stimulates the formation of collateral vessels in a rabbit model of unilateral extremity ischemia. To distinguish the effects of ischemia alone from those of ischemia combined with angiogenic stimulation in the same animals, a rabbit model of bilateral hind limb ischemia was used.

Methods.—Severe ischemia compatible with a viable extremity was produced in both hind limbs of 11 rabbits by ligating arterial vessels above the inguinal ligament and excising the common and superficial femoral arteries. An 8-mg dose of ECGF in saline was injected into 1 extremity 10 days later, and saline alone was injected into the other. A total of 5 doses were administered. Systolic blood pressure was measured in the calves 10, 30, and 50 days after operation. Angiography was done to quantify formation of collateral vessels on day 50, and samples of muscle were taken to determine capillary density.

Results.—The mean calf systolic blood pressures were similar in the 2 extremities on day 10, but on days 30 and 50 the pressures were significantly higher in the ECGF-treated extremities. Collateral vessels were significantly more numerous in actively treated extremities on day 50, as were capillaries.

Conclusions.—The value of administering a mitogen that stimulates angiogenesis as a treatment for severe extremity ischemia was affirmed. This approach could be used in conjunction with direct bypass procedures and also to salvage ischemic tissue in patients with diffuse disease of small vessels that is not amenable to direct operative treatment.

▶ Endothelial cell growth factor is attracting tremendous attention for its potential to enhance collateral blood vessel formation. In this article, the authors attempt to convince us that injection of ECGF into one ischemic rabbit hind limb resulted in a markedly enhanced collateral development compared with no injection being administered into the control ischemic hind limb. Experiments such as this one inherently confuse me because of predictable spillover of the intramuscularly injected substance into the opposite leg. Nonetheless, the results are impressive, and we are definitely going to hear more about this.

Consistent Responses of the Human Vascular Smooth Muscle Cell in Culture: Implications for Restenosis

Munro E, Chan P, Patel M, Betteridge L, Gallagher K, Schachter M, Sever P, Wolfe J (St Mary's Hosp, London; Imperial College of Science, Technology and Medicine, London)

J Vasc Surg 20:482–487, 1994   145-96-1–54

Background.—Restenosis is the most important single factor limiting the success of invasive vascular interventions, but how restenoses develop at particular vascular sites remains uncertain. Recent observations have

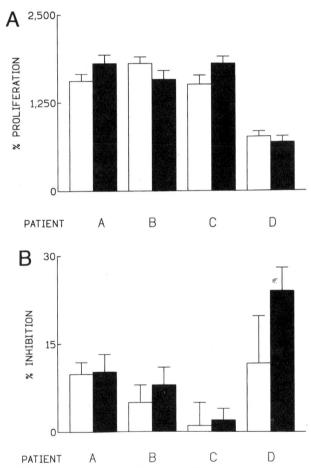

Fig 1–24.—(A) Mean 14-day percentage proliferation and (B) mean 14-day heparin inhibition of 15% fetal calf serum–stimulated vascular smooth muscle cells derived from paired artery (*filled bars*) and saphenous vein (*open bars*) samples from 4 patients. Variations in proliferation rates and in heparin inhibitions between artery and vein samples within each pair were not significantly different from interreplicate variance. (Courtesy of Munro E, Chan P, Patel M, et al: *J Vasc Surg* 20:482–487, 1994.)

indicated that vascular smooth muscle cells (VSMCs) from patients whose grafts have stenosed resist the growth-inhibiting effect of heparin.

Methods.—The VSMCs from the proximal, middle, and distal segments of long saphenous veins from 7 patients having coronary bypass surgery were cultured in 15% fetal calf serum (FCS), with or without heparin added in a concentration of 100 µg/mL. Cell proliferation was monitored for 2 weeks. Cells from up to 6 passages were cultured, as were samples from paired arteries and veins of 4 other patients.

Results.—There were no significant differences between vein segment cultures of individual veins in either cellular proliferation or the inhibitory response to heparin. Repeated passage did not alter this finding. There were, however, significant inter-patient differences in the sensitivity of VSMCs to inhibition by heparin (Fig 1–24). The paired artery-vein samples did not differ significantly in proliferation or heparin inhibition.

Conclusions.—The growth pattern of VSMC differs between individuals and is maintained in culture. Cultures of human VSMCs should prove helpful in evaluating pharmacologic measures for preventing restenosis.

▶ For some years, Dr. John Wolfe has attempted to convince us that veins from some patients differ from veins from other patients. Specifically, the VSMCs in some patients' veins appear uniformly sensitive to heparin inhibition of proliferation, whereas VSMCs from others appear to be uniquely unresponsive to heparin inhibition. Dr. Wolfe goes on to suggest that patients who have recurrent vein graft stenosis are in the group of heparin nonresponders. Although this may be true, it does not immediately suggest a therapeutic alternative for the nonresponders.

Detection of Active Cytomegalovirus Infection in Inflammatory Aortic Aneurysms With RNA Polymerase Chain Reaction
Tanaka S, Komori K, Okadome K, Sugimachi K, Mori R (Kyushu Univ, Fukuoka, Japan)
J Vasc Surg 20:235–243, 1994   145-96-1–55

Background.—Past studies have implicated cytomegalovirus and other herpesviruses in the pathogenesis of inflammatory vascular disorders. Accordingly, herpesviruses were sought in tissue samples from 7 inflammatory aortic aneurysms, 37 atherosclerotic aneurysms, and 16 normal aortas.

Methods.—The DNA polymerase chain reaction technique was used to detect herpes simplex viruses types 1 and 2, cytomegalovirus, and Epstein-Barr virus. Viral transcripts were detected by ribonucleic acid (RNA) polymerase chain reaction.

Results.—Cytomegalovirus was identified in 86% of inflammatory aneurysms, 65% of atherosclerotic aneurysms, and 31% of normal aortas. The respective figures for herpes simplex virus were 29%, 27%, and 6%.

No aneurysmal or normal specimen yielded Epstein-Barr virus. Cytomegaloviral transcripts were found in 71% of inflammatory aneurysms but not in the other groups.

Conclusion.—Proliferation of cytomegalovirus in the aortic wall may lead to formation of an inflammatory aneurysm.

▶ These investigators have expanded their previous work (1) concerning the possible involvement of herpesvirus in the production of inflammatory aneurysms. Using sophisticated DNA and RNA polymerase chain reactions, they concluded that the human cytomegalovirus, one of the herpesviruses, may indeed be involved in the pathogenesis of inflammatory aneurysms. Other investigators have shown a rather consistent lymphoid infiltration in inflammatory aneurysms, which on MRI, has a peculiar "bull's-eye" appearance. The preponderance of evidence appears to be suggesting an infectious component, and I suppose cytomegalovirus is as good a candidate as any.

Reference

1. 1994 YEAR BOOK OF VASCULAR SURGERY, p 218.

Aberrant Expression of Membrane Cofactor Protein and Decay-Accelerating Factor in the Endothelium of Patients With Systemic Sclerosis: A Possible Mechanism of Vascular Damage
Venneker GT, van den Hoogen FHJ, Boerbooms AMT, Bos JD, Asghar SS
(Univ of Amsterdam; Univ Hosp, Nijmegen, The Netherlands)
Lab Invest 70:830–835, 1994   145-96-1–56

Introduction.—Vascular damage is a prominent feature of systemic sclerosis (SSc), although its mechanism is unknown. The complement regulatory molecules—membrane co-factor protein (MCP), decay-accelerating factor (DAF), and CD59—normally protect endothelial cells from damage by autologous complement. If these molecules are deficient or persistently downregulated in patients with SSc, their vascular endothelium would likely be susceptible to damage from physiologically or pathologically activated complement. Skin endothelial specimens both from patients with diffuse and limited SSc and from normal subjects were tested for the expression of MCP, DAF, and CD59.

Methods.—Punch biopsy specimens of normal skin were obtained from 11 subjects, and those of lesional and nonlesional skin were obtained from 5 patients with diffuse SSc and 5 patients with limited SSc. Serial sections were subjected to immunoperoxidase staining using 4 monoclonal antibodies directed to different epitopes of DAF, 4 to different epitopes of MCP, 1 to CD59, and 1 to von Willebrand's factor, which served as an endothelial cell marker. Control specimens of lesional skin from patients with systemic lupus erythematosus and other inflammatory and proliferative diseases were also studied.

Results.—Normal skin endothelium strongly expressed MCP, DAF, and CD59. In contrast, the endothelium of lesional and nonlesional skin from all 10 patients with SSc had a decreased or undetectable expression of MCP and DAF. Some patients with SSc had normal CD59 expression, whereas others had subnormal expression of this protein. Specimens from patients with other inflammatory, connective tissue, and proliferative diseases showed no aberrant expression of MCP, DAF, or CD59.

Conclusions.—Membrane co-factor protein and decay-accelerating factor are virtually absent from the endothelium of patients with SSc. Because these proteins protect self cells against autologous complement, their deficiency in patients with SSc may play a role in vascular damage, leading to intimal proliferation and fibrosis. The mechanism of these deficiencies must now be discovered.

▶ For years, we have been searching for an explanation for the vascular damage seen in many patients with SSc (scleroderma). Many pathologists have observed that this does not appear to be a typical arteritis, such as that seen in most other vasculitides. In this sophisticated study, the authors searched for the presence of a group of proteins that normally protect endothelial cells from damage by complement. They concluded that patients with scleroderma with arterial lesions have either decreased or undetectable amounts of these proteins. They interpreted this finding as suggesting that deficiency of these proteins contributes to vascular damage in scleroderma. This is long-awaited new information.

2 Endovascular

Angioplasty

Femoropopliteal Angioplasty in Patients With Claudication: Primary and Secondary Patency in 140 Limbs With 1–3-Year Follow-Up
Matsi PJ, Manninen HI, Vanninen RL, Suhonen MT, Oksala I, Laakso M, Hakkarainen T, Soimakallio S (Kuopio Univ Hosp, Finland; Central Hosp of Joensuu, Finland)
Radiology 191:727–733, 1994   145-96-2–1

Series.—Percutaneous transluminal angioplasty of the femoropopliteal arteries was performed in a prospective series of 106 patients with claudication who had changes of chronic ischemia. A total of 208 lesions were treated in 140 extremities. The patients were followed up for 1–3 years after angioplasty.

Results.—The success rate of the procedure was 88%. Angioplasty was technically successful in treating 91% of the stenoses and 83% of the occlusions. The overall hemodynamic success rate for the 140 treated extremities was 89%. Primary patency rates were 47% at 1 year and 42% at both 2 and 3 years of follow-up. Secondary patency rates were 63% at 1 year and 59% subsequently (Fig 2–1). Primary patency mainly depended on the number of affected vessels, the state of runoff after angioplasty, and the total length of lesions treated. Half of the failures occurred within 3 months after angioplasty. Angioplasty was repeated in 28 extremities, and surgery was done on 10% of the limbs that were managed primarily by angioplasty. Major complications occurred in 4% of all angioplasties.

Conclusion.—Percutaneous femoropopliteal angioplasty can provide acceptable long-term results in selected patients with claudication.

▶ A technical success rate of 88% is noted in these patients. Although the authors are a bit murky about how they define success, even they claim a respective primary patency at 1, 2, and 3 years of only 47%, 41% and, interestingly, 43%. It is a bit difficult to imagine a Kaplan-Meier life-table going up as time passes.

These authors repeat a traditional error of failing to give any objective documentation of the patients' claudication other than the radiologist's presumptive diagnosis. No preoperative Doppler pressures or treadmill results were presented. Even with loading the boat in this fashion, they have

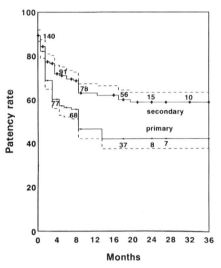

Fig 2–1.—Results of survival analysis (Kaplan-Meier method) for the primary and secondary patency rates for all 140 treated limbs. *Solid lines* indicate estimated patency rate, and *dotted lines* indicate estimated patency rate plus or minus 1 standard error of the estimate. The numbers indicate the number of cases remaining under evaluation as a function of time since angioplasty. (Courtesy of Matsi PJ, Manninen HI, Vanninen RL, et al: *Radiology* 191:727–733, 1994.)

been able to produce extremely mediocre patency results. I consider this to be approximately the state of the art for femoropopliteal angioplasty, which indicates that the procedure should rarely be considered and, even more rarely, undertaken. Any disagreement?

Hospital Costs of Revascularization Procedures for Femoropopliteal Arterial Disease

Hunink MGM, Cullen KA, Donaldson MC (Harvard Medical School, Boston)
J Vasc Surg 19:632–641, 1994   145-96-2-2

Introduction.—Revascularization procedures have been shown to be effective in the management of patients who have peripheral arterial disease with claudication or ischemia. A 1984 study reported that percutaneous transluminal angioplasty (PTA) was considerably more cost-effective than bypass. However, both the therapeutic value and cost-effectiveness of revascularization procedures have been questioned, indicating the need for more recent data. The hospital costs associated with PTA and with bypass in patients with femoropopliteal disease were analyzed and compared.

Methods.—Patients who were treated with femoropopliteal PTA or bypass between 1985 and 1991 were prospectively studied. Treatment choices were made on the basis of diagnostic evaluation. The hospital costs, excluding physician fees, related to PTA and bypass were compared for all admissions. They were then compared for admissions with and without unrelated additional procedures and with and without related vascular procedures, including débridement or amputation. Multiple linear regression analyses examined the factors that influenced costs.

Results.—The primary indication for admission was disabling claudication in the PTA group and critical ischemia in the bypass group. Additional major procedures were performed in 7% of each group. The patients in the PTA group required additional bypass and thrombolysis (34% and 16%) more often than patients in the initial bypass group (3% and 7%). The mean hospital costs for all admissions were $16,341 for the PTA group and $17,076 for the bypass group (table). Among patients who did not require unrelated procedures, the mean hospital costs were $14,852 for PTA and $14,288 for bypass. Among patients who required neither additional unrelated or related vascular procedures, the mean hospital costs were $8,019 for PTA and $13,439 for bypass. When excluding all additional procedures and comparing indications for admission, PTA costs were significantly lower than bypass costs for patients with claudication, but the cost differences were only of borderline significance for patients with critical ischemia. Hospital costs were influenced significantly by the primary procedure, additional unrelated procedures, additional related vascular procedures, and whether débridement or amputation was required.

Components of the Mean Hospital Costs Per Admission for Femoropopliteal Percutaneous Transluminal Angioplasty (*PTA*) and Bypass

	Mean cost in 1990 U.S. dollars (% of total cost)			
	Claudication		*Critical ischemia*	
	PTA	*Bypass*	*PTA*	*Bypass*
Component	*(n = 25)*	*(n = 96)*	*(n = 14)*	*(n = 110)*
Procedural costs				
Diagnostic angiography/interventional radiology	5,008 (81)	2,340 (20)	4,358 (38)	2,120 (14)
Operating room and anesthesia	0 (0)	3,800 (33)	283 (3)	4,325 (29)
Hotel costs				
Routine room and board	814 (13)	4,077 (35)	3,694 (33)	5,575 (37)
Intermediate/intensive care	0 (0)	144 (1)	428 (4)	890 (6)
Supportive				
Diagnostic radiology (other than angiography)	32 (<1)	144 (1)	93 (1)	243 (2)
Clinical laboratory services*	87 (1)	262 (2)	434 (4)	485 (3)
Patient laboratory services†	97 (2)	194 (2)	216 (2)	293 (2)
Pharmacy and blood bank‡	101 (2)	482 (4)	1,497 (13)	799 (5)
Miscellaneous other§	13 (<1)	136 (1)	351 (3)	328 (2)
Total	6,152	11,582	11,353	15,059

Notes: Excluding admissions associated with additional major procedures (additional bypass, additional angiography, thrombolysis, coronary artery bypass grafting, percutaneous heart valvuloplasty, carotid endarterectomy, abdominal aortic aneurysm repair, and other major surgery). Physicians' professional fees are excluded from the analysis.
* Includes chemistry, hematology, and microbiology.
† Includes noninvasive testing and electrocardiography.
‡ Includes medications, IV solutions, and transfusions.
§ Includes inpatient rehabilitation, hemodialysis, and respiratory therapy.
(Courtesy of Hunink MGM, Cullen KA, Donaldson MC: *J Vasc Surg* 19:632–641, 1994.)

Discussion.—Because PTA is not as cost-effective as it was believed to be and because questions exist regarding patient outcome after PTA, perhaps the indications for PTA should be reevaluated.

▶ It is important to remember when reading any article on reported hospital costs that such costs are imaginary figures with little basis in fact. Consider the vast "indirect" costs that are always factored into hospital expense. This is an imprecise exercise at best. Nonetheless, the authors tell us that for all admissions for leg ischemia, the angioplasty admissions and the bypass admissions cost the same. Of course, stratifications are added, but they really contribute little.

When one considers that the hospital costs and the mortality and morbidity of angioplasty and bypass are the same, the only benefit that can be defined for angioplasty is a shorter patient recovery time. Ninety percent of my patients are retired and intend to stay that way, and whether they recover at 2 weeks, 4 weeks, or 3 months appears to be monumentally irrelevant. Therefore, it is critical to compare the patency of the procedures. At best, a well-performed angioplasty below the inguinal ligament yields a 1-year primary patency rate of 50%, whereas well-performed bypass surgery for a similar period yields a primary patency rate in excess of 90%. I am sorry, but I am simply unable to perceive the glowing benefits of angioplasty that almost everyone else seems to recognize without difficulty.

Treatment of Recurrent Femoral or Popliteal Artery Stenosis After Percutaneous Transluminal Angioplasty
Treiman GS, Ichikawa L, Treiman RL, Cohen JL, Cossman DV, Wagner WH, Levin PM, Foran RF (Cedars-Sinai Med Ctr, Los Angeles)
J Vasc Surg 20:577–587, 1994   145-96-2-3

Background.—Although many patients with localized occlusive disease in the superficial femoral or popliteal artery benefit from percutaneous transluminal angioplasty (PTA), a significant proportion have recurrent stenosis develop in the treated arterial segment. Repeat PTA was compared with arterial reconstruction and noninvasive treatment in 93 patients with recurrent femoropopliteal stenosis after PTA of the superficial femoral or popliteal artery. Seventy-two patients were treated for claudication, 9 for rest pain, and 12 for ischemic ulceration.

Methods.—The PTA procedure was repeated in 35 patients. Thirty-six others underwent arterial bypass surgery, whereas 22 patients were managed by exercise and medication. The results were assessed by duplex scanning and monitoring of the ankle-brachial index. The mean follow-up was 42 months.

Results.—The clinical and hemodynamic success rates in patients who had repeat PTA were 41% at 1 year, 20% at 2 years, and 11% at 3 years. The respective primary graft patency rates in patients who had arterial bypass were 84%, 72%, and 72%, and the secondary patency rates were 94%, 88%, and 88%, respectively. Cumulative patency was substantially

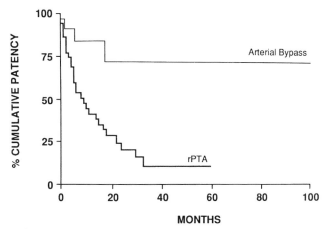

Fig 2–2.—Life-table plot of benefit after repeat percutaneous transluminal angioplasty (*rPTA*) or operation. (Courtesy of Treiman GS, Ichikawa L, Treiman RL, et al: *J Vasc Surg* 20:577–587, 1994.)

greater after bypass than after repeat PTA (Fig 2–2). All patients whose grafts remained patent were free of symptoms, whereas all those who were managed noninvasively continued to be symptomatic, but none required amputation. In both the repeat PTA and bypass groups, patients who were treated for claudication did better than those who had rest pain or ischemic ulceration.

Conclusion.—Arterial bypass is a more effective and safe treatment of recurrent superficial femoral or popliteal artery stenosis than repeat angioplasty. Repeat PTA should be limited to patients who have contraindications to surgery or whose life expectancy is limited.

▶ In this study, the authors carefully compared the outcome of the treatment of recurrent stenosis after PTA of the superficial femoral or popliteal arteries with arterial reconstruction, repeat angioplasty, or noninvasive treatment. They concluded that repeat PTA produces dismal results, arterial bypass gives good results, and noninvasive therapy gives fairly good results. The 1-year rate of patency with bypass of 84% compared with 1-year rate of patency with repeat angioplasty of 41% speaks volumes and supports the previous 2 comments (Abstracts 145-96-2–1 and 145-96-2–2).

Percutaneous Transluminal Angioplasty of Infrainguinal Vein Graft Stenosis: Long-Term Outcome
Dunlop P, Varty K, Hartshorne T, Bell PRF, Bolia A, London NJM (Leicester Royal Infirmary, England)
Br J Surg 82:204–206, 1995   145-96-2–4

Objective.—The long-term outcome of percutaneous transluminal angioplasty (PTA) was studied prospectively in patients with infrainguinal vein graft stenosis who had PTA as first-line treatment.

Methods.—Thirty-three stenoses were detected by graft surveillance in 44 months. The median follow-up after PTA was 39 months.

Results.—Nineteen stenoses resolved after a single angioplasty, but 14 recurred after a median interval of 8½ months. Seven restenoses occurred more than 1 year after initial PTA. Recurrent stenosis tended to involve the distal third of the graft. Restenosis was more frequent in in situ vein grafts than in reverse vein grafts.

Conclusion.—There is a substantial risk of recurrent stenosis after PTA when the distal third of an infrainguinal vein graft is involved. Continued surveillance is important after stenoses at this site are treated by angioplasty.

▶ Although the authors are to be commended for attempting to document the long-term follow-up of PTA for infrainguinal vein graft stenoses, the data in this article are difficult to interpret. Recurrence of stenosis was documented in 14 of 33 (42%) vein graft lesions that were treated with PTA in 30 patients. An additional 9 grafts had stenosis develop in at least 1 other site after the first angioplasty. The locations of these lesions were not identified in the article, and the authors chose not to consider them in their statistical evaluation, because the lesions were considered new events. Presumably, these lesions, which developed at a mean interval of 17 months after the first angioplasty, were not present at the time of the initial PTA, although perhaps they should be considered a complication of the endovascular procedure.

Intimal injury resulting from catheter manipulation in the vein graft is a potential etiology of such stenoses. If these stenoses are figured into the data, the recurrence rate for vein graft stenoses after PTA is at least 70%. The authors stratified the rate of recurrent stenosis on the basis of the location of the lesion, and they determined that distal vein graft lesions did not respond well to PTA. I agree with this conclusion and add that the literature supports operative revision of a distal anastomotic vein graft stenosis with graft extension to a more distal artery.—E.S. Weinstein, M.D.

▶ The results of PTA for vein graft stenosis are lousy.—J.M. Porter, M.D.

Controlled Trial of High- Versus Low-Dose Aspirin Treatment After Percutaneous Transluminal Angioplasty in Patients With Peripheral Vascular Disease

Ranke C, Creutzig A, Luska G, Wagner H-H, Galanski M, Bode-Böger S, Frölich J, Aveuarius H-J, Hecker H, Alexander K (Medizinische Hochschule Hannover, Germany; Zentralkrankenhaus Links der Weser, Bremen, Germany)

Clin Investigator 72:673–680, 1994   145-96-2-5

Background.—Patients with atherosclerotic lesions of the aortoiliac or femoropopliteal system can realize long-term hemodynamic improvement from percutaneous transluminal angioplasty. Aspirin often is given in high doses to prevent reocclusion; however, if it is effective, a low dose would be preferable to limit side effects.

Objective.—In a double-blind, randomized trial, high or low doses of aspirin were given to 359 patients who had peripheral vascular lesions that were suitable for angioplastic treatment. Aspirin was given to 175 patients in a daily dose of 900 mg for 1 year, starting at the time of angioplasty; the 184 remaining patients took 50 mg of aspirin each day.

Results.—Angiography confirmed restenosis at the site of angioplasty in 39 of 317 patients who were evaluated an average of 9 months after angioplasty. The patency rates were 85% in the high-dose group and 84% in the low-dose group at 1 year (Fig 2–3). Nine patients in the high-dose group and 2 patients in the low-dose group had serious gastrointestinal side effects.

Conclusion.—In patients who had angioplasty for peripheral vascular disease in a lower extremity, a 50-mg daily dose of aspirin prevented restenosis as effectively as a 900-mg dose and was much safer.

▶ It is widely agreed that patients who are undergoing balloon agioplasty should be taking aspirin. However, the complications of long-term aspirin therapy are well known and have been vividly demonstrated in several recent studies, including carotid ones.

This comparison, which examines 2 doses of aspirin—50 mg vs. 900 mg—indicates that the 2 are equally effective. This is important support for our preconceived position that patients who require long-term aspirin therapy are best served by a daily dose of 80 mg. I have found no persuasive evidence that higher doses of aspirin are any more effective in our vascular surgery patients.

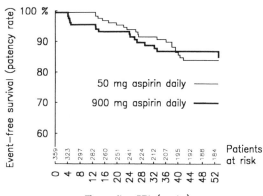

Fig 2–3.—Kaplan–Meier curves for the outcome event of restenosis or reocclusion at the angioplasty site, by treatment. The *x-axis* represents the number of patients at risk during follow-up. (Courtesy of Ranke C, Creutzig A, Luska G, et al: Controlled trial of high- versus low-dose aspirin treatment after percutaneous transluminal angioplasty in patients with peripheral vascular disease. (Figure 1.) *Clin Investigator* 72:673–680, 1994. Copyright 1994 Springer Verlag.)

Stents

Stent Placement in Coeliac and Superior Mesenteric Arteries to Restore Vascular Perfusion Following Aortic Dissection

Connell DA, Thomson KR, Gibson RN, Wall AJ (Univ of Melbourne, Australia; Royal Melbourne Hosp, Parkville, Victoria, Australia)
Australas Radiol 39:68–70, 1995   145-96-2-6

Background.—Percutaneous intravascular placement of an expandable metallic stent.has been an effective approach to treating renal artery stenosis and creating a communication between the portal and systemic venous systems to decompress the liver. In a patient with visceral ischemia secondary to aortic dissection, both the celiac and superior mesenteric arteries—sheared off the abdominal aorta—were cannulated, and a Wal-stent was placed across the false lumen.

Case Report.—Woman, 72, had epigastric pain radiating to the back. Gastroscopy revealed engorged submucosal veins in the stomach. Progressive acidosis and disseminated intravascular coagulopathy ensued. Liver function was grossly abnormal. Aortography showed poor filling of the splanchnic vessels (Fig 2–4), and an

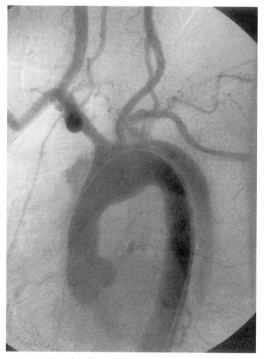

Fig 2–4.—Arch aortogram. Pigtail catheter placed at aortic root. Intimal flap arising proximal to the brachiocephalic trunk with delayed contrast transit through dissection. (Courtesy of Connell DA, Thomson KR, Gibson RN, et al: *Australas Radiol* 39:68–70, 1995.)

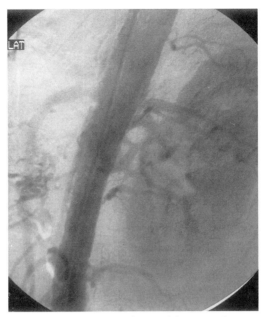

Fig 2–5.—Abdominal aortogram. Delayed opacification of the anterior dissection with poor perfusion of the superior mesenteric artery. (Courtesy of Connell DA, Thomson KR, Gibson RN, et al: *Australas Radiol* 39:68–70, 1995.)

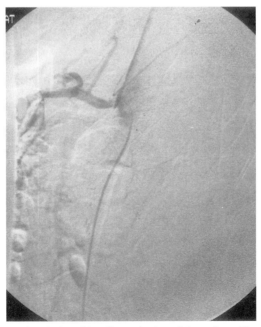

Fig 2–6.—Selective catheterization of the celiac trunk using a Cobra catheter. (Courtesy of Connell DA, Thomson KR, Gibson RN, et al: *Australas Radiol* 39:68–70, 1995.)

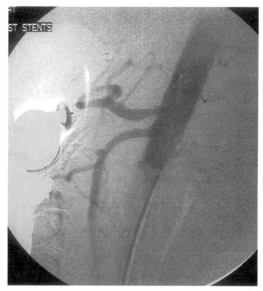

Fig 2–7.—Walstent in place across the false lumen of the celiac and superior mesenteric arteries. Reperfusion has been established. (Courtesy of Connell DA, Thomson KR, Gibson RN, et al: *Australas Radiol* 39:68–70, 1995.)

arch study demonstrated an intimal tear arising from the innominate origin (Fig 2–5). The celiac (Fig 2–6) and superior mesenteric arteries were entered with a Cobra catheter, and after passing the false lumen with a steerable guide wire, angioplasty was done and Walstents were placed across the false lumen (Fig 2–7). The patient improved initially, but she died 3 days later. Autopsy showed the stents were enmeshed across the false lumen, with perfusion restored. The bowel was ischemic but not infarcted.

▶ This case report shows excellent angiograms of the restoration of visceral vascular perfusion after aortic dissection with stent placement. As I have noted previously (1), I believe that this currently is the initial procedure of choice to restore impaired visceral or reduce extremity circulation caused by acute aortic dissection.

Reference

1. 1994 YEAR BOOK OF VASCULAR SURGERY, p 71.

Endovascular Stents in Subclavian and Innominate Vein Stenosis
Gibson M, Al-Kutoubi A (St Mary's Hospital, London)
J Intervent Radiol 9:113–120, 1994   145-96-2-7

Introduction.—Endovascular stents appear to offer an alternative to percutaneous transluminal angioplasty (PTA) in the treatment of subclavian and innominate vein stenoses. There is a high rate of restenosis with PTA, and the stenosis sometimes resists balloon dilation. The outcome was reported for 14 patients who received endovascular stents across 16 subclavian and innominate stenoses.

Patients and Methods.—The patients ranged in age from 33 to 79 years. The causes of stenosis were hemodialysis in 10 cases, radiotherapy in 2, breast carcinoma in 1, and thoracic inlet syndrome in 1. The primary venous approach was from the ipsilateral arm in all patients. Two patients had bilateral stenting. The wallstent was used in all but 2 patients. Antiplatelet therapy was used in all patients, but only 3 who had stent thrombosis received anticoagulation. Venography was performed at 3 and 12 months after stent placement whenever possible.

Case Report.—Man, 58, was receiving hemodialysis and experienced a swollen left arm after creation of an arteriovenous fistula. A tight stenosis of the left innominate vein and a mild stenosis of the distal cephalic vein draining the fistula were demonstrated at venography. Total relief of signs and symptoms was achieved after a 16-mm wallstent was placed across the innominate vein. Although the patient was asymptomatic at 8-month follow-up, a venogram showed recurrence of the stenosis through the stent (Fig 2–8). The symptoms of venous obstruction

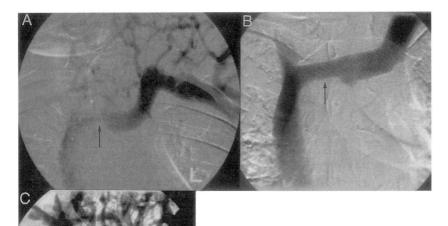

Fig 2–8.—A, tight stenosis of the left innominate vein (*arrows*). B, wallstent has been placed through the stenosis, which is now widely patent (*arrow*). C, stenosis has developed within the stent (*arrow*). (Courtesy of Gibson M, Al-Kutoubi A: *J Intervent Radiol* 9:113–120, 1994.)

subsequently developed and balloons were used to dilate stenoses in the stent and the cephalic vein. Recurrence of symptoms at 18 months necessitated a further PTA.

Results and Discussion.—The stents achieved initial technical success, which was defined as a wide lumen with less than 50% residual stenosis, in all patients. Despite symptomatic relief, 5 patients required secondary or tertiary intervention. Follow-up venograms, which were obtained in 11 patients, showed that 6 stents had restenosed, 3 had thrombosed, and 2 were widely patent. Eight of the 10 patients undergoing hemodialysis had follow-up venograms that showed 6 restenoses, 1 thrombosis, and 1 widely patent stent. Overall, the metallic endovascular stents were successful in relieving symptoms in subclavian and innominate vein stenoses; however, like PTA, they had a high incidence of restenosis.

▶ This potpourri of case reports demonstrates the high initial success rates that can be achieved with endovascular stenting of subclavian and innominate vein stenoses, as well as the high rates of recurrence that occur after the procedure, particularly in patients with proximal arteriovenous fistulas. Several technical points need to be emphasized. First, the use of balloon-expandable stents in this location should be avoided because it is likely, particularly in cases where there is external compression, that arm and shoulder abduction could recompress the stent. Second, this procedure can provide excellent palliation in patients with superior vena cava syndrome resulting from malignancy, where it obviates the need for an operative procedure and long-term patency is not an issue. Third, in patients undergoing hemodialysis, the examples of subclavian vein stenoses that have occurred, presumably secondary to the use of temporary dialysis catheters, stress that use of these catheters should be avoided whenever possible. If catheters are required, they should not be placed in the subclavian position if another route, such as the IJ is available.—E.S. Weinstein, M.D.

Transluminal Placement of Endovascular Stent-Grafts for the Treatment of Descending Thoracic Aortic Aneurysms
Dake MD, Miller DC, Semba CP, Mitchell RS, Walker PJ, Liddell RP (Stanford Univ, Calif)
N Engl J Med 331:1729–1734, 1994   145-96-2–8

Introduction.—Thoracic aortic aneurysms have traditionally been managed with surgical placement of a graft. The mortality has been estimated at 12% for patients undergoing elective surgical repair and more than 50% for patients undergoing emergency surgical repair. An alternative, less invasive, and less costly management approach for these patients is the transluminally placed endovascular stent-graft prosthesis, a technique that has been used in the repair of descending thoracic aortic aneurysms in 13 patients.

Methods.—The 11 men and 2 women received transluminal endovascular grafts to treat thoracic aortic aneurysms. The selection criteria included an aneurysm neck of less than 4 cm, a relatively localized or false aneurysm, an aneurysm neck that did not involve the origin of the left subclavian artery or celiac axis, and aneurysm with morphological and anatomical characteristics that could accommodate placement of a stent-graft, adequate peripheral arterial access, or contraindications for a second surgical approach. Four true aneurysms and 9 false aneurysms of the thoracic aorta were treated. An atherosclerotic degenerative process was responsible in 9 cases.

Endovascular Technique.—A fluoroscopically guided wire was placed from the femoral artery (or the infrarenal abdominal aorta) to the aortic arch. After an initial aortogram was obtained, a 24-F Teflon sheath and dilator were introduced along the guide wire until the sheath was positioned across the aneurysm. The dilator was then removed, and the custom-designed endovascular stent-graft that was composed of stainless steel covered with woven Dacron graft material was advanced using a Teflon pusher under fluoroscopic guidance. Vasodilator and β-blocker drugs were given to reduce the arterial pressure and minimize the risk of dislodging the stent-graft. The sheath was removed, and the femoral arteriotomy was repaired.

Results.—The stent-graft was technically deployed successfully in all 13 patients. The aneurysm surrounding the stent-graft achieved complete thrombosis in 12 patients and partial thrombosis in 1. Small tracts to the aneurysms appeared initially, but they thrombosed within 2 months in 2 patients. Four patients had residual filling and required 2 stent-graft prostheses for the large aneurysm that resulted. The patient who had only partial thrombosis of her extensive chronic type A dissection required surgical repair 4 months after the procedure. No patients died or had paraplegia, stroke, distal embolization, or infection during an average follow-up of 11.6 months.

Discussion.—A transluminally placed endovascular stent-graft appears to be a feasible management approach for highly selected patients with aneurysms of the descending thoracic aorta. More study is warranted.

▶ This article summarizes early experience with the use of transluminal endovascular stent grafts for the treatment of descending thoracic aortic aneurysms. The technique is well described and the results, which have a mean follow-up of approximately 11 months, are encouraging. In the initial 13 patients, there were no neurologic deficits and no deaths. On long-term follow-up, 1 patient required additional reconstruction because of continued dissection through the distal opening of the false lumen.

The information provided at the end of the article describes an additional 20 patients who have been treated in a similar fashion. Among them, there have been 2 deaths and 3 cases of neurologic deficit. This underscores one of the drawbacks of endovascular repair of thoracoabdominal aneurysms, i.e., the inability to reimplant important intercostal vessels. Nevertheless, this is a promising technique for selected patients, and as experience grows, the selection criteria are likely to improve. The less invasive nature, potential decrease in cost, and patient acceptance will doubtless continue to fuel enthusiasm to further refine this approach. Nevertheless, until adequate follow-up is available to demonstrate long-term effectiveness, endovascular repair of aneurysmal disease should only be done under established protocols, where strict surveillance can be ensured so that important information on the long-term outcome of this approach can be obtained.—W. Quiñones-Baldrich, M.D.

▶ Please note the last sentence in Dr. Quiñones-Baldrich's commentary. It is critically important.—J.M. Porter, M.D.

Transfemoral Endoluminal Repair of Abdominal Aortic Aneurysm with Bifurcated Graft
Yusuf SW, Baker DM, Chuter TAM, Whitaker SC, Wenham PW, Hopkinson BR (Univ Hosp, Nottingham, England; Columbia Univ, New York)
Lancet 344:650–651, 1994   145-96-2–9

Background.—Endoluminal repair is an alternative to the conventional open method of repairing abdominal aortic aneurysms. It is a minimally invasive means of excluding the aneurysm and placing a graft transfemorally, which precludes the need for laparotomy, retroperitoneal dissection, and clamping of the aorta.

Methods.—In the endoluminal technique, the graft, rather than being sutured to the aorta, is secured by a self-expanding metal stent that is deployed under angiographic control. Twenty-nine consecutive patients who had an abdominal aortic aneurysm greater than 5.5 cm in diameter were considered for endoluminal repair. An additional patient had a 3.2-cm aneurysm and bilateral iliac stenoses. No patient had a nonaneurysmal segment of aorta between the aneurysm and the bifurcation so that a straight graft could be placed. In only 5 cases was it practical to use the bifurcated system. The most common findings that precluded use of the bifurcated system were a short aneurysmal neck, a wide neck, and the presence of iliac aneurysms.

Results.—A bifurcated aortoiliac graft was successfully inserted in all 5 patients. All remained hemodynamically stable during the procedure. In 2 cases it proved necessary to expose the common iliac artery extraperitoneally on 1 side to accurately deploy the bottom stent. There were no major complications.

Conclusion.—Hopefully, modifications in the endoluminal repair technique will make it more widely applicable in treating abdominal aortic aneurysms.

▶ Dr. Chuter and his associates have led the way in obtaining experience with endoluminal repair of aortic aneurysms using the bifurcated graft system. It is interesting that only 5 of 29 patients who were evaluated were suitable for the procedure, which appeared to be successful in all patients. The authors wisely observe that only limited follow-up is available, and even they urge some caution in adopting this technique.

My experience in this area also suggests caution. I am old enough to remember the early enthusiastic reports resulting from the use of the McGovern sutureless aortic valve prosthesis, which, with time, had such a high incidence of paravalvular leak because of unstable fixation that use of the device was abandoned. I have grave reservations about the permanence of the stent-induced graft to aortic wall adhesion. I believe that, using current technology, remote filling of the aneurysm sac is not only possible but predictable. I note a recent report of 2 delayed aneurysm ruptures that caused death after apparently successful endoluminal aneurysm graft placement (1). I am not optimistic about the future of these devices.

Reference

1. Lumsden AB, et al: Delayed rupture of aortic aneurysms following endovascular stent grafting. *Am J Surg* 170:174–179, 1995.

Tantalum-Dacron Coknit Stent for Endovascular Treatment of Aortic Aneurysms: A Preliminary Experimental Study
Piquet P, Rolland P-H, Bartoli J-M, Tranier P, Moulin G, Mercier C (Hôpital de la Timone, Marseille, France; Université d'Aix-Marseille II, France)
J Vasc Surg 19:698–706, 1994   145-96-2–10

Background.—It is generally agreed that any abdominal aortic aneurysm larger than 5 cm should be removed, but an alternative to direct reconstruction is needed for patients whose associated conditions put them at high operative risk. The results of induced aneurysmal thrombosis with axillobifemoral bypass have been unsatisfactory.

Methods.—The use of an intraluminal tantalum-Dacron co-knit stent was evaluated in mini-pigs by replacing a segment of the infrarenal aorta with a fusiform-shaped conduit made of crimped woven Dacron. The artificial aneurysm was 4 cm long and 3 cm in maximal transverse diameter. After 2 weeks, a balloon-expandable co-knit stent mounted on a balloon catheter was inserted through the femoral artery to the site of the "aneurysm." The stent and aneurysm were removed after intervals of 1 day to 12 weeks and examined by scanning electron microscopy.

Results.—The aneurysm was immediately excluded by stent placement, and all the stents remained patent. The entire stent lumen appeared to be endothelialized after 6 weeks.

Conclusion.—The tantalum-Dacron co-knit stent should prove clinically useful in the management of aortic aneurysms in poor risk patients if stents of adequate size are developed and a suitable delivery system is devised.

▶ These authors propose the use of an interesting device in which the stent apparently extends the entire length of the graft. It seemed to work well in preliminary animal studies. I also note the Sydney attachment system proposed by Professor May in Australia. I have no idea whether any of these modified attachment systems are superior to the single stent attachment proximally and distally.

Repair of Abdominal Aortic Aneurysm by Transfemoral Endovascular Graft Placement
Moore WS, Vescera CL (Univ of California, Los Angeles)
Ann Surg 220:331–341, 1994   145-96-2-11

Background.—Direct repair of an abdominal aortic aneurysm through excision and graft replacement has become standard practice. Despite the high rate of success for this procedure, approximately 15,000 patients die of ruptured abdominal aortic aneurysms each year in the United States. This high incidence of rupture occurs because surgery is sometimes withheld because of the patient's increased risk of operation compared with a relatively small aneurysm size. Approved by the Food and Drug Administration for clinical investigation, a new device allows for the repair of an abdominal aortic aneurysm by a transfemoral endovascular graft placement. It permits a more aggressive approach in the management of patients with smaller aneurysms or high-risk patients.

Method.—Sixty-nine patients with abdominal aortic aneurysms were screened, and 10 were found to have suitable anatomical and clinical characteristics for the endovascular graft system (EGS). Repair was performed with the patient under general anesthesia. One femoral artery was surgically exposed, and the EGS, which consisted of an introducer sheath and a catheter-based delivery system containing a graft of appropriate size with fixation devices at each end (Fig 2–9) was inserted through an open arteriotomy with fluoroscopic control. Postoperative evaluation included documentation of the anatomical position of the graft, as seen by the radiopaque self-expanding fixation devices at each graft extremity and examination of a color-flow duplex scan indicating flow through the graft and showing evidence of perianastomotic reflux into the aneurysm. Fi-

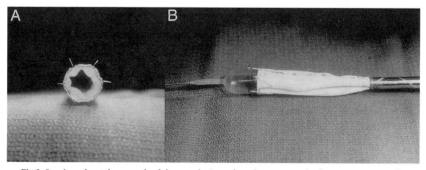

Fig 2–9.—A, end-on photograph of the prosthetic graft to demonstrate the fixation pins in profile. B, the balloon within the graft is being inflated; this demonstrates how the pins will be driven into the wall of the aorta. (Courtesy of Moore WS, Vescera CL: *Ann Surg* 220:331–341, 1994.)

nally, a CT scan was obtained to ensure the position of the graft, its function, and the presence or absence of contrast-enhanced blood within the aneurysm sac.

Results.—Eight of the 10 grafts were considered to be immediate successes and were entered in the follow-up protocol. Two graft deployments were considered to be failures and required conversion to an open repair. At follow-up, 7 of the 8 patients who underwent successful implantation were still alive. Four of the 8 patients had normal completion angiography at the time of surgery, with no sign of perianastomotic reflux. Follow-up CT scans showed no evidence of contrast enhancement with the aneurysm sac, and color-flow duplex scans demonstrated normal graft flow without perianastomotic reflux. Six of the 8 patients had completely normal functioning grafts without any function of the thrombosed aneurysms. Two patients continued to show some evidence of perianastomotic reflux but not of aneurysm expansion.

Conclusion.—Transfemoral endovascular graft placement appears to be safe and effective. Long-term follow-up studies of this procedure are now required.

▶ Dr. Moore presents his initial experience with 10 patients with the EVT endovascular graft repair system. He notes that he screened 69 patients to find the 10 who were suitable for inclusion in this study. Two of the 10 were tried with the EVT but required conversion to open repair. The 8 endoluminal graft patients have been followed; 2 of the 8 show evidence of perianastomotic leak into the aneurysm sac. As Dr. Moore sagely notes, long-term follow-up studies are now required.

I note that shortly after this report, implantation of the EVT devices was suspended because of broken hooks on the stents. As of summer 1995, ongoing clinical studies remain suspended. I do not know when implantation with the EVT devices will start again. At least 2 other manufacturers in the United States are contemplating endoluminal graft clinical trials, but I do not yet have information as to when they are actually going to begin. The promise of endoluminal aneurysm repair is attracting an avalanche of attention with, as yet, precious few results, and even those are far from perfect. Stay tuned.

Endovascular Femoropopliteal Bypass: Early Human Cadaver and Animal Studies

Ahn SS, Reger VA, Kaiura TL (UCLA Ctr for the Health Sciences, Los Angeles; The Portland Clinic, Ore)
Ann Vasc Surg 9:28–36, 1995   145-96-2–12

Background.—Femoropopliteal bypass still is the standard approach to occlusive disease of the superficial femoral artery. An endovascular bypass procedure might provide a less invasive means of achieving results as durable as those expected from a standard bypass.

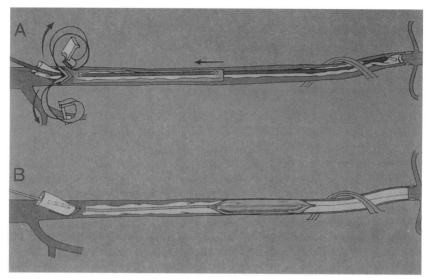

Fig 2–10.—A, removal of the peel-away sheath while holding the PTFE graft in place with the Graft Inserter. B, balloon dilatation of the graft. (Courtesy of Ahn SS, Reger VA, Kaiura TL: *Ann Vasc Surg* 9:28–36, 1995.)

Technique.—The femoral artery is exposed by a small groin incision, and a guide wire is passed to mechanically dilate the diseased superficial femoral artery. A semi-closed endarterectomy is then performed using an expandable metal catheter that engages the atheroma. A thin-walled 6-mm polytetrafluoroethylene graft is placed, and a balloon is dilated to press the graft against the arterial wall (Fig 2–10.) Finally, the proximal graft is joined end to end to the femoral artery (Fig 2–11). The operative specimen is shown in Figure 2–12.

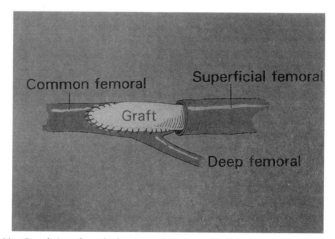

Fig 2–11.—Completion of standard end-to-end anastomosis of the proximal graft to the common femoral artery. (Courtesy of Ahn SS, Reger VA, Kaiura TL: *Ann Vasc Surg* 9:28–36, 1995.)

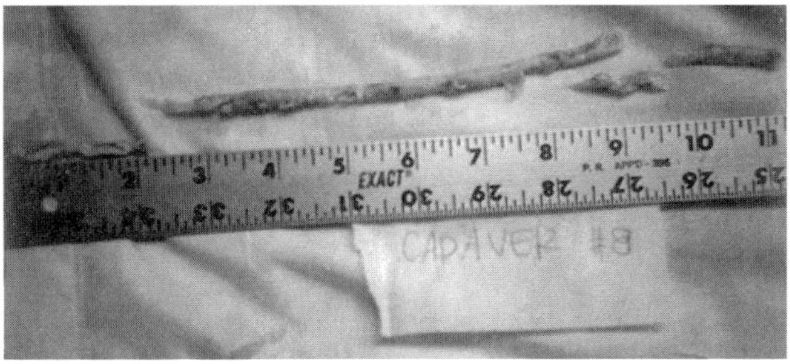

Fig 2–12.—Endarterectomized specimen revealing intima, atheromatous plaque, and media. (Courtesy of Ahn SS, Reger VA, Kaiura TL: *Ann Vasc Surg* 9:28–36, 1995.)

Results.—The technique was used in 13 fresh cadaver extremities, 5 of which had stenotic lesions of the superficial femoral artery averaging 7.6 cm in length, and 4 had occlusive lesions averaging 26.8 cm. The procedure was successfully completed in 10 extremities. Completion angiography demonstrated a widely patent graft and a smooth interface with the popliteal artery in 9 limbs. In one, a size mismatch had resulted in a fold in the distal part of the graft. The procedure was also performed in 6 large dogs, except that endarterectomy was omitted. It was technically successful in all animals and angiographically successful in 4. In 2 cases, a size mismatch had caused a longitudinal fold near the distal end of the graft.

Conclusion.—It appears to be technically feasible to perform endovascular femoropopliteal bypass grafting through a single groin incision.

▶ Here we have a real prize winner. Who said things could not be made more difficult?

Endoluminal Aortic Aneurysm Repair Using a Balloon-Expandable Stent-Graft Device: A Progress Report
Parodi JC, Criado FJ, Barone HD, Schönholz C, Queral LA (Instituto Cardiovascular de Buenos Aires, Argentina; Maryland Vascular Inst, Baltimore)
Ann Vasc Surg 8:523–529, 1994   145-96-2–13

Objective.—Twenty-four patients with an abdominal aortic aneurysm underwent 25 endoluminal repair procedures with the use of a stent-graft device. All but 4 were considered to be at high risk for conventional operative repair.

Methods.—Sixteen patients received an aortoaortic stent-graft, and 8 received a unilateral aortoiliac stent-graft. At reoperation, 1 patient received an ilioiliac graft to repair a separate common iliac artery aneurysm. Seven of the 8 unilateral repairs entailed a concomitant femorofemoral bypass (Fig 2–13). An iliac pull-down maneuver (Fig 2–14) proved to be an effective measure in several cases. If marked angulation and severe iliac artery disease are present, a temporary prosthetic graft can be attached to

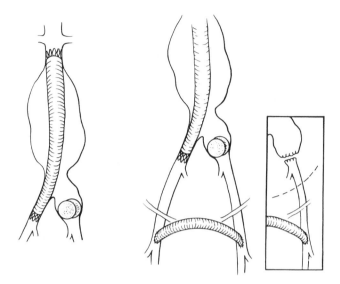

Fig 2–13.—A tapered endoluminal aortoiliac unilateral graft. Crossover grafting and contralateral iliac exclusion, either transluminally or by surgical ligation (*inset*) complete the procedure. (Courtesy of Parodi JC, Criado FJ, Barone HD, et al: *Ann Vasc Surg* 8(6):523–529, 1994.)

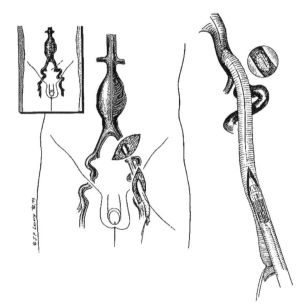

Fig 2–14.—An iliac pull-down maneuver by extensive circumferential dissection of common femoral and external iliac arteries. (Courtesy of Parodi JC, Criado FJ, Barone HD, et al: *Ann Vasc Surg* 8(6):523–529, 1994.)

the common iliac artery through a limited retroperitoneal incision. The graft is passed beneath the inguinal ligament and used as a conduit for the endoluminal device (Fig 2–15.)

Results.—One patient with a tortuous aneurysm required numerous transluminal reentries that led to distal embolization of the aneurysm contents, severe disseminated intravascular coagulation, and fatal intracerebral bleeding. One patient required secondary deployment of a distal stent 4 months after the initial procedure and subsequently underwent surgical replacement.

Conclusion.—Although the method has to be improved, aneurysmal exclusion with an endoluminal stent-graft is likely to become an important alternative to operative repair.

▶ This article from the originator of the stenting technique is of interest, but the authors should not suggest that this technique might be safer and cheaper than conventional repair. The so-called conversion rates to ordinary operation worldwide approach 20%, and it is in the unfit patient where this is likely to be necessary. Similarly, as far as costs are concerned, it has yet

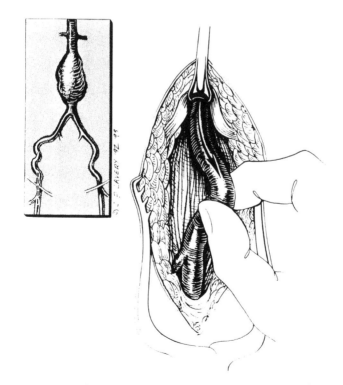

Fig 2–15.—A retroperitoneal exposure of the common iliac artery and anastomosis of a 10-mm Dacron tube used for transluminal delivery of the device. After the implantation, the Dacron iliac graft is cut and oversewn almost flush with the iliac artery. (Courtesy of Parodi JC, Criado FJ, Barone HD, et al: *Ann Vasc Surg* 8(6):523–529, 1994.)

to be proven that this technique is cheaper than conventional repair, bearing in mind that a number of stent manufacturers are now selling this device for more than $6,000 before other costs are taken into consideration. Mortality in this particular series was acceptable at 4%.

Since this article was published, longer-term results and complications have been presented at the Phoenix meeting in January 1995. These articles indicate that the results are much worse than cited here. A controlled trial is essential, with the costs, complications, and all criteria determined before claims can be made about the utility of this procedure.—P.R.F. Bell, M.D.

Thrombolysis

Thrombolytic Therapy for Arterial Occlusion: A Mixed Blessing

Smith CM, Yellin AE, Weaver FA, Ming KA, Siegel AE (Univ of Southern California, Los Angeles; LAC+USC Med Ctr, Los Angeles)
Am Surg 60:371–375, 1994   145-96-2–14

Introduction.—The results of thrombolytic therapy with the use of intra-arterial urokinase were reviewed in 41 patients with severe peripheral vascular disease who received treatment in 42 lower extremities. The occluded sites included 21 superficial femoral, 20 infrapopliteal, 11 popliteal, and 6 iliac artery segments.

Methods.—Urokinase was infused regionally, usually in a loading dose of 250,000 units, followed by a continuous infusion of approximately 100,000 units per hour for as long as 72 hours. Heparin was administered at the same time.

Results.—Arterial occlusions resolved at least partially in 26 (62%) of the treated extremities. Endovascular procedures were necessary in 19 extremities after clot lysis. In 22 of the 26 technical successes a return of a distal pulse or an increase in the angle brachial index of greater than 0.1 occurred. All 4 patients who were considered clinical failures and all 16 in whom the procedure failed technically required revascularization or a major amputation. Major complications occurred in 43% of patients (table), 2 of whom died. The occurrence of major bleeding could not be related either to the dose of urokinase or to the duration of thrombolytic treatment.

Conclusion.—Although thrombolysis combined with endovascular treatment when appropriate may help some patients with major extremity ischemia, lethal complications can develop. Hopefully, prospective studies will show which patients are best managed in this way and which should have primary operative treatment.

Major Complications of Thrombolytic Procedures

Complication	Success	Failure	Total (%)
Thromboembolic	3	4	7 (17)
Dissection	1	1	2 (5)
Hemorrhage	5	4	9 (21)
Death	0	2	2 (5)
Total	9	11	20

(Courtesy of Smith CM, Yellin AE, Weaver FA, et al: *Am Surg* 60:371–375, 1994.)

▶ The message of this article is repetitious and boring: Early occlusion of lower extremity arteries that is promptly treated with urokinase will result in a resolution of the thrombotic process in about two thirds of patients, a number of whom will require concomitant procedures to retain patency. Despite this, the 1-year patency rate has been extremely disappointing, being in the range of 30% to 40% in the series reported to date.

As the authors note, significant complications invariably occur in thrombolytic series. Almost 20% of patients had bleeding that was sufficient to require transfusions, and some had devastating intracranial bleeding. On balance, whereas thrombolytic therapy may be of limited value in the occasional carefully selected patient with thrombosis of endogenous arteries, I find no reason to use it in thrombosed grafts.

Results of a Prospective Randomized Trial Evaluating Surgery Versus Thrombolysis for Ischemia of the Lower Extremity: The STILE Trial

The STILE Investigators (Cleveland Clinic Found, Ohio; Temple Univ, Philadelphia; Saint Sacrement Hosp, Quebec)
Ann Surg 220:251–268, 1994   145-96-2-15

Introduction.—Catheter-directed thrombolysis has been used to manage patients with acute and chronic arterial and graft occlusions, but its therapeutic efficacy has been questioned. Relative effectiveness of catheter-directed thrombolysis or standard surgical intervention was assessed in patients with lower limb ischemia caused by nonembolic arterial and bypass graft occlusion.

Methods.—Patients with worsening limb ischemia and nonembolic arterial or bypass graft occlusion identified by angiography were stratified for native artery occlusion or bypass graft occlusion and randomly assigned to 1 of 3 treatment groups: surgical revascularization or catheter-directed thrombolysis with either recombinant tissue plasminogen activator (rt-PA) or urokinase (UK). At 30 days after treatment, composite clinical outcome was assessed, including occurrence of ongoing or recurrent ischemia, death, major amputation, and major morbidity.

Results.—Patients in the thrombolysis group had a 61.7% adverse event rate; 36.1% of the surgical patients had adverse events. Thrombolysis patients had a significantly higher incidence of ongoing or recurrent ischemia (54% vs. 25.7%), life-threatening hemorrhage (5.6% vs. .7%), and vascular complications (9.7% vs. 3.5%) than surgical patients. Overall, rates of mortality and major amputation were comparable in the groups. Thrombolysis with rt-PA or UK was equally effective and had comparable bleeding complications. In the thrombolysis group, the overall composite clinical outcome was similar among patients with native arterial or graft occlusions. In the surgical group, those with graft occlusions tended to have a higher amputation rate; those with native arterial occlusions tended to have a higher mortality rate. Overall, outcome was not influenced by duration of ischemia.

Conclusion.—Patients with acute ischemia are optimally managed with catheter-directed thrombolysis, and patients with chronic ischemia are optimally managed with surgical revascularization.

▶ It appears that the STILE (Surgery vs. Thrombolysis for Ischemia of the Lower Extremity) investigators designed and performed a prospective study but then based one of their important and controversial conclusions on retrospective data analysis. The STILE trial was not originally designed to answer the question of optimal treatment for *acute* limb ischemia. Candidates were required to have worsening limb ischemia within 6 months of SVS/ISCVS classification for *chronic* limb ischemia.

It is noteworthy that the study was terminated by the Safety Monitoring Committee at the first interim analysis, with significantly greater ongoing/recurrent ischemia, life-threatening hemorrhage, and more vascular complications in patients with thrombolysis compared with surgery patients. However, with a retrospective, post hoc analysis it was determined that among patients who had ischemic deterioration from 0 to 14 days before randomization there were significantly fewer amputations at 6 months in the thrombolysis group. Unfortunately, patients were not prospectively stratified on the basis of the duration of ischemia, nor were they categorized according to the SVS/ISCVS classification for *acute* limb ischemia. The STILE investigators' post hoc data analysis is interesting, but it may prove profoundly misleading and cannot be used as conclusive proof that initial thrombolysis is superior to surgery for patients with acute limb ischemia.—R. Yeager, M.D.

▶ Dr. Yeager's comments are too kind. A clinical trial has prospective end points that are the only ones that can be used for hypothesis-proving analysis. The authors have retrospectively defined another end point: post hoc analysis (also known as data dredging). This can only be used as an hypothesis-seeking exercise, never an hypothesis-proving exercise. I confer on the authors the prestigious Camel Dung Award.—J.M. Porter, M.D.

Is Thrombolysis of Occluded Popliteal and Tibial Bypass Grafts Worthwhile?
Hye RJ, Turner C, Valji K, Wolf YG, Roberts AC, Bookstein JJ, Plecha EJ (Univ

of California, San Diego; VA Med Ctr, San Diego)
J Vasc Surg 20:588–597, 1994   145-96-2–16

Background.—Some vascular surgeons have recommended thrombolysis of occluded infrainguinal bypass grafts. Although this intervention has been highly successful in reestablishing flow through the graft, the long-term outcomes are unclear. The results of thrombolysis of occluded infrainguinal bypass grafts were reviewed.

Methods.—The retrospective study included 40 episodes of graft thrombosis that were treated over 62 months at 1 center. These episodes occurred in 33 grafts of 31 patients. The short- and long-term patency results were assessed, including the effects of graft age, material, and anatomy, as well as patient symptoms, treatment, anticoagulation, and duration of occlusion. The dose and duration of therapy were also examined when using the pulse-spray thrombolysis technique.

Results.—Graft patency was successfully reestablished by thrombolysis in 92% of cases. The mean lysis time was 118 minutes, and the mean urokinase dose was 607,000 units. In 35 of 37 cases, angioplasty or surgery allowed identification and treatment of the responsible lesions. The postthrombolysis patency rate was 28% at 30 months (Fig 2–16), and the 18-month secondary patency rate was 46%. Patency was unaffected by the duration of occlusion, symptoms, treatment, graft anatomy, or previous graft revision. The mean secondary patency was 22 months for grafts that had been in place for more than 1 year compared with 7 months for grafts that had been in place for a shorter time. Polytetrafluoroethylene grafts were associated with a better mean secondary patency than vein grafts: 24 vs. 8 months. The 30-month extremity salvage rate was 84%, and the 42-month patient survival was 84%.

Conclusion.—For patients with occluded infrainguinal grafts, the pulse-spray technique of thrombolysis can provide quick and effective recanali-

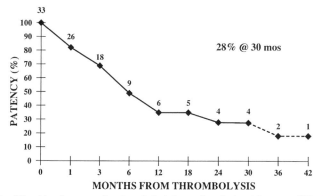

Fig 2–16.—Life-table of patency after thrombolysis for graft occlusion. (Courtesy of Hye RJ, Turner C, Valji K, et al: *J Vasc Surg* 20:588–597, 1994.)

zation. Thrombolysis and revision should be used only in grafts that have been in place for more than 1 year, whereas grafts that fail within the first year should probably be replaced. Thrombosed vein grafts have worse long-term patency than thrombosed synthetic grafts.

▶ The lousy patency rate of 28% at 30 months in thrombolysed grafts is about what one has come to expect on the basis of the available data. The authors recommend that grafts that fail in the first year be replaced with new grafts and thrombolysis be reserved for failed grafts more than 1 year old. I agree with the former but not the latter. If a graft fails, let it go and replace it with a new graft if the patient requires regrafting. Thrombolysis is simply not a durable choice for treatment of leg graft thrombosis.

A Comparison of Thrombolytic Therapy With Operative Revascularization in the Initial Treatment of Acute Peripheral Arterial Ischemia
Ouriel K, Shortell CK, DeWeese JA, Green RM, Francis CW, Azodo MVU, Gutierrez OH, Manzione JV, Cox C, Marder VJ (Univ of Rochester, NY)
J Vasc Surg 19:1021–1030, 1994   145-96-2–17

Background.—Intra-arterial thrombolytic therapy has come into widespread use for patients with peripheral arterial occlusion, because of its perceived advantages over surgical intervention. However, no randomized trials have compared the efficacy of these 2 approaches. Intra-arterial thrombolysis was compared with surgical revascularization for the initial treatment of acute peripheral arterial ischemia in a randomized trial.

Methods.—One hundred fourteen patients with limb-threatening ischemia that lasted less than 1 week participated in the study. They were randomly assigned in equal numbers to receive intra-arterial catheter-directed urokinase or surgical revascularization. Anatomical lesions, disclosed by thrombolysis were managed either by balloon dilation or surgery.

Results.—Urokinase dissolved the occluding thrombus in 70% of patients, but 67% of patients assigned to the thrombolysis group had some type of surgical intervention afterward. The 12-month cumulative limb salvage rate was 82% in both groups. However, at the same time, cumulative survival was 84% in the thrombolysis group and 58% in the surgical group. Cardiopulmonary complications occurred in the hospital in 16% of the thrombolysis group and in 49% of the surgical group; this appeared to account for the difference in mortality. The median length of hospital stay was 11 days in both groups. The median hospital costs were $15,672 with thrombolysis and $12,253 with surgery. Both groups had a 1-year patency rate of less than 60% (Fig 2–17).

Conclusion.—For patients with acute peripheral arterial occlusion, intra-arterial thrombolytic therapy with urokinase decreased in-hospital cardiopulmonary complications while it increased patient survival. The benefits of thrombolysis accrued with no increase in the duration of hospital stay and only a moderate increase in hospital costs. Thrombolytic therapy

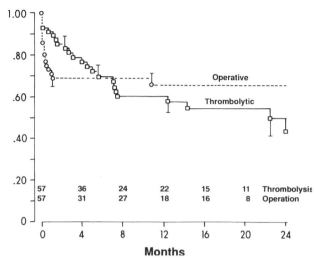

Fig 2–17.—Kaplan-Meier curves for patency rates according to assigned treatment. Data are expressed in terms of primary patency of revascularization, defined as the interval between the restoration of arterial continuity by means of thrombolysis or surgical reconstruction and subsequent thrombotic failure of revascularized segments. Numbers of patients at risk are shown at bottom of graph; *error bars* represent SEM at representative follow-up intervals. (Courtesy of Ouriel K, Shortell CK, DeWeese JA, et al: *J Vasc Surg* 19:1021–1030, 1994.)

appears to be safe and effective for the initial management of patients with acute, limb-threatening peripheral arterial ischemia.

▶ Although I admire the authors' intent to conduct a prospective random-ized study, this particular study admitted apples, oranges, pomegranates, and grapefruit; no 2 patients were the same. In the important group with occluded bypass grafts, 1-year patency was identical in both the throm-bolytic and the surgical arm. The peculiar benefit of an increased patient survival rate with thrombolytic therapy is a classic example of post hoc analysis. If you do enough post hoc analyses, 1 of every 20 will be positive by chance alone. I notice that in the TOPAS Trial, of which Dr. Ouriel is one of the principal investigators, no such reduction in mortality has been claimed.

Local Thrombolysis for Occluded Arterial Grafts: Is the Yield Worth the Effort?
Lacroix H, Suy R, Nevelsteen A, Verheyen L, Stockx L, Wilms G, Verhaeghe R (Univ Hosp Gasthuisberg, Leuven, Belgium)
J Cardiovasc Surg 35:187–191, 1994   145-96-2–18

Introduction.—The many small studies of local thrombolysis for the treatment of occluded vascular grafts have yielded inconsistent results.

After some surprisingly severe complications, experience with local thrombolytic therapy in 50 occluded grafts was reviewed.

Methods.—Fifty recently occluded arterial grafts in 41 patients were treated by local thrombolysis. The patients had acute, severe ischemia that was still reversible, and most had infrainguinal synthetic grafts. Thrombolysis was performed with the use of an intra-arterial catheter with alteplase in 38 patients, streptokinase in 11, and urokinase in 1.

Results.—The rate of complete angiographic lysis was 72%, and the rate of partial lysis was 12%. Alteplase yielded 89%, the highest lysis rate. Seventeen patients required complementary endovascular or surgical interventions, or both, to manage an underlying stenosis or to salvage the extremity. The complication rate was 30%; there were 8 cases of bleeding (3 of which were fatal) and 4 of distal embolization. All but 2 of the patients with bleeding complications were taking aspirin on a chronic basis. The 6-month primary patency rate in successfully lysed grafts was only 19% (Fig 2–18), and the 6-month salvage rate was only 64%.

Conclusion.—Because of the poor late results, local thrombolysis is not the optimal form of management for occluded arterial grafts. The difficulty in this situation is not in restoring patency but in maintaining it.

▶ The title of this article by LaCroix and colleagues succinctly summarizes the dilemma faced by vascular surgeons: Thrombolysis of occluded grafts is feasible but, as the authors suggest, it is often of limited long-term benefit. Advocates of thrombolytic infusion can point to several flaws in this article, which is a retrospective, nonsequential review of an experience involving 3 lytic agents. From 1980 to 1985, streptokinase or urokinase was used on 12 grafts, whereas tissue plasminogen activator was used in 39 cases that

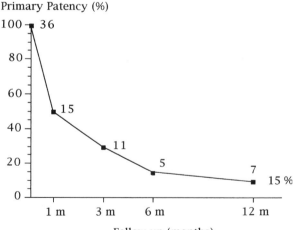

Fig 2–18.—Actuarial primary patency of the 36 grafts that were successfully lysed with or without adjuvant endovascular or surgical intervention. The numbers include grafts at risk. (By permission of LaCroix H, Suy R, Nevelsteen A, et al: Local thrombolysis for occluded arterial grafts: Is the yield worth the effort? *J Cardiovasc Surg* 35:187–191, 1994.)

were treated between 1990 and 1992. The overall results were negatively influenced by the use of streptokinase in the early experience and by the limited use of adjunctive procedures (in only 10 cases), the majority of which were percutaneous transluminal angioplasty. In this context, the high rate of early thrombosis reported by the Leuven group is hardly unexpected.

Despite these criticisms, the results reported in this article are disturbingly familiar: a major complication rate of 30%, including 2 cases of death resulting from intracerebral hemorrhage. The majority of cases of bleeding, including both intracranial hemorrhages, occurred in patients receiving tissue plasminogen activator. The mortality rate seen for therapeutic arterial lysis is consistent with rates from major series reported in the literature and remains a cause for concern. As the authors note in their discussion, application of thrombolysis as primary therapy for graft thrombosis has disappointed those who hoped it would lead to improved early or late patency. This has led us to depend increasingly on secondary vascular reconstruction and spare the use of thrombolytic agents.—J. Ricotta, M.D.

Intra-Arterial Thrombolytic Therapy in the Initial Management of Thrombosed Popliteal Artery Aneurysms
Garramone RR Jr, Gallagher JJ Jr, Drezner AD (Univ of Connecticut, Hartford)
Ann Vasc Surg 8:363–366, 1994   145-96-2–19

Introduction.—Three patients with acute, limb-threatening ischemia of the lower extremity secondary to a thrombosed popliteal artery aneurysm received urokinase intra-arterially before definitive surgery was performed. In each patient, infrapopliteal runoff improved, permitting successful arterial reconstruction.

Case 1.—Man, 56, had paresthesias in the left foot 24 hours earlier, which progressed rapidly to marked claudication and rest pain. The left lower limb was ischemic; angiography showed an occluded popliteal artery with intraluminal thrombus and below-knee runoff by collaterals only. Repeat arteriography after a 24-hour intra-arterial infusion of urokinase demonstrated a 2-cm popliteal aneurysm that was partly filled with thrombus, and patent peroneal and anterior tibial arteries. An in situ femoral to below-knee popliteal bypass was followed by adequate perfusion of the foot. Symptoms of ischemia were absent 7 months postoperatively.

Case 2.—Man, 68, who was known to have atrial fibrillation, was seen with a cold, cyanotic, pulseless left foot. The superficial femoral artery was occluded, and there was little infrapopliteal runoff. A thrombectomy was performed, and urokinase was infused for 48 hours, after which the popliteal artery was patent and there was runoff by a patent proximal anterior tibial artery. The latter vessel provided collateral flow to a distal peroneal artery that was patent to the foot. Revascularization was done using a polytetrafluoroethylene interposition graft, excluding the aneurysm. The patient had no ischemic symptoms 3 years later; the ankle/brachial index was 0.96.

Case 3.—Man, 56, suddenly experienced paresthesias and nocturnal rest pain in the left lower limb. The foot was cold and pulseless, and the superficial femoral artery was occluded. The peroneal artery was patent to the ankle, and the anterior tibial artery was patent proximally. The patient improved clinically after 6 hours of urokinase infusion, after which the superficial femoral artery was widely patent. Thrombus was evident within a popliteal artery aneurysm. An in situ femoral to peroneal and posterior tibial artery bypass rendered the patient free of ischemic symptoms 21 months later, when the ankle/brachial index was 1.0.

Conclusion.—In patients with a thrombosed popliteal arterial aneurysm, intra-arterial thrombolysis should improve the chances of achieving long-term patency and limit limb loss.

► This represents a genuine exception to my prejudice against lytic therapy. If a patient appears with a thrombosed popliteal aneurysm and no detectable runoff and a foot that does not require emergent vascular surgery, intra-arterial thrombolysis is extremely helpful to assist in defining an outflow tract. In fact, Dr. Taylor and I presented one of the very early case reports in this area (1).

Reference

1. Taylor LM, Porter JM: *Am J Surg* 147:583–588, 1984.

3 Vascular Lab and Imaging

Carotid

Reappraisal of Duplex Criteria to Assess Significant Carotid Stenosis With Special Reference to Reports From the North American Symptomatic Carotid Endarterectomy Trial and the European Carotid Surgery Trial
Neale ML, Chambers JL, Kelly AT, Connard S, Lawton MA, Roche J, Appleberg M (Royal North Shore Hosp, Sydney, Australia)
J Vasc Surg 20:642–649, 1994   145-96-3–1

Background.—Duplex scanning is now the most widely used method of evaluating extracranial disease in the carotid and vertebral arteries. No consistent set of hemodynamic criteria has been adopted, and there are also different methods of estimating the degree of angiographic stenosis.

Methods.—The extent of agreement between 2 commonly used methods of assessing carotid stenosis by duplex scanning and between 2 methods of angiographic interpretation was determined in a series of 120 carotid bifurcations. The duplex criteria established by Zwiebel and by Strandness were compared, as were the angiographic methods used in the North American Symptomatic Carotid Endarterectomy Trial and the European Carotid Surgery Trial. Receiver operating characteristic curves were derived from the duplex data to detect stenoses exceeding 70% from the angiographic method used in the North American trial.

Results.—The accuracy of the duplex criteria depended on the method used to report the angiograms. The Zwiebel criteria agreed more closely with the angiographic method used in the European trial (accuracy, 88%), whereas the Strandness criteria agreed more with the angiographic method used in the North American trial (accuracy, 89%). A peak systolic velocity greater than 270 cm/sec and an end-diastolic velocity greater than 110 cm/sec were 96% sensitive, 91% specific, and 93% accurate in detecting stenoses exceeding 70%.

Conclusion.—When validating the duplex criteria used to assess carotid stenosis, vascular laboratories should validate them against a standard angiographic method.

▶ There has been a spate of articles attempting to define precise duplex criteria for both the North American Symptomatic Carotid Endarterectomy Trial (NASCET) 70% and the ACAS 60% stenosis. I note that the current effort, which looks fairly good with regard to sensitivity and specificity, has a positive predictive value of only 74%, which, on balance, is disappointing. I wonder whether such detailed criteria-seeking really makes sense. Is a patient with 65% stenosis functionally different from one with 70% stenosis? I think we may be kidding ourselves in trying to calibrate these criteria so precisely, because there is clear variation in the machinery and in tests of the same patient done by the same technologist on different occasions. References 1 and 2 contain both the NASCET and the ACAS criteria from our laboratory.

References

1. Moneta GL, et al: *J Vasc Surg* 17:152–159, 1993.
2. Moneta GL, et al: *Arch Surg* 128:1117–1123, 1993.

Clinical Outcome in Patients With Mild and Moderate Carotid Artery Stenosis
Johnson BF, Verlato F, Bergelin RO, Primozich JF, Strandness DE Jr (Univ of Washington, Seattle)
J Vasc Surg 21:120–126, 1995   145-96-3–2

Objective.—An attempt was made to determine the natural course of mild carotid artery stenosis, defined as narrowing of less than 50%, and moderate (50% to 79%) stenosis using duplex ultrasonography.

Methods.—A total of 232 patients who had a carotid bruit and less than 80% luminal narrowing at the outset, and who had no associated symptoms, underwent bilateral carotid duplex studies annually for up to 10 years. Sufficient data for a 7-year life-table analysis were collected.

Results.—The degree of stenosis increased in 23% of the patients during follow-up. Nearly half of those patients progressed to severe (80% or greater) stenosis or occlusion (Fig 3–1). The risk of progression to severe disease was significantly greater when moderate, rather than mild, stenosis was present at initial evaluation. The cumulative risk of stroke after 7 years was 6% in patients with mild initial stenosis and 11% in those with moderate initial stenosis. Twenty-seven patients underwent carotid endarterectomy, 14 because of asymptomatic high-grade stenosis and 13 because of an ipsilateral ischemic event.

Conclusion.—Monitoring the course of initially asymptomatic carotid stenosis by duplex ultrasonography permits a realistic assessment of the risk of an ischemic cerebrovascular event.

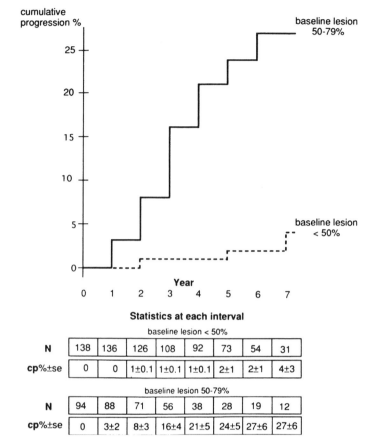

cumulative progression %

baseline lesion 50-79%

baseline lesion < 50%

Year

Statistics at each interval

baseline lesion < 50%

N	138	136	126	108	92	73	54	31
cp%±se	0	0	1±0.1	1±0.1	1±0.1	2±1	2±1	4±3

baseline lesion 50-79%

N	94	88	71	56	38	28	19	12
cp%±se	0	3±2	8±3	16±4	21±5	24±5	27±6	27±6

Fig 3–1.—Cumulative progression to 80% to 99% diameter-reducing lesion. (Courtesy of Johnson BF, Verlato F, Bergelin RO, et al: *J Vasc Surg* 21:120–126, 1995.)

▶ Natural history studies are interesting, although the results are impossible to apply to the individual patient. On balance, about 25% of carotids progressed during a life-table 7-year observation and, in general, the more stenosis the patient had at entry, the more likely he or she was to have disease progress to 80% to 99% stenosis or complete occlusion. The problem with this study, of course, is that it was not a prospective study with unselected patients. Instead, the patients were highly selected as those referred to the vascular laboratory for some reason. Whether the behavior of these patients is the same as patients in the general population is unknown, although I suspect that it is *not* the same. Studies like this one may be of modest value in helping us plan duplex screening protocols, but the relatively low rate of progression and the wide variation among patients will make this exercise quite imprecise.

Carotid Artery Stenosis: Clinical Efficacy of MR Phase-Contrast Flow Quantification as an Adjunct to MR Angiography

Vanninen RL, Manninen HI, Partanen PLK, Vainio PA, Soimakallio S (Kuopio Univ Hosp, Finland)
Radiology 194:459–467, 1995   145-96-3–3

Background.—It has been proposed that carotid endarterectomy may be based on the MR angiographic findings alone. This imaging method is, however, sensitive to artifacts produced by slow, turbulent flow in severely stenosed vessels. Also, carotid MR angiography tends to overestimate the stenosis.

Methods.—The usefulness of quantifying blood flow was examined in 55 patients who were referred for MR angiography and in 10 healthy controls. In addition to Doppler ultrasonography and three-dimensional time-of-flight MR angiography, phase-contrast flow quantification was done to estimate peak systolic velocity (PSV) and the volumetric flow rate (VFR) in the common and internal carotid arteries distal to the site of stenosis.

Results.—Both PSV and VFR were significantly reduced in internal carotid arteries that were stenosed by 70% or more (table). The ratio of VFR values in the internal and common carotid arteries was 91% accurate in detecting severe stenosis. When flow data were combined with the findings of MR angiography, the method was totally sensitive, with only a modest loss of specificity. Doppler and MR estimates of PSV in the common carotid artery were correlated at a level of .64 in the patients and .73 in controls. Peak systolic velocity values in the common carotid artery were significantly greater in controls than in patients, but this parameter did not distinguish among patients with varying degrees of bifurcational disease (Fig 3–2).

Carotid Peak Systolic Velocity (*PSV*) and Volumetric Flow Rate (*VFR*)					
		No. of Bifurcations at MR Angiography			
	Group 1 Normal (*n* = 20)	Group 2 Mild Stenosis (<30%) (*n* = 69)	Group 3 Moderate Stenosis (30%–69%) (*n* = 13)	Group 4 Severe Stenosis (70%–99%) (*n* = 17)	Group 5 Occluded (*n* = 7)
PSV (cm/sec)					
Internal carotid artery	51 ± 15	36 ± 11	35 ± 14	18 ± 9	0
Common carotid artery	77 ± 14	48 ± 15	41 ± 14	30 ± 14	32 ± 14
PSV ratio*	0.67 ± 0.17	0.78 ± 0.29	0.88 ± 0.29	0.51 ± 0.39	0
VFR (mL/min)					
Internal carotid artery	251 ± 38	226 ± 90	204 ± 94	109 ± 83	0
Common carotid artery	391 ± 54	371 ± 102	312 ± 114	293 ± 124	132 ± 71
VFR ratio†	0.65 ± 0.11	0.61 ± 0.19	0.72 ± 41	0.39 ± 0.30	0

Note: Values are mean ± 1 SD.
* *PSV ratio* represents the PSV internal carotid artery/PSV common carotid artery.
† *VFR ratio* represents the VFR internal carotid artery/VFR common carotid artery.
(Courtesy of Vanninen RL, Manninen HI, Partanen PLK, et al: *Radiology* 194:459–467, 1995.)

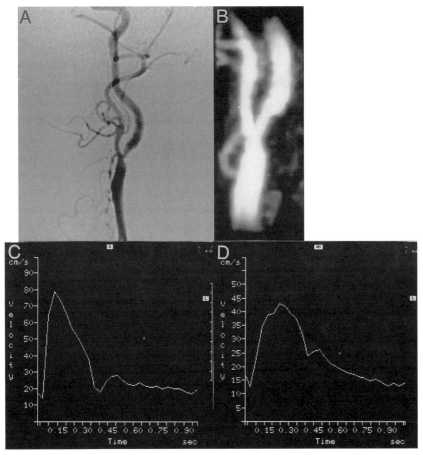

Fig 3–2.—Digital subtraction angiographic image (A) and MR angiographic image (B) of a moderately stenosed left internal carotid artery. Velocity curves of the common carotid artery (C) and internal carotid artery (D) show almost normal peak systolic velocity. (Courtesy of Vanninen RL, Manninen HI, Partanen PLK, et al: *Radiology* 194:459–467, 1995.)

Conclusion.—Quantitative MR flow studies can indicate whether carotid stenoses are hemodynamically significant, and they may help in distinguishing between critical stenosis and occlusion.

► These authors present a detailed description of the use of phase-contrast flow quantification in the carotid arteries. This is a good review of technical MRI material. Clearly, MRI can be used to accurately quantitate volumetric flow. However, I am not at all certain it is going to be better than simple velocity data. See the commentary after Abstract 145-96-3–4.

Hemodynamic Effects of Carotid Endarterectomy by Magnetic Resonance Flow Quantification

Vanninen R, Koivisto K, Tulla H, Manninen H, Partanen K (Kuopio Univ Hosp, Finland)

Stroke 26:84–89, 1995   145-96-3–4

Objective.—The method of MR phase-contrast flow quantification was used to assess blood flow before and 3 days after carotid endarterectomy in a prospective series of 25 patients having 27 operations.

Methods.—Volumetric flow rates and peak systolic velocities were recorded in the internal and common carotid arteries and the vertebral artery. Complete flow data were available from 16 patients who had surgery on 18 vessels.

Results.—The preoperative rate of blood flow in the internal carotid artery were inversely correlated with the degree of angiographic stenosis to a highly significant degree. Postoperatively, mean flow in the ipsilateral internal carotid artery increased from 143 to 233 mL/min as the mean peak systolic flow velocity increased from 23 to 37 cm/sec (table). No significant changes in flow were noted in the contralateral carotid artery or the vertebral arteries. The mean total blood flow increased by 81 mL/min. Flow rates improved the most in severely stenosed vessels.

Conclusions.—Carotid blood flow significantly improves after successful carotid endarterectomy. Quantitative MR flow monitoring is a useful means of following the hemodynamic effects of this surgery.

▶ The phase-contrast methodology used in conjunction with MR allows the measurement of volumetric flow, which has been shown to correlate well with electromagnetic flow measurements. This study shows the expected increase in internal carotid artery flow after endarterectomy. I note with interest that the use of volumetric flow determined noninvasively with either

Volumetric Flow Rates in the Internal and Common Carotid and Vertebral Arteries by MR Phase-Contrast Flow Quantification

Variable	Preoperative Measurement	Postoperative Measurement	P*
Operated ICA, mL/min	143 ± 76	233 ± 88	<.001
Contralateral ICA, mL/min	206 ± 94	201 ± 98	.82
Operated CCA, mL/min	274 ± 125	350 ± 116	.07
Contraleteral CCA, mL/min	355 ± 126	371 ± 134	.72
Vertebral arteries, sum of both sides, mL/min	233 ± 114	230 ± 109	.70
TBF, mL/min	583 ± 161	664 ± 188	.08
Operated ICA/TBF, %	25 ± 11	35 ± 11	<.001

Note: Data represent the preoperative and postoperative measurements of 16 neurologically symptomatic patients undergoing 18 carotid endarterectomies. Values are mean ± SD.
* Difference between preoperative and postoperative values tested by paired *t*-test.
Abbreviations: ICA, internal carotid artery; *CCA*, common carotid artery; *TBF*, total blood flow, calculated as the sum of the measured volumetric flow rates of both the ICAs and the vertebral arteries.
(Courtesy of Vanninen R, Koivisto K, Tulla H, et al: *Stroke* 26:84–89, 1995.)

MRI or the duplex technique has really achieved little standing in vascular surgery. We continue to rely on Doppler-determined intravascular pressure and flow velocities; to date, most of us have limited confidence in volumetric flow determinations. I wonder whether, in the future, information on volumetric flow will prove superior to today's information on velocity flow?

Arterial Wall Thickness is Associated With Prevalent Cardiovascular Disease in Middle-Aged Adults: The Atherosclerosis Risk in Communities (ARIC) Study
Burk GL, for the ARIC Study Group (Univ of North Carolina, Chapel Hill; ARIC Ultrasound Reading Ctr, Winston-Salem, NC; National Heart, Lung, and Blood Institute, Bethesda, Md; et al)
Stroke 26:386–391, 1995   145-96-3–5

Objective.—The prevalence of cardiovascular disease was related to arterial wall thickness in a population of 13,870 middle-aged adults in the United States. Participants included black and white men and women, 45 to 64 years of age, who were participants in the Atherosclerosis Risk in Communities (ARIC) Study.

Methods.—Prevalent coronary heart disease, cerebrovascular disease, and peripheral vascular disease were ascertained by self-report, baseline ECG and fasting blood glucose, and a history of medication use. Intimal-medial thickness (IMT) was measured in the carotid and popliteal arteries by B-mode ultrasonography.

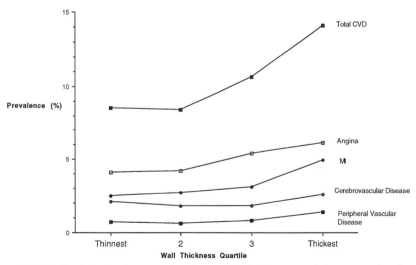

Fig 3–3.—Graph showing disease prevalence by carotid wall thickness quartile (age; race; and gender-adjusted) in middle-aged adults. *Abbreviations: CVD*, cardiovascular disease; *MI*, myocardial infarction. (Courtesy of Burk GL, for the ARIC Study Group: *Stroke* 26:386–391, 1995.)

Results.—For all racial and gender groups, the mean IMT of the far carotid artery wall was consistently greater in individuals with clinical cardiovascular disease than in those free of disease (Fig 3–3). The most marked differences in carotid IMT were seen in participants with symptomatic peripheral vascular disease. Both carotid and popliteal IMT were related to clinically manifest disease of the coronary, cerebral, and peripheral arteries.

Conclusion.—Prevalent cardiovascular disease was related to increased arterial wall thickness in a population-based sample of middle-aged adults.

▶ The ARIC study is a massive population-based study that is producing important information concerning the epidemiology of atherosclerosis. In this important study, the authors conclude that carotid IMT is an excellent predictor of generalized atherosclerosis and, in fact, is quantitatively related to the clinical severity of associated cardiovascular disease. Although it has been noted in a previous YEAR BOOK (1) that carotid IMT is a valid marker of atherosclerosis, this article extends these observations to a much larger population.

Reference

1. 1995 YEAR BOOK OF VASCULAR SURGERY, p 111.

Carotid Artery Occlusion: Positive Predictive Value of Duplex Sonography Compared With Arteriography
Kirsch JD, Wagner LR, James EM, Charboneau JW, Nichols DA, Meyer FB, Hallett JW (Mayo Clinic and Found, Rochester, Minn)
J Vasc Surg 19:642–649, 1994   145-96-3–6

Background.—Duplex ultrasonography is known to be an accurate noninvasive means of evaluating atherosclerotic stenosis of the extracranial carotid vessels, but its ability to accurately detect carotid occlusion has not been established. This is an important question because high-grade stenoses are treated operatively, whereas patients with occlusive disease are managed nonoperatively.

Methods.—The ability of duplex ultrasonography to distinguish carotid occlusion from high-grade stenosis was examined in 158 patients seen over 6.5-years, who had a total of 174 occluded carotid artery segments. Angiographic correlation was available in all cases.

Results.—Duplex sonography had a positive predictive value of 92.5% in detecting carotid artery occlusion; the rate of false positive results was 7.5%. Seven of 13 false positive studies were caused by very high-grade stenoses with slow flow or a "slim sign" (Fig 3–4). False positive results became significantly less frequent in the latter part of the review (table). The addition of color Doppler flow imaging to high-resolution B-mode scanning and pulsed Doppler spectral analysis did not improve the results significantly.

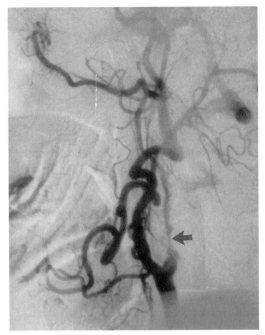

Fig 3–4.—Subtraction arteriogram in a patient with a false positive ultrasound diagnosis of internal carotid artery occlusion. Lateral view of injection of the right carotid artery reveals very high-grade stenosis ("slim sign") in the proximal internal carotid artery (*arrow*). (Courtesy of Kirsch JD, Wagner LR, James EM, et al: *J Vasc Surg* 19:642–649, 1994.)

Conclusion.—In most cases, duplex ultrasonography is a reasonably accurate means of detecting carotid artery occlusion. Arteriography may be limited to those symptomatic patients who are candidates for operative repair.

▶ This careful study indicates that the best duplex carotid examination has a false positive rate in detecting carotid artery occlusion that ranges between 3.5% and 7.5%, generally depending on the experience of the technologist. This is a very important point. One of the worst errors a vascular laboratory can make is to diagnose carotid occlusion when, in fact, there is

False Positive Rates for the Ultrasonographic Diagnosis of Carotid Artery Occlusion During 3 Periods

Portion of study	Date of examination	False positive results, no.	Correlated examinations, no.	False positive rate (%)
First third	1/85–2/87	3	29	10.3
Middle third	3/87–4/89	7	57	12.3
Last third	5/89–7/91	3	88	3.4
Total		13	174	

(Courtesy of Kirsch JD, Wagner LR, James EM, et al: *J Vasc Surg* 19:642–649, 1994.)

99% stenosis with string patency and potential for a successful endarterectomy. In our vascular laboratory, we have adopted the policy of adding this statement to the end of our reading of a carotid artery occlusion: "The vascular laboratory is not 100% accurate in differentiating carotid occlusion from 99% stenosis. A contrast arteriogram is required for this purpose and should be considered if warranted by clinical circumstances." In our clinical practice, we will obtain arteriograms in such patients, and we do, on occasion, find string patency permitting successful endarterectomy.

Assessment of Carotid Artery Stenosis by Ultrasonography, Conventional Angiography, and Magnetic Resonance Angiography: Correlation With Ex Vivo Measurement of Plaque Stenosis

Pan XM, Saloner D, Reilly LM, Bowersox JC, Murray SP, Anderson CM, Gooding GAW, Rapp JH (San Francisco VA Med Ctr; Univ of California, San Francisco)

J Vasc Surg 21:82–89, 1995   145-96-3–7

Background.—A number of attempts have been made to correlate the findings of Doppler ultrasonography (DUS), carotid angiography, and MR angiography (MRA) in patients with stenosis of the carotid bifurcation. Because the studies have lacked a true control in the form of the actual lesion, conclusions regarding diagnostic accuracy are necessarily tentative.

Methods.—Lesion size was estimated by all 3 of these methods in 28 patients who underwent 31 elective carotid endarterectomies. In each case, the imaging findings were compared with the carotid atheroma present in the en bloc operative specimen. All studies were done within one month before thromboendarterectomy. Standard flow criteria were used to estimate stenosis size by DUS. For carotid angiography and MRA, stenosis was defined as the ratio of the residual luminal diameter to the estimated normal diameter. Actual stenosis was estimated by high-resolution ex vivo MRI and by injecting the specimen with acrylic under pressure.

Results.—The results of ex vivo MRI correlated with estimates of size made in acrylic specimen casts at a level of 0.92. The ex vivo estimates generally correlated well with the results of all modalities (table), but correlation was better for DUS (0.80) and MRA (0.76) than for carotid angiography (0.56).

Agreement of Stenosis With Specimen			
	MRA (%)	DUS (%)	XRA (%)
Overestimate	17	14	6
Match	76	75	57
Underestimate	7	11	37

Abbreviations: MRA, MR angiography; *DUS*, Doppler ultrasonography; *XRA*, x-ray angiography.
(Courtesy of Pan XM, Saloner D, Reilly LM, et al: Assessment of carotid artery stenosis by ultrasonography, conventional angiography, and magnetic resonance angiography: Correlation with ex vivo measurement of plaque stenosis. *J Vasc Surg* 21:82–89, 1995.)

Conclusion.—These findings support the use of DUS to screen for carotid stenosis. Magnetic resonance angiography is suitable when another method is needed to determine the degree of bifurcational stenosis.

▶ These authors compare the ability of a two-dimensional imaging technique (angiography), a three-dimensional imaging technique (MRA), and a hemodynamic methodology (Doppler frequency analysis) to accurately detect severe arterial stenosis. The methodology was precise, and the comparison was both prospective and blinded, with the intact endarterectomy specimen used as the reference standard. Refreshingly, the least expensive, least invasive modality, DUS, provided the best results. Angiography underestimated the degree of stenosis seen in the specimen in 11 of 23 cases (48%) with critical stenosis, an observation that is of great importance when taken in the context of the recently reported endarterectomy trials. This study provides further evidence against using angiography as the "gold standard" in the evaluation of carotid bifurcation lesions, and in view of its expense and complication rate (1.3% in ACAS), this is a point worthy of emphasis. This paper also provides an elegant methodology for evaluating excised specimens by MR technique. However, as the authors note in their manuscript and discussion, MRA has not yet developed to the point where it can be routinely used for clinical decision-making.—J. Ricotta, M.D.

Clinical Relevance of Intraoperative Embolization Detected by Transcranial Doppler Ultrasonography During Carotid Endarterectomy: A Prospective Study of 100 Patients
Gaunt ME, Martin PJ, Smith JL, Rimmer T, Cherryman G, Ratliff DA, Bell PRF, Naylor AR (Leicester Royal Infirmary, England)
Br J Surg 81:1435–1439, 1994   145-96-3–8

Background.—Several studies have shown that transcranial Doppler ultrasonography (TCD) monitoring of the ipsilateral middle cerebral artery during carotid endarterectomy is able to detect embolization in different phases of surgery. However, these studies were not specifically designed to assess clinical outcomes. Thus, the clinical relevance of embolization detected by TCD remains unclear.

Methods.—The clinical significance of TCD-detected microembolization was investigated by determining the quantity and nature of the emboli and by correlating them with the neurologic and psychometric outcome, fundoscopy, automated visual field testing, and CT brain scans. One hundred consecutive patients who were undergoing carotid endarterectomy were studied.

Findings.—Embolization was found in 92% of successfully monitored procedures. Most emboli were characteristic of air, unassociated with adverse clinical outcomes (Fig 3–5). However, a significant deterioration in postoperative cognitive function was associated with more than 10 particulate emboli during initial carotid dissection (Fig 3–6). Persistent par-

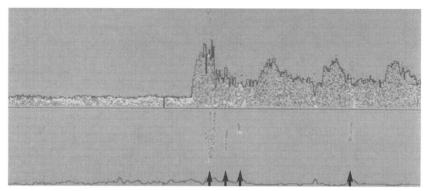

Fig 3–5.—Series of air emboli occurring at clamp release. Extraspectral overload is evident (*arrows*). (Courtesy of Gaunt ME, Martin PJ, Smith JL, et al: Clinical relevance of intraoperative embolization detected by transcranial Doppler ultrasonography during carotid endarterectomy: A prospective study of 100 patients. *Br J Surg* 81:1435–1439, 1994. Reproduced with permission of Blackwell Science, Ltd.)

ticulate embolization in the immediate postoperative period was associated with both incipient carotid artery thrombosis and the development of major neurologic deficits.

Conclusions.—Embolization detected by TCD during carotid endarterectomy appears to be clinically significant. In particular, TCD can provide an early warning of incipient carotid thrombosis in the immediate postoperative period. Early intervention may decrease the morbidity and mortality associated with this serious complication. Also, TCD can alert surgeons to potentially harmful embolization occurring during dissection of the carotid artery.

▶ If you, for some reason, wish to attach a TCD over the middle cerebral artery during carotid endarterectomy, you undoubtedly will be rewarded by lots of whooshing noises. Some of these noises apparently represent air,

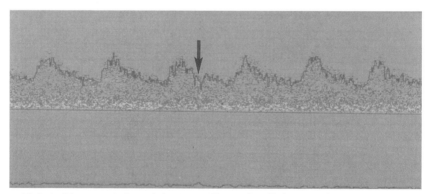

Fig 3–6.—Discrete particulate embolus (*arrow*). The signal is of high intensity but there is no overload. (Courtesy of Gaunt ME, Martin PJ, Smith JL, et al: Clinical relevance of intraoperative embolization detected by transcranial Doppler ultrasonography during carotid endarterectomy: A prospective study of 100 patients. *Br J Surg* 81:1435–1439, 1994. Reproduced with permission of Blackwell Science, Ltd.)

whereas others represent particulate matter. These investigators found that the number of particulate emboli were closely correlated with postoperative neurologic dysfunction and, in the immediate postoperative period, with incipient carotid artery thrombosis. They speculated that the careful use of this diagnostic methodology has the potential to significantly assist patient management. I wonder.

Is Transcranial Doppler a Worthwhile Addition to Screening Tests for Cerebrovascular Disease?
Comerota AJ, Katz ML, Hosking JD, Hashemi HA, Kerr RP, Carter AP (Temple Univ Hosp, Philadelphia; Univ of North Carolina, Chapel Hill)
J Vasc Surg 21:90–97, 1995   145-96-3–9

Background.—Carotid duplex imaging is the standard diagnostic evaluation for patients with suspected cerebrovascular disease. Transcranial Doppler (TCD) ultrasonography expands the noninvasive diagnostic capabilities, allowing investigation of the intracranial arteries. The role of routine TCD examination in patients referred for noninvasive cerebrovascular evaluation was considered.

Patients.—Between 1991 and 1993, 670 of 976 patients underwent TCD examination as part of their routine noninvasive cerebrovascular examination. Almost half (48%) of the patients had hemispheric symptoms, 34% had no symptoms, and 18% had nonhemispheric symptoms. Transcranial Doppler examinations were considered abnormal in the presence of intracranial stenosis, collateral pathways, greater than 30% velocity difference between sides, flow reversal, and velocities ±2 SD from normal. Severity of carotid artery disease was classified as less than 50% stenosis, 50% to 79%, 80% to 99%, and occlusion.

Results.—Only 45% of patients had an interpretable TCD examination. The ability to insonate the basal cerebral arteries through the temporal bone was significantly reduced in women, black patients, and older patients. Although 56% of patients had notable findings on the TCD examination, the results did not alter the diagnostic or therapeutic plan of any patients. In patients whose TCD examinations could be interpreted, 44% had normal results, 19% showed side-to-side velocity differences, 11% had intracranial collateral pathways, 11% had velocity measurements ±2 SD, 10% demonstrated intracranial stenosis, and 4% had reversed flow pattern.

Implications.—Transcranial Doppler ultrasonography provides little objective value as part of the routine noninvasive cerebrovascular examination in patients with suspected cerebrovascular disease. A large proportion of patients do not have an adequate examination and, although the number of positive findings is reasonably high, the results have no impact diagnostically or therapeutically. The selection criteria for TCD examinations should be refined, and TCD should not be incorporated as part of the "routine" noninvasive cerebrovascular examination.

▶ One must indeed question the utility of a screening test if its results have no direct impact on patient management. From this paper it would seem that for those patients with carotid symptoms, TCD examination provides no useful additional information. Although other authors have demonstrated a higher success rate in obtaining technically adequate studies (which may be a reflection of their patient mix rather than their technical expertise), and although some use this examination intraoperatively to determine the need for a shunt, I concur with Comerota et al. that TCD examination information has little or no impact on the management of patients with carotid artery disease. Clearly, this test *does* have a role in neurosurgical patients in identifying vasospasm and determining brain death, and it may provide useful information in patients with vertebrobasilar symptoms.—E.S. Weinstein, M.D.

Asymptomatic Carotid Artery Stenosis and Stroke in Patients Undergoing Cardiopulmonary Bypass
Schwartz LB, Bridgman AH, Kieffer RW, Wilcox RA, McCann RL, Tawil MP, Scott SM (Asheville VA Med Ctr, NC; Duke Univ, Durham, NC)
J Vasc Surg 21:146–153, 1995   145-96-3–10

Objectives.—The incidence and natural history of carotid artery atherosclerosis in symptom-free patients undergoing cardiopulmonary bypass (CPB) procedures were investigated.

Patients.—Between 1989 and 1993, all patients undergoing CPB were offered carotid artery ultrasound screening as part of an investigative protocol. The typical patient is a man who is undergoing heart surgery and has a high incidence of comorbid conditions. The mean patient age was 62 years.

Results.—Of the 582 patients who underwent carotid artery ultrasound screening, 22% had greater than 50% stenosis or occlusion of 1 or both internal carotid arteries, and 12% had 80% or greater stenosis or occlusion of 1 or both arteries. Twelve (2.1%) patients had in-hospital stroke, and 36 (6.2%) died. Of the 5 patients with global strokes, none had evidence of carotid artery stenosis. In contrast, 5 of 7 patients with hemispheric strokes had significant 50% or greater stenosis or occlusion of the internal carotid artery ipsilateral to the hemispheric stroke. The risk of hemispheric stroke in patients without significant stenosis was 0.34% compared with 3.8% in patients with 50% or greater stenosis or occlusion. Furthermore, the risk of hemispheric stroke in patients with unilateral 80% to 99% stenosis, bilateral 50% to 99% stenosis, or unilateral occlusion with contralateral 50% or greater stenosis was 5.3%, which was significantly greater than the risk of stroke in patients with less severe disease patterns (0.59%). None of the patients with unilateral 50% to 79% stenosis had a stroke.

Conclusion.—Carotid atherosclerosis is a risk factor for hemispheric stroke in patients undergoing CPB. Until the long-term benefit of carotid endarterectomy for asymptomatic lesions is conclusively demonstrated, simultaneous endarterectomy and CPB can only be justified if a reduction in perioperative stroke rates can be achieved.

▶ I agree with these authors that the presence of significant carotid artery stenosis before other major operations, such as CPB, presents an increased risk of hemispheric stroke in the postoperative period. I believe that significant carotid stenoses detected before elective surgery should lead to a strong consideration of prophylactic endarterectomy before the other scheduled surgery. The information contained in this article provides modest scientific support for this position, although I notice that other large population screening studies have not provided support. Nonetheless, this is my opinion, and I am going to stick to it.

Aortic Aneurysm

Screening for Abdominal Aortic Aneurysm: A Single Scan Is Enough
Emerton ME, Shaw E, Poskitt K, Heather BP (Gloucestershire Royal Hosp, England; Cheltenham Gen Hosp, England; Nuffield Orthopaedic Centre, Headington, Oxford, England)
Br J Surg 81:1112–1113, 1994   145-96-3–11

Background.—It has been suggested that all men who reach 65 years of age should be screened for abdominal aortic aneurysm, but the risk of an aneurysm developing and rupturing later is not known.

Methods.—Follow-up ultrasound scanning was performed after 5 years in 223 men who, at 65 or 66 years of age, had an abdominal aortic diameter smaller than 2.6 cm.

Results.—None of the 27 deaths were known to have resulted from aneurysmal rupture. In the 189 subjects who were rescanned, there was no change in mean aortic diameter, and 166 of 189 repeat measurements were within 3 mm of the original aortic diameter (table). Only 2 individuals had an aortic diameter of 3 cm or larger at follow-up.

Comparison of Aortic Diameter in 189 Repeat Ultrasonographic Scans
Done in 1993 With That Observed in Original 1988 Scan

Year	Mean (s.d.) diameter (cm)	Median (range) diameter (cm)
1988	1·88 (0·23)*	1·9 (1·3–2·5)
1993	1·90 (0·28)*	1·9 (1·3–3·1)

* P = .38 (paired *t*-test).
(Courtesy of Emerton ME, Shaw E, Poskitt K, et al: Screening for abdominal aortic aneurysm: A single scan is enough. *Br J Surg* 81:1112–1113, 1994. Reproduced with permission of Blackwell Science, Ltd.)

Conclusions.—A single ultrasound study at 65 years of age will identify all but a minority of men who are likely to die of a ruptured abdominal aortic aneurysm. Follow-up scanning is appropriate if the baseline aortic diameter is 2.6 cm or larger.

▶ This useful piece of work confirms that a single scan at the age of 65 need not, if normal, be repeated, as the patient is unlikely to have an aneurysm develop.—P.R.F. Bell, M.D.

MR Imaging (Including MR Angiography) of Abdominal Aortic Aneurysms: Comparison With Conventional Angiography
Kaufman JA, Geller SC, Petersen MJ, Cambria RP, Prince MR, Waltman AC
(Massachusetts Gen Hosp, Boston; Univ of Michigan, Ann Arbor)
AJR 163:203–210, 1994   145-96-3–12

Introduction.—Although diagnosis of abdominal aortic aneurysm (AAA) can usually be accomplished with noninvasive imaging techniques, determining its extent, the number of renal arteries involved, and the presence of visceral, renal, and iliac occlusive disease to plan surgery has often required conventional angiography. A recently developed imaging technique, MR angiography, may be able to evaluate noninvasively the extent of stenotic disease in these patients. The results of conventional angiography and MR angiography were compared in the evaluation of patients with AAA in a prospective, blinded study.

Methods.—Twenty-seven patients with confirmed AAA underwent both MRI, including MR angiography, and conventional angiography. The MR images included sagittal and coronal T1-weighted spin-echo abdominal images, axial MR angiograms centered on the renal arteries, and coronal MR angiograms centered on the aorta with contrast. The observers who interpreted the MR studies and the conventional angiograms were blinded to the results of the other study. The imaging findings were then compared with the surgical findings.

Results.—In the detection and grading of celiac stenoses of greater than 50%, MR angiography had a sensitivity of 100% and a specificity of 91% (Fig 3–7 A and B). The MR angiograms visualized 100% of the main renal arteries and 78% of the accessory renal arteries visualized by conventional angiography. In detecting renal artery stenoses of greater than 50%, MR angiography had a sensitivity of 89% and a specificity of 98% (Fig 3–7 C–F). However, it had 100% sensitivity and specificity in detecting renal artery stenosis of greater than 75%. The location of the aneurysm was correctly identified by MRI in all 26 patients who underwent surgery, but its proximal extent was incorrectly identified by conventional angiography in 2 patients. In detection of focal aneurysms of the common iliac arteries, MRI had a sensitivity of 100% and a specificity of 94%. In identifying greater than 50% stenoses of the common or external iliac arteries, MR angiography had 100% sensitivity and specificity.

Discussion.—Magnetic resonance angiography can image and detect stenoses in the celiac, superior mesenteric, renal, and pelvic runoff arteries in patients with AAA. The role of MR angiography in the preoperative evaluation of AAA should be studied further with larger patient samples.

▶ On balance, these careful comparative results suggest that MRI is as good as contrast arteriography in the detailed evaluation of AAA, including recognition of visceral stenosis, associated aneurysms, and the proximal extent of aneurysmal disease. The ability to reformat the images and view them from any direction is a real advantage. I continue to believe that, in the immediate future, MRI is going to replace contrast arteriography in all but a few diagnostic studies for which contrast angiography is currently the standard.

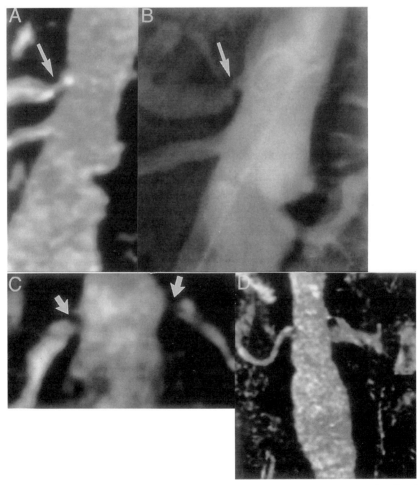

(continued)

Fig 3–7 (cont)

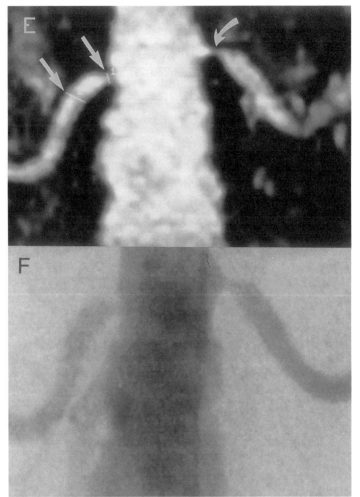

Fig 3–7.—Man, 77 with an abdominal aortic aneurysm (AAA). **A,** reformatted sagittal view of coronal dynamic contrast-enhanced 3-dimensional time-of-flight (3D TOF) MR angiogram shows moderate stenosis at the origin of the celiac artery (*arrow*). **B,** lateral view of conventional aortogram confirms moderate stenosis at the origin of the celiac artery (*arrow*). **C,** coronal maximum-intensity projection (*MIP*) of axial multiple overlapping thin-slab 3D TOF MR angiogram shows single renal arteries with bilateral proximal stenoses, severe on left and moderate on right (*arrows*). **D,** MIP of coronal 3D TOF dynamic contrast-enhanced MR angiogram shows infrarenal AAA that extends into the right common iliac artery. Left renal vein partially obscures the proximal left renal artery. A prominent mesenteric vessel is presented in the right lower quadrant. **E,** anteroposterior MIP of 3D TOF dynamic contrast-enhanced MR angiogram that depicts bilateral stenoses of the proximal part of the renal artery, severe on the left side (*curved arrow*) and moderate on the right side. On the *right*, the diameter of the stenotic lumen measured 2 mm, and the diameter of the normal segment of the vessel measured 5 mm (*straight arrows*). Distal part of the left renal artery is obscured by the left renal vein. **F,** conventional digital subtraction angiogram shows single renal arteries with bilateral severe stenoses. (Courtesy of Kaufman JA, Geller SC, Petersen MJ, et al: MR imaging [including MR angiography] of abdominal aortic aneurysms: Comparison with conventional angiography. *AJR* 163:203–210, 1994.)

MR Angiography as the Sole Method in Evaluating Abdominal Aortic Aneurysms: Correlation with Conventional Techniques and Surgery
Ecklund K, Hartnell GG, Hughs LA, Stokes KR, Finn JP (Harvard Med School, Boston)
Radiology 192:345–350, 1994   145-96-3–13

Objective.—Forty patients known to have an abdominal aortic aneurysm (AAA) had MR angiography to determine whether this method, by itself, can provide all the information needed to repair the aneurysm. The results were compared with those of conventional imaging methods, including conventional angiography and digital subtraction angiography, as well as with the surgical findings.

Technique.—Two-dimensional time-of-flight MR angiography was done using maximum-intensity projections. Imaging extended from the posterior to the renal arteries and through the entire aneurysm to include the aortic bifurcation and iliac arteries. Three-dimensional projectional angiograms were reconstructed from the two-dimensional images.

Results.—Diagnostic images were acquired in all 40 patients. In the 30 patients who had surgery, MR angiography accurately showed the location of the aneurysmal neck relative to the origin of the renal artery and also showed the best site for cross-clamping. Seven of 8 renal artery stenoses exceeding 50% were detected by MR angiography. No iliac stenosis detected by conventional angiography was missed on the MR study. In 4 patients, MR angiography provided anatomical information that was not evident from conventional angiography.

Conclusions.—In most cases, it is feasible to use multiplanar MR angiography as the sole means of evaluating AAAs before surgery. The technique is less invasive and less costly than conventional angiography, and it requires no contrast medium or ionizing radiation.

▶ This paper reaches substantially the same conclusions as those in Abstract 145-96-3–12 concerning aneurysm imaging.

Intravenous Digital Subtraction Angiography *Versus* Computed Tomography in the Assessment of Abdominal Aortic Aneurysm
Salaman RA, Shandall A, Morgan RH, Fligelstone L, Davies WT, Lane IF (Univ Hospital of Wales, Cardiff; Royal Gwent Hosp, Newport, Wales)
Br J Surg 81:661–663, 1994   145-96-3–14

Objective.—The preoperative imaging findings were compared with the operative findings in 127 patients having an aortic aneurysm repaired electively after receiving both CT scanning and intravenous digital subtraction angiography (DSA).

Results.—Ten of 12 suprarenal aneurysms were correctly predicted by preoperative CT scanning, but 11 studies had false positive results. Computed tomography was 83% sensitive and 90% specific for suprarenal

Preoperative Diagnosis of Proximal Extent of Aneurysm Compared With
Operative Findings

Operative finding	Computed tomography			Intravenous digital subtraction angiography		
	Suprarenal	Infrarenal	Total	Suprarenal	Infrarenal	Total
Suprarenal	10	2	12	6	4	10
Infrarenal	11	95	106	1	92	93
Total	21	97	118	7	96	103

(Courtesy of Salaman RA, Shandall A, Morgan RH, et al: Intravenous digital subtraction angiography *versus* computed tomography in the assessment of abdominal aortic aneurysm. *Br J Surg* 81:661–663, 1994. Reproduced with permission of Blackwell Science, Ltd.)

aneurysm, and it had a positive predictive value of 48% (table). In comparison, 6 of 10 suprarenal aneurysms were correctly predicted by DSA; only 1 study had a false positive result. Digital subtraction angiography was 60% sensitive, 99% specific, and had a positive predictive value of 86%. Computed tomography was 56% sensitive and 88% specific in diagnosing aneurysmal iliac arteries, with a positive predictive value of 60%. The respective figures for DSA were 75%, 79%, and 53%. In addition, DSA yielded useful information about occlusive disease in the renal and peripheral arteries.

Conclusion.—Both CT and DSA are relatively noninvasive methods that may be used on an outpatient basis. They provide useful information on the extent of abdominal aortic aneurysms. The studies should be viewed as complementary: When 1 fails, the other frequently succeeds.

▶ This interesting paper compares the accuracy of preoperative CT and intravenous DSA with the surgical findings in 127 patients who underwent elective aortic aneurysm repair over 3 years. Computed tomography had a rather poor positive predictive value and sensitivity for suprarenal aneurysms. Also, DSA had only a 60% sensitivity for suprarenal aneurysms and a positive predictive value of 86%. It appears that, in this study, neither CT nor DSA performed nearly as well as MR angiography, as discussed in the previous 2 papers (Abstracts 145-96-3–12 and 145-96-3–13).

High-Attenuating Crescent in Abdominal Aortic Aneurysm Wall at CT: A Sign of Acute or Impending Rupture
Mehard WB, Heiken JP, Sicard GA (Washington Univ, St Louis, Mo)
Radiology 192:359–362, 1994   145-96-3–15

Background.—The CT signs of abdominal aortic aneurysm (AAA) rupture have been studied extensively, but only those criteria relating to size are able to recognize impending rupture. Previous investigators have reported a high-attenuating crescent a long the aortic margin in dissected AAA, which they ascribe to intramural hematoma without intimal rupture. A similar sign in AAAs has been observed on unenhanced CT scans of patients initially seen for back pain. The value of this finding as a sign of impending rupture was evaluated retrospectively.

Methods.—A total of 149 consecutive patients who were undergoing surgery for AAA and had undergone preoperative unenhanced CT were studied. Seventy-six percent of the patients had aneurysm repair surgery within 1 month of the CT scan, and those with a high-attenuating crescent sign had repair within 2 weeks. The finding of a peripheral high-attenuating crescent sign was correlated with the surgical findings of acute mural hematoma, acute rupture, or contained rupture. The aneurysmal diameter was also correlated with the presence or absence of pain at the time of CT scanning, a high-attenuating crescent, and aneurysmal complications.

Results.—Thirteen percent of the patients had a high-attenuating crescent sign on CT (Fig 3–8). Three of these 19 patients also had CT evidence of rupture (Fig 3–9); surgery, which was done the same day, documented the occurrence of frank rupture. Another 3 patients were found to have contained rupture; 3 were found to have acute intramural hematoma; and 1 was found to have had rupture in the interval between CT and surgery. The other 9 patients with a high-attenuating crescent sign were found to have uncomplicated aneurysms at surgery. Of the 130 patients with no high-attenuating crescent sign, 4 were eventually found to have frank ruptures and 2 to have small contained ruptures.

As an indicator of complicated aneurysm, the high-attenuating crescent sign had a sensitivity of 77%, a specificity of 93%, and a positive predic-

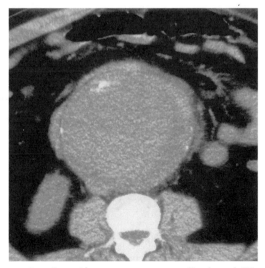

Fig 3–8.—Symptomatic patient without aneurysm rupture. Unenhanced CT scan shows a high-attenuating crescent in the anterolateral abdominal aortic aneurysm (AAA) wall (*arrow*) in this patient with surgically documented acute intramural hemorrhage. A bowel loop (*arrowheads*) is draped over the AAA. (Courtesy of Mehard WB, Heiken JP, Sicard GA: High-attenuating crescent in abdominal aortic aneurysm wall at CT: A sign of acute or impending rupture. *Radiology* 192:359–362, 1994.)

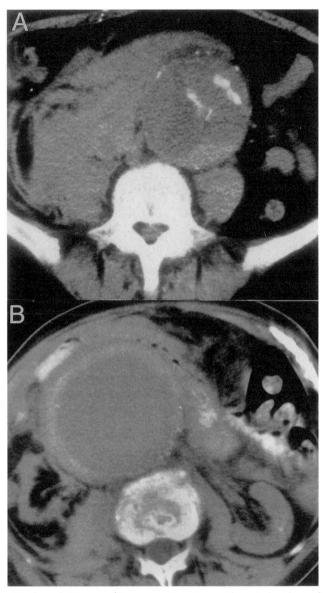

Fig 3–9.—Unenhanced CT scans of 2 symptomatic patients with surgical evidence of rupture. **A,** high-attenuating crescent is present in the posterior abdominal aortic aneurysm (AAA) wall (*arrow*). Note the higher attenuating calcification within mural thrombus and the large right retroperitoneal hematoma. **B,** nearly circumferential high-attenuating crescent is present in the AAA wall. There is a small amount of perirenal blood adjacent to the psoas muscle. (Courtesy of Mehard WB, Heiken JP, Sicard GA: High-attenuating crescent in abdominal aortic aneurysm wall at CT: A sign of acute or impending rupture. *Radiology* 192:359–362, 1994.)

tive value of 53%. Significant correlations were noted between the presence of this sign and large aneurysm size and pain at the time of CT scanning.

Conclusions.—The presence of a high-attenuating crescent sign on unenhanced CT in patients without evidence of frank aneurysm leakage should be considered a sign of impending AAA rupture. This sign is particularly important in patients with pain. The peripheral high attenuation may result from acute hematoma within the aneurysmal wall or within adjacent mural thrombus.

▶ We need an accurate way to detect early or impending rupture of an AAA. I firmly believe that painful but unruptured aneurysms should not be operated upon emergently because of the inevitable combination of an unprepared patient, tired surgeons, and random on-call anesthesiologists. In my opinion, it is better to operate on these patients electively, at the next opening in your schedule. Like everyone else, we use CT to detect blood outside the lumen, and I believe our radiologists are quite good at this.

The material presented in this article suggests that a rather specific crescent appearance on the unenhanced CT scan of the aorta may represent an intramural hematoma and appears to be a valid sign of impending rupture. If confirmed by others, this may prove to be a useful, early objective sign of aortic rupture, and it may help us identify those patients who really need emergency surgery.

Computed Tomography Scanning Findings Associated With Rapid Expansion of Abdominal Aortic Aneurysms
Wolf YG, Thomas WS, Brennan FJ, Goff WG, Sise MJ, Bernstein EF (Scripps Clinic and Research Found, La Jolla, Calif; Naval Hosp, San Diego, Calif)
J Vasc Surg 20:529–538, 1994   145-96-3–16

Background.—Ideally, abdominal aortic aneurysms (AAAs) that are likely to expand will be repaired at an early stage. Preliminary observations have suggested that CT demonstrates a relatively large area of thrombus in expanding aneurysms.

Methods.—The CT findings were reviewed in 80 patients having an AAA more than 3 cm in diameter. These patients had abdominopelvic CT scanning twice at an interval of 6 months or longer. Computerized measurements of minimal and maximal diameter and aneurysmal area were recorded, as were the dimensions of luminal thrombus and the degree of arc of the aneurysmal wall that was covered by thrombus (TARC).

Results.—The average initial aneurysmal diameter was 4.4 cm. The mean expansion during an average interval of 22 months was 0.26 cm per year. The rate of expansion was significantly correlated with the mean TARC, the thrombus volume fraction, the TARC on the largest cross-section of the aneurysm, and the thrombus area fraction. Fifteen aneurysms (19%) expanded at a rate of more than 0.5 cm per year. Rapid expansion was related to both the mean TARC and the presence of carotid artery disease.

Conclusions.—The more thrombus is present in an AAA, the more likely it is that the aneurysm will expand rapidly. A large load of thrombus in a small AAA should prompt consideration of early repair or, at a minimum, frequent measurement of the aneurysm.

▶ This interesting study attempts to determine the features on CT scans of AAA that predict rapid expansion. The authors conclude that both the volume of intraluminal thrombus and the TARC accurately predict aneurysmal expansion. They reach the interesting conclusion that an increased AAA thrombus load is associated with an increased likelihood of rapid expansion and may be an indication to recommend earlier surgical repair. Interestingly, the presence of significant carotid artery disease also predicted more rapid expansion. Although they are interesting, I have reservations about the conclusions of this study.

Abdominal Aortic Aneurysms: Evaluation With Variable-Collimation Helical CT and Overlapping Reconstruction
Zeman RK, Silverman PM, Berman PM, Weltman DI, Davros WJ, Gomes MN (Georgetown Univ Med Ctr, Washington DC)
Radiology 193:555–560, 1994   145-96-3–17

Objective.—The value of using variable collimation and overlapping reconstruction was examined in 23 patients clinically suspected of having an abdominal aortic aneurysm who underwent helical CT scanning.

Methods.—Computed tomography scanning was performed from the celiac axis to the iliac bifurcation before and after injection of iohexol. Fixed 5-mm collimation was used in 9 cases, whereas in 14 cases, 3-mm and 7-mm collimation techniques were combined. One set of images was reconstructed without overlap, and a second set was constructed with overlap.

Results.—When nonoverlapping sections were read, the extent of the aneurysm was accurately determined in 17 of 23 cases. In 9 of these cases, ancillary findings such as accessory arteries and stenoses were missed. Nineteen aneurysms were accurately evaluated using overlapping sections (Fig 3–10), and there were only 4 ancillary errors. There were 5 errors with fixed collimation and 3 errors when variable collimation was used.

Conclusion.—When abdominal aortic aneurysms are evaluated by helical CT scanning, it is best to use variable collimation and to reconstruct overlapping images.

▶ This study presents another means of imaging an aortic aneurysm: helical CT with overlapping reconstruction. Although these images look fairly re-

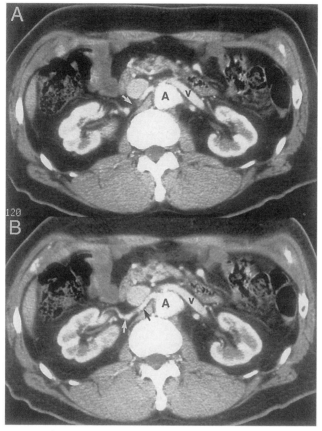

Fig 3–10.—Improved renal artery visualization with overlapping reconstruction. **A,** helical CT scan obtained with 5-mm collimation and reconstructed at 5-mm intervals fails to show the entire right renal artery. The origin (*arrowhead*) and midportion of the renal artery (*arrow*) were not clearly identified on either of the contiguous sections. **B,** section reconstructed 3 mm above the section shown in **A** demonstrates the entire length of the right renal artery (*arrows*). With reconstruction of the overlapping sections, the right renal artery is better visualized in this patient. *Abbreviations: A,* aorta; *v,* left renal vein. (Courtesy of Zeman RK, Silverman PM, Berman PM, et al: Abdominal aortic aneurysms: Evaluation with variable-collimation helical CT and overlapping reconstruction. *Radiology* 193:555–560, 1994.)

spectable, I continue to have little use for the helical CT. I have yet to define an area where this modality produces important new information that is not readily available otherwise.

Abdominal Aortic Aneurysm Morphology: CT Features in Patients With Ruptured and Nonruptured Aneurysms

Siegel CL, Cohan RH, Korobkin M, Alpern MB, Courneya DL, Leder RA (Univ of Michigan, Ann Arbor; Henry Ford Hosp, Detroit; Duke Univ, Durham, NC)
AJR 163:1123–1129, 1994   145-96-3–18

Objective.—Because the CT appearances of a ruptured abdominal aortic aneurysm (AAA) may be subtle, the internal architecture of both ruptured and nonruptured aneurysms was examined to find features that could help identify rupture when there is no obvious retroperitoneal hematoma.

Methods.—The CT findings in 52 patients with a ruptured AAA were compared with those in 56 asymptomatic patients who had a nonruptured aneurysm greater than 4.5 cm in diameter.

Findings.—There were no significant group differences in age and gender, and the ruptured and nonruptured lesions were similar in length. Ruptured aneurysms averaged 7.4 × 7.9 cm in size, whereas nonruptured aneurysms measured 5.9 × 6.1 cm. More thrombus surrounded nonruptured aneurysms, and calcified thrombus was twice as frequent in these cases. Homogeneous thrombus and a periluminal halo were similarly

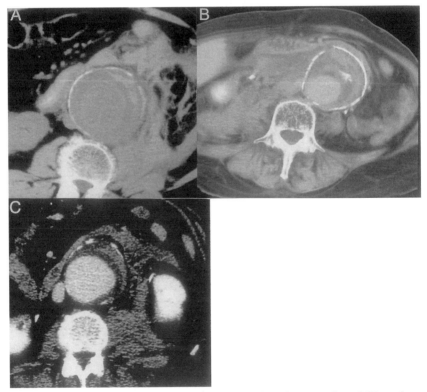

Fig 3–11.—A, man, 70, with severe left lower quadrant pain for 24 hours. Unenhanced CT scan shows crescent of high attenuation. B, woman, 84, with right lower quadrant pain and fever. Enhanced CT scan shows crescent sign, thrombus calcification, and focal break anteriorly in the thick, continuously calcified aortic wall. Blood surrounds the aorta and inferior vena cava, predominantly involving the right side of the retroperitoneum. C, man, 87, with left lower quadrant pain. Enhanced CT scan shows crescent of high attenuation in the outer perimeter of the aneurysm thrombus. (Courtesy of Siegel CL, Cohan RH, Korobkin M, et al: Abdominal aortic aneurysm morphology: CT features in patients with ruptured and nonruptured aneurysms. *AJR* 163:1123–1129, 1994.)

frequent in the 2 groups, but a diffusely heterogeneous pattern was more prevalent in nonruptured aneurysms. A crescent of increased attenuation (Fig 3–11) was seen only in ruptured aneurysms, and the same was true of a focal discontinuity in otherwise circumferential calcification of the aortic wall. The respective frequencies of these findings in patients with ruptured aneurysms were 21% for the crescent and 8% for the focal discontinuity.

▶ These investigators took the novel approach of retrospectively reviewing CT scans of aneurysms subsequently shown to be ruptured and comparing them with scans of nonruptured aneurysms to determine the CT features more frequently associated with ruptured aneurysm. Their finding that 21% of the ruptured aneurysms had a crescent of increased attenuation is fascinating and is hauntingly similar to the material presented in Abstract 145-96-3–15. A few ruptured aneurysms had focal discontinuity of circumferential calcification, but I question just how helpful this finding will be. These investigators also theorize that the crescent is the result of internal dissection or leakage of blood into the thrombus or the wall of the aneurysm. Based on the findings of this paper and of Abstract 145-96-3–15, we shall certainly look for this sign in the future.

Leg Arterial

Lower Extremity Spiral CT Angiography Versus Catheter Angiography
Lawrence JA, Kim D, Kent KC, Stehling MK, Rosen MP, Raptopoulos V (Beth Israel Hosp, Boston; Harvard Med School, Boston)
Radiology 194:903–908, 1995   145-96-3–19

Purpose.—Spiral CT permits rapid acquisition of data that can be timed to allow visualization of arterial blood flow, thereby opening the way to CT angiography. Although CT angiography has been used to demonstrate many arterial systems and the peripheral venous system, it has not previously been used to evaluate the peripheral arterial system. Catheter and spiral CT angiography was done on the lower extremity vasculature in 6 patients with symptomatic peripheral vascular disease.

Findings.—The 2 angiographic techniques were used to study 48 arteries, which were independently evaluated for the presence of arterial stenoses and occlusions. Catheter arteriography detected segmental occlusions and stenoses of more than 50% in 28 arteries. These lesions were correctly depicted in 26 arteries by CT angiography, which had a sensitivity of 93%, a specificity of 96%, and an overall accuracy of 96%.

Conclusions.—Computed tomographic angiography is a potentially valuable technique for identifying and grading stenoses of the lower extremity arteries. Conventional angiography offers better image resolution. However, CT angiography has the advantages of noninvasiveness, short examination time, and ability for three-dimensional imaging. More studies to evaluate the applications of CT angiography and larger clinical trials are required to compare the findings with those of duplex ultrasonography and MR angiography.

▶ A 95.5% accuracy of lower extremity spiral CT angiography compared with conventional angiography sounds pretty good, especially when one considers that spiral CT is less invasive. Unfortunately, the image resolution of spiral CT angiography is inferior, and patients with extensive arterial calcification remain a serious problem. It is noteworthy that, in this study, CT angiography required 200 mL of contrast material (power injected into an antecubital vein), and the arteries were visualized only from the inguinal ligament to the proximal calf. That is not much information for such a large volume of contrast. What about the critical mid- and distal calf and foot arteries? In addition, because CT angiography does not involve an arterial puncture, there is no opportunity to measure pull-back iliac artery pressure gradients or to perform intra-arterial balloon dilatation or other catheter-based interventions simultaneously. In sum, I find it unlikely that I will use lower extremity spiral CT angiography in my vascular surgical practice.—R. Yeager, M.D.

Limitations of Ultrasonic Duplex Scanning for Diagnosing Lower Limb Arterial Stenoses in the Presence of Adjacent Segment Disease
Allard L, Cloutier G, Durand L-G, Roederer GO, Langlois YE (Hôpital Hôtel-Dieu de Montréal)
J Vasc Surg 19:650–657, 1994   145-96-3–20

Background.—There have been few in vivo studies of the performance of duplex scanning in diagnosing lower limb arterial stenoses in patients with multisegment disease. A quantitative analysis was done to determine the effects of adjacent segment lesions on the duplex ultrasound classification of lower limb arterial disease.

Background.—The study sample comprised 55 patients who were referred for arteriography of the lower limb arteries. All underwent arterial duplex scanning from the distal aorta to the popliteal artery. In "blinded" fashion, the visual interpretations of Doppler spectra were compared with the angiographic measurements. Severe arterial stenoses were defined as those reducing diameter by 50% to 100%.

Results.—In any arterial segment, duplex scanning detected severe stenoses with a sensitivity of 74% and a specificity of 96%. When there were no severe stenoses in adjacent segments, the sensitivity increased to 80% and the specificity to 98%. When there was at least 1 severe stenosis in the adjacent segments, the sensitivity decreased to 66% and the specificity to 94% (table). There were 48 instances in which duplex scanning underestimated or overestimated the degree of arterial stenosis, and 63% of the misclassifications involved segments with 1 or more severe stenoses in adjacent segments. Proximal and distal arterial lesions were most frequently associated with the popliteal arteries and the common and deep

Duplex Scanning vs. Angiography in Detecting 0% to 49% and 50% to 100% Diameter-Reducing Stenoses for Arterial Segments Studied as a Function of Adjacent Segment Status

Adjacent segment status	Correctly classified 0%–49%	50%–100%	Misclassified 0%–49%	50%–100%	Accuracy/sensitivity/specificity (%)
0%–49%	313	47	12	6	95/80/98
50%–100%	203	31	16	14	89/66/94
All	516	78	28	20	93/74/96

Total number of arterial segments is 642.
(Courtesy of Allard L, Cloutier G, Durand L-G, et al: Limitations of ultrasonic duplex scanning for diagnosing lower limb arterial stenoses in the presence of adjacent segment disease. *J Vasc Surg* 19:650–657, 1994.)

femoral arteries. Eighty-six percent of misclassifications in these sites involved proximal or distal severe stenoses.

Conclusions.—The ability of duplex ultrasound scanning to detect and measure arterial lesions of the lower limb is limited by the presence of stenoses in adjacent segments. To overcome this problem, new objective and quantitative criteria derived from the Doppler spectra will likely be needed.

▶ I have always regarded the methodical plotting of duplex patterns from aortic bifurcation to the ankle to be a matter fit for clinical research but of limited value in the daily practice of vascular surgery. These authors make a convincing case that adjacent disease may severely affect the accuracy of duplex segmental determinations. I think they are correct. Although I can easily see how a significant proximal stenosis may cause one to underestimate distal disease, at least based on velocity criteria, I am a bit hard-pressed to understand how significant proximal disease would cause one to over-call a distal lesion. The authors' suggestion of turbulent flow coming in through collaterals is not very convincing. Overall, the overwhelming majority of our leg bypasses are done for limb salvage, and most of these patients have multisegmental disease. If the results of this paper are correct, and I suspect they are, the inescapable conclusion is that duplex scanning may be of limited value in determining the precise characterization of lower extremity disease in patients selected for surgery.

Falsely Elevated Ankle Pressures in Severe Leg Ischaemia: The Pole Test. An Alternative Approach
Smith FCT, Shearman CP, Simms MH, Gwynn BR (Stafford District Gen Hosp, Birmingham, England; Selly Oak Hosp, Birmingham, England)
Eur J Vasc Surg 8:408–412, 1994   145-96-3-21

Background.—The ankle-brachial pressure index (ABPI), measured using a sphygmomanometer and Doppler probe, is an accepted measure of chronic ischemia in the lower extremity. If the tibial artery is sclerosed or calcified, however, the resultant decrease in compliance leads to falsely increased cuff occlusion pressures. Arterial cannulation is an invasive procedure. An alternative means of measuring systolic pressure at the ankle is to elevate the foot and note the height at which the Doppler signal disappears.

Method.—An 8-MHz Doppler unit and a calibrated pole (Fig 3–12) were used to measure the ABPI in 49 severely ischemic legs of 40 patients. The index was derived by dividing the ankle systolic pressure by the brachial pressure.

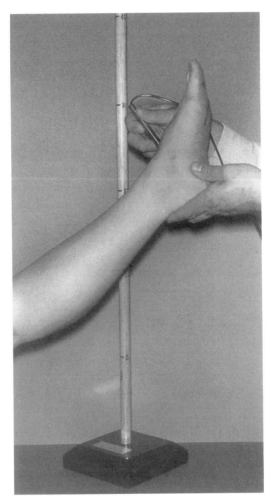

Fig 3–12.—Use of an 8-MHz Doppler probe and calibrated pole to assess ankle systolic pressure. Systolic pressure in mm Hg is determined from the pole as a function of height above the left ventricle at which the Doppler signal is lost on leg elevation. (Courtesy of Smith FCT, Shearman CP, Simms MH, et al: Falsely elevated ankle pressures in severe leg ischaemia: The pole test. An alternative approach. *Eur J Vasc Surg* 8:408–412, 1994.)

Results.—The median ABPI, as measured by sphygmomanometry, was 0.46, and the median index obtained by leg elevation was 0.21—a significantly lower value. Twenty patients having direct transducer pressure measurements in connection with vein bypass grafting had a median ABPI of 0.15, which was not significantly different from the pole-derived index of 0.2. The median sphygmomanometric index was 0.37. The elevation- and transducer-derived indices were correlated at a level of 0.88 compared with 0.69 for the transducer- and cuff-derived indices.

Conclusion.—The leg elevation method provides more accurate ABPI measurements than does sphygmomanometry in patients with severe lower limb ischemia. However, the method may only be used for pressures less than approximately 60 mm Hg.

▶ The problems of measuring accurate ankle pressures in patients with diabetes and those with sclerosed peripheral arteries are well known. One way around these problems is to measure the toe pressure, which is always difficult to determine and is by no means universally available. The other way is to use this test suggested by Smith and his colleagues—the pole test, which is based on the clinical Buerger's symptom, i.e., foot pallor on elevation and rubor on dependency. Pressures measured this way were closer to those measured at surgery than were pressures measured with conventional APBI. This is a useful test and should help to identify patients with critical ischaemia more easily.—P.R.F. Bell, M.D.

▶ We have begun to use this test regularly in patients with calcified arteries, and we have found it very helpful.—J.M. Porter, M.D.

Venous

A Comparison of the Cuff Deflation Method With Valsalva's Maneuver and Limb Compression in Detecting Venous Valvular Reflux
Markel A, Meissner MH, Manzo RA, Bergelin RO, Strandness Jr DE (Univ of Washington, Seattle)
Arch Surg 129:701–705, 1994   145-96-3-22

Objective.—Two commonly used methods for detecting venous valvular reflux—Valsalva's maneuver and limb compression—were compared with the standing cuff inflation-deflation method in 67 patients who had had an episode of deep venous thrombosis.

Methods.—The reflux tests were evaluated by pulsed Doppler recordings of the common femoral, superficial femoral, popliteal, and posterior tibial veins. Reflux was signified by the appearance of retrograde venous flow on reversal of the normal transvalvular pressure gradient. The cuff test involves inflating appropriate-sized cuffs on the thigh, calf, and foot at respective pressure levels of 80, 100, and 120 mm Hg with the patient standing. Inflation is completed within 3 seconds, and deflation is completed within 0.3 second. Valsalva's maneuver and limb compression tests were done with the patient supine.

Sensitivity and Specificity of Supine Maneuvers

	Valsalva's Maneuver		Method, % Manual		Combined*	
Segment	Sensitivity	Specificity	Sensitivity	Specificity	Sensitivity	Specificity
CFV	75	86	21	98	79	86
GSV	67	100	10	100	67	100
SFV	83	97	50	97	88	93
PPV	49	98	73	88	76	88
PTV	20	99	30	92	30	92

* Combined indicates supine Valsalva's and manual compression maneuvers. In this case, reflux is considered to be present if either individual maneuver is positive.
Abbreviations: CFV, common femoral vein; GSV, greater saphenous vein; SFV, superficial femoral vein; PPV, popliteal vein; and PTV, posterior tibial vein.
(Courtesy of Markel A, Meissner MH, Manzo RA, et al: A comparison of the cuff deflation method with Valsalva's maneuver and limb compression in detecting venous valvular reflux. *Arch Surg* 129:701–705, 1994. Copyright 1994/95, American Medical Association.)

Results.—Both limb compression and Valsalva's maneuver elicited reflux, but they proved difficult to standardize (table). The results of the cuff inflation-deflation test were more readily quantified and appeared to be consistent in all segments of the venous system. In 95% of normal subjects, the time to valve closure was less than 0.5 seconds.

Conclusion.—The standing cuff inflation-deflation test is a reliable means of detecting reflux in the superficial and deep veins of the lower extremity.

▶ These authors note that the method of detecting reflux has not been standardized. Variable methods have been used, including Valsalva's maneuver, thigh compression with a cuff, and distal limb manual compression and release. Markel et al. present rather convincing evidence that cuff deflation in the standing, non–weight-bearing position produces the most reliable results. They are probably correct. There is a need for various vascular laboratories to standardize the method of reflux detection so the results obtained will be comparable.

Bilateral Lower Extremity US in the Patient With Unilateral Symptoms of Deep Venous Thrombosis: Assessment of Need

Sheiman RG, McArdle CR (Beth Israel Hosp, Boston; Harvard Med School, Cambridge, Mass)
Radiology 194:171–173, 1995   145-96-3-23

Background.—Gray-scale ultrasonography with compression and color Doppler has become the major objective screening examination for symptomatic patients with lower extremity deep venous thrombosis (DVT). Evaluation of both the symptomatic and asymptomatic legs is often requested in patients with unilateral symptoms, possibly because of the historically poor sensitivity of physical examination. To assess the need for bilateral ultrasound evaluation, regardless of predisposing factors, results in patients with unilateral symptoms were studied prospectively.

Study Design.—Two hundred six patients who had unilateral lower extremity symptoms suggestive of DVT underwent bilateral lower extremity ultrasound. Data concerning predisposing factors for DVT, including underlying malignancy, previous DVT, pregnancy, prolonged travel or immobility, and recent surgery, were collected.

Results.—Acute DVT was identified in 37 (18%) patients; all had thrombosis in the symptomatic leg. Twenty-five of these patients had predisposing factors. None of the patients had thrombosis in the asymptomatic extremity. The sensitivity and specificity for detection of DVT with ultrasound were both greater than 90%, indicating that the difference between DVT detection in the symptomatic extremity and that in the asymptomatic extremity was statistically significant.

Conclusion.—Ultrasound screening for DVT in the lower extremities should be limited to the symptomatic extremity in patients with unilateral symptoms, regardless of predisposing factors. This protocol would reduce scanning time and cost without a decline in the DVT detection rate.

▶ These radiologists are addressing the need for bilateral lower extremity ultrasound in the evaluation of a patient for DVT, regardless of unilateral symptoms. Overall, 18% of the patients referred to the authors' laboratory to rule out DVT actually had DVT, which is approximately the right number. The authors noted that no DVT was found in any asymptomatic extremity, which led them to conclude that ultrasound screening for DVT in the lower extremity should be limited to the symptomatic side in patients with unilateral symptoms. I consider the conclusions of this paper totally incorrect. Please see the next paper (Abstract 145-96-3–24) for the correct conclusion concerning this contentious question.

Does the Asymptomatic Limb Harbor Deep Venous Thrombosis?
Lohr JM, Hasselfeld KA, Byrne MP, Deshmukh RM, Cranley JJ (Good Samaritan Hosp, Cincinnati, Ohio)
Am J Surg 168:184–187, 1994   145-96-3–24

Introduction.—The clinical diagnosis of deep venous thrombosis (DVT) is difficult, because its occurrence cannot be reliably predicted on the basis of the patient's symptoms, history, or risk factors. A large series of bilateral lower extremity duplex ultrasound scans were reviewed to identify a population in which a unilateral scan might be appropriate.

Methods and Results.—Bilateral venous scans of 2,511 patients were reviewed. Forty-three percent showed DVT, which was unilateral in 30% of cases and bilateral in 14%. In 64% of patients for whom information regarding the side of the symptoms was available, the symptoms were referable to the involved extremity. In the other 36%, however, the symptoms were referable to the contralateral extremity. The lower extremities were asymptomatic in 362 patients, 35% of whom had DVT. Another 263 patients with a symptomatic extremity were found to have clots in the contralateral, asymptomatic extremity. On logistic regression analysis, no combination of symptoms and risk factors could predict DVT.

Conclusions.—Patients suspected of having DVT should undergo bilateral lower extremity duplex ultrasound scanning. This approach will not only detect asymptomatic DVT, but it will also allow an anatomical comparison of the extremities and avoid aberrant false negative studies.

▶ The Cranley Vascular Laboratory has had a more than 35-year interest in the noninvasive diagnosis of DVT, and it was an early pioneer in the use of duplex scanning for establishing the presence of DVT. A major reason for studying both limbs in a patient suspected of having DVT is to alter clinical management, i.e., to have the patient receive anticoagulation. This study confirms an earlier ascending phlebographic study by Browse (1), in which 10% to 30% of the limbs contralateral to established DVT, although asymptomatic, harbored a DVT. The data are powerful and draw on a registry containing more than 2,500 patients.

As emphasized in many previous studies, Lohr and associates emphasize the weak predictive nature of clinical factors for establishing the presence of DVT. In the asymptomatic group of 2,149 patients, 43% were positive for DVT and, therefore, would undergo anticoagulation. The most interesting group was that comprising 362 patients who were asymptomatic in both limbs, 128 (35%) of whom had DVT by duplex scan. Forty-eight (13%) would be treated, however, because of a co-existing pulmonary embolism. The remainder of the asymptomatic group were patients undergoing screening after orthopedic and neurosurgical procedures, 16% of whom had DVT.—T. O'Donnell, M.D.

Reference

1. Browse N: Diagnosis of deep-vein thrombosis. *Br Med Bull* 34:163, 1978.

▶ Study both legs in all patients with suspected DVT.—J.M. Porter, M.D.

Prediction of Long Saphenous Vein Graft Adaptation
Davies AH, Magee TR, Hayward JK, Baird RN, Horrocks M (Bristol Royal Infirmary, Bristol, England)
Eur J Vasc Surg 8:478–481, 1994   145-96-3–25

Background.—Autogenous vein is the preferred conduit for use in infrainguinal arterial reconstruction below the knee. If the extent to which veins adapt by dilating could be predicted, smaller veins could be used. A Duplex ultrasonographic technique is now used in place of saphenography to predict the functional size of vein grafts 2 months after surgery.

Methods.—Duplex studies of the long saphenous vein were done in 60 patients having femorodistal popliteal or infrapopliteal bypass. The vein diameter was estimated at the groin, mid-thigh, and knee, both at rest and with a thigh cuff inflated to 100 mm Hg. The measurements were begun 1 week postoperatively and were repeated at 3, 6, 9, and 12 months.

Results.—At mid-thigh level, the mean vein diameter was 4.2 mm Hg at rest; it increased to 5.1 mm with occlusion. At 1 year, the mean diameter was 5.5 mm. Comparable changes occurred at the level of the knee. If a minimal internal vein diameter of 3 mm at rest was taken as indicating suitability for bypass, 22% more veins would have been used.

Conclusion.—Simple Duplex ultrasound measurements can accurately predict the adaptation of saphenous vein grafts over 1 year.

▶ The authors' assertion that postoperative vein graft diameter can be predicted by vein mapping preoperatively with a tourniquet is probably correct. They have previously published this information (1). In this fine example of salami slicing from Bristol, they have thinly sliced a piece of salami between 2 months' follow-up and 12 months' follow-up and have added 16 patients. That their conclusions remained exactly the same did not dissuade them from squeezing yet another manuscript out of these meager data. For such repeated publication (in the same journal!), they are presented the coveted Camel Dung Award.

Reference

1. Davies AH, Magee TR, Jones DR, et al: The value of duplex scanning and venous occlusion in the preoperative prediction of femoro-distal vein bypass graft diameter. *Eur J Vasc Surg* 5:633–636, 1991.

Preoperative Duplex Venous Mapping: A Comparison of Positional Techniques in Patients With and Without Atherosclerosis
Blebea J, Schomaker WR, Hod G, Fowl RJ, Kempczinski RF (Univ of Cincinnati, Ohio)
J Vasc Surg 20:226–234, 1994   145-96-3–26

Objective.—The greater saphenous vein is sized and evaluated by duplex venous mapping to confirm its suitability for use in infrainguinal bypass surgery. The best mapping method and the optimal peak venous diameter were sought in patients with and others without atherosclerotic disease.

Methods.—The preoperative findings in 10 patients with either disabling claudication or tissue loss secondary to atherosclerosis were compared with those in 20 controls 26–51 years of age and 10 others aged 60–78 years. The patients ranged from 44 to 75 years in age. Two experienced vascular technologists used a duplex ultrasound scanner to measure peak internal venous diameters from just beyond the saphenofemoral junction to just above the medial malleolus. The measurements were repeated with the patient supine in bed, in the 20-degree reversed Trendelenburg position, sitting on the bed, standing, and supine with a low-pressure tourniquet applied to the upper thigh.

Results.—The younger controls had progressive increases in vein diameter at all levels of the leg as they assumed increasingly erect positions.

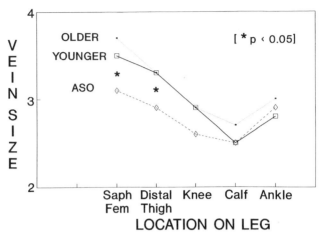

Fig 3–13.—Greater saphenous vein diameter (in mm) as function of position along the length of the leg with subjects in the supine position: older controls (*filled squares*), younger controls (*open squares*), and patients with atherosclerosis (*ASO*) (*diamonds*). (Courtesy of Blebea J, Schomaker WR, Hod G, et al: Preoperative duplex venous mapping: A comparison of positional techniques in patients with and without atherosclerosis. *J Vasc Surg* 20:226–234, 1994.)

Neither the older controls nor the patients with atherosclerosis exhibited such positional change in vein diameter. The patients had significantly smaller veins than either group of controls (Fig 3–13). Application of a tourniquet significantly increased the patients' vein diameters to the level seen in older controls (Fig 3–14).

Conclusion.—Vein mapping is best performed with the patient in a supine position. Veins may be maximally distended in atherosclerotic patients by applying a low-pressure tourniquet to the upper thigh.

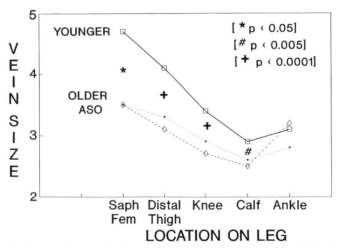

Fig 3–14.—Greater saphenous vein diameter (in mm) as function of position along the length of the leg with application of a high-thigh tourniquet. (Courtesy of Blebea J, Schomaker WR, Hod G, et al: Preoperative duplex venous mapping: A comparison of positional techniques in patients with and without atherosclerosis. *J Vasc Surg* 20:226–234, 1994.)

► This careful study of vein mapping agrees with the importance of the high thigh cuff, a position repeatedly taken by Davies et al. (Abstract 145-96-3–25). This study does not compare the preoperative vein size to any postoperative determined values. As more and more of our lower extremity bypass patients require repeat surgery, we increasingly rely upon vein mapping to guide us in our vein harvest. At present, approximately 25% of our lower extremity bypasses consist of portions of arm vein, and we are able to get important information about the quality and size of arm veins from preoperative venous mapping. Vein mapping is becoming more difficult to obtain as so many of our surgical patients have to be admitted on the same day because of case management requirements. Therefore, the vein mapping has to be obtained in a prehospital visit, which requires additional authorization from the HMO, frequently coming only after a long and heated debate with an HMO case manager. I suspect many of you are facing similar problems.

Intravascular Ultrasound

Intravascular Ultrasound Imaging in Acute Aortic Dissection
Weintraub AR, Erbel R, Görge G, Schwartz SL, Ge J, Gerber T, Meyer J, Hsu T-L, Bojar R, Iliceto S, Carella L, Rizzon P, Vilacosta I, Goicolea J, Zamorano J, Alfonso F, Pandian NG (Tufts Univ, Boston; The Univ of Mainz, Germany; Univ of Bari, Italy; et al)
J Am Coll Cardiol 24:495–503, 1994   145-96-3–27

Background.—Intravascular ultrasound imaging is a new technique designed to display cross-sectional images of the arterial interior in real time. To date, it has been used mainly in the coronary and peripheral arteries.

Methods.—Intravascular ultrasonography of the aorta, using a 20-MHz ultrasound catheter, was performed in 28 patients suspected of having aortic dissection. The aorta was imaged from the level of the aortic root to the bifurcation in an average of 10 minutes. Dissection was diagnosed from the appearance of a curvilinear structure, the flap, that moved rapidly and often chaotically and separated the aorta into true and false lumens. All patients had contrast angiography as well. Computed tomography was done in 7 patients, and transesophageal echocardiography was done in 22.

Results.—There were no complications. Dissection was identified in 23 of the 28 patients. In addition to showing the intimal flap and the false lumen, intravascular sonography demonstrated the extent of dissection, involvement of branch vessels, and the presence of hematoma in the aortic wall. The ultrasound study defined the distal extent of dissection in some cases where aortography did not provide this information.

Conclusions.—Intravascular ultrasound imaging is a rapid, safe, and accurate means of identifying aortic dissection and associated pathology. It may be especially useful when transesophageal echocardiography is not feasible.

► Intravascular ultrasound is a fascinating and potentially powerful diagnostic tool. In this study, 28 patients with suspected aortic dissection underwent a detailed intravascular ultrasound examination from the aortic root to the bifurcation in a commendable average of 10 minutes. Dissection was actually present in 23 patients, and each intravascular ultrasound examination demonstrated the intimal flap and the true and false lumens. The extent of the aortic dissection and the involvement of the branch vessels were clearly identified. The investigators actually found intravascular ultrasound to be, in some respects, superior to aortography. On balance, I believe that this technique will become progressively applicable to patients. With rare exceptions, I suspect this will be performed by radiologists and not by vascular surgeons.

Preliminary Results From Attenuation-Slope Mapping of Plaque Using Intravascular Ultrasound
Wilson LS, Neale ML, Talhami HE, Appleberg M (Ultrasonics Laboratory, Chatswood, Australia; Royal North Shore Hosp, Sydney, Australia)
Ultrasound Med Biol 20:529–542, 1994   145-96-3–28

Background.—The findings of both mechanical modeling and in vitro studies suggest that it is necessary to have a detailed idea of plaque pathology to confidently predict the outcome of balloon angioplasty and other treatments. Intravascular ultrasound imaging can view lesions without other tissue—apart from blood itself—intervening. Most studies that have been done are based on estimating ultrasonic attenuation, which is known to vary in a number of pathologic states and is relatively easily studied.

Methods.—Excised segments of femoral and iliac arteries were evaluated by intravascular ultrasound imaging using a 20-MHz device. They were then examined histologically. Radiofrequency (RF) data were recorded digitally and used to calculate attenuation slope locally throughout the tissue, using a frequency-domain technique. In addition, the RF data were reconstructed into conventional ultrasound images in which the attenuation-slope data appeared as a thresholded color overlay.

Results.—In general, areas of degenerative plaque corresponded to regions of high attenuation slope and were readily apparent from the color pattern on combined images. Lipid pooling, cholesterol clefts, necrosis, and both microcalcification and gross calcification presented in this way. Most of these changes were not unequivocally identified in gray-scale images.

Conclusions.—Intravascular ultrasonography with mapping of attenuation slope values probably is able to distinguish between normal vessel wall and both fibrous plaque and degenerative plaque. This method should prove helpful in selecting and implementing treatment and in predicting the success of various procedures.

▶ As noted previously (in the commentary after Abstract 145-96-1–11), one of the hottest current topics in atherosclerotic disease is characterization of the atherosclerotic plaque in an attempt to identify plaques at risk for rupture. Although I am monumentally uninformed regarding the engineering and physics involved in this complex paper, in which ultrasound examinations with different RF pulses were used for calculating values of attenuation throughout atherosclerotic tissue using a frequency-domain technique, I do admire the results. These authors have preliminary data indicating that they may be able to identify a degenerating plaque by finding areas with a high attenuation-slope clearly different from what is seen in plaques without degenerative characteristics. If we indeed are able to identify plaques at risk for rupture that are in the prerupture state, this will represent a monumental advance. The results presented in this article are fascinating.

Graft Surveillance

Duplex Scan Surveillance of Infrainguinal Prosthetic Bypass Grafts
Lalak NJ, Hanel KC, Hunt J, Morgan A (St George Hosp and Hurstville Community Vascular Lab, Kogarah, Australia)
J Vasc Surg 20:637–641, 1994   145-96-3–29

Background.—Postoperative surveillance of infrainguinal vein bypass grafts by Duplex ultrasound scanning is an accepted procedure, but whether surveillance of prosthetic grafts at this site is equally useful remains uncertain.

Methods.—In a prospective, 4-year follow-up study, 69 polytetrafluoroethylene infrainguinal grafts in 56 patients were evaluated every 6 months by full duplex scan mapping of the grafts along with the inflow and outflow arteries. Peak flow velocity was estimated at mid-graft level and, in addition, standard ankle pressure measurements were made.

Results.—Twenty-seven of the 69 prosthetic grafts (39%) became occluded during follow-up, with no warning from the duplex scan findings. Of the 42 grafts that remained patent, only 4 had stenoses develop that were amenable to treatment. Neither altered ankle pressures nor changes in mid-graft flow velocity predicted graft failure.

Conclusion.—The infrequency with which duplex scanning reveals correctable changes in prosthetic infrainguinal bypass graft precludes its use for routine surveillance.

▶ Detailed information on postoperative leg graft surveillance has been derived only from vein grafts. Frequently, physicians send patients with prosthetic grafts to the vascular laboratory for graft surveillance. We have always told these physicians that we have no idea whether the same rules applied to prosthetic grafts. The authors of this interesting study addressed this issue and concluded that the failure of prosthetic grafts is not predicted by duplex scan surveillance. I believe this to be an accurate conclusion, although I have limited experience with prosthetic graft surveillance.

140 / Vascular Surgery

The Origin of Infrainguinal Vein Graft Stenosis: A Prospective Study Based on Duplex Surveillance

Mills JL, Bandyk DF, Gahtan V, Esses GE (Univ of South Florida, Tampa)
J Vasc Surg 21:16–25, 1995   145-96-3-30

Background.—Intrinsic vein graft stenosis is the most prominent cause of failed infrainguinal vein bypass surgery. It accounts for about 60% of all vein graft thromboses.

Objective.—Color duplex imaging was done postoperatively in a prospective series of 135 infrainguinal vein bypass operations to learn the causes of vein graft lesions and assess the risk of their progression.

Methods.—In addition to 116 greater saphenous vein grafts, 13 spliced, 5 cephalic, and 1 superficial femoral vein grafts were evaluated. Duplex studies were done at the time of surgery, 1 and 6 weeks afterward, 3 and 6 months afterward, and then at 3- to 6-month intervals. Identified lesions were graded on peak systolic flow velocity and velocity ratio.

Results.—Only 2 of 91 grafts that appeared normal 3 months postoperatively (2.2%) became stenotic and required revision. Forty-four other grafts had a peak systolic velocity exceeding 150 cm/second or a velocity ratio greater than 1.5 in either the body of the graft or the anastomotic region. In 14 grafts, the flow abnormality normalized. Ten grafts had persistent stenosis of moderate degree. In all 20 instances in which grafts developed high-grade stenosis and were revised, a residual flow abnormality had been present after bypass or within 6 weeks of surgery (Fig 3-15).

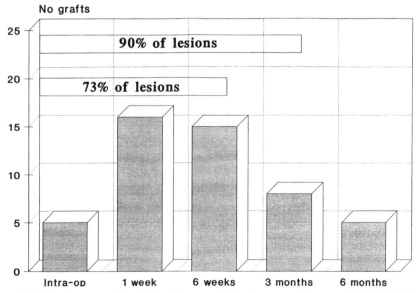

Fig 3–15.—Appearance time of index (first-appearing) graft stenoses. (Courtesy of Mills JL, Bandyk DF, Gahtan V, et al: The origin of intrafrainguinal vein graft stenosis: A prospective study based on duplex surveillance. *J Vasc Surg* 21:16–25, 1995.)

The overall rate of graft failure during an average follow-up of 1 year was 4.4%. Two of the 6 failures followed revision.

Conclusions.—Graft stenosis does not often develop after infrainguinal vein bypass surgery. Most stenoses develop at sites of unrepaired defects or abnormalities noted shortly after surgery. Early abnormalities should be closely watched because they frequently progress to high-grade stenosis.

▶ This excellent group at the University of South Florida followed a significant number of vein grafts with detailed postoperative duplex surveillance in an effort to determine the incidence and origin of vein graft lesions. Sixty-seven percent of the vein grafts were normal on early scans, and only 2% of these later developed stenoses. Forty-four grafts had an early abnormal scan; of these, 14 normalized, 10 persisted, and 20 progressed. These authors report a 12-month patency of 95.6%, which is, indeed, an excellent result. Dr. Mills concluded that early graft flow normality conveyed immortality on these grafts, a position not agreed upon by the discussant, Dr. Moneta, who is from our staff. At Oregon Health Sciences University, about 20% to 25% of GFV abnormalities are first detected after 12 months.

Miscellaneous

MR Imaging of Edematous Limbs in Lymphatic and Nonlymphatic Edema

Fujii K (Kinki Univ, Osaka, Japan)
Acta Radiol 35:262–269, 1994   145-96-3–31

Objective.—Because MR images reflect the water content of tissue, this method might prove useful in diagnosing various types of edema. Accordingly, edematous limbs were imaged in 48 patients with lymphatic edema and 12 with nonlymphatic edema.

Methods.—Both T1- and T2-weighted spin-echo sequences were used, as well as short inversion time inversion recovery sequences. Thickness and signal intensity were evaluated in the skin, subcutis, and subfascia.

Results.—A consistent finding in patients with lymphatic edema was the presence of trabecular structures in the swollen subcutis, which presumably represented dilated collateral lymph vessels (Fig 3–16). Similar findings were noted in 2 patients with nephrotic syndrome. In 6 patients with venous edema, MR images demonstrated fat intensity in the subfascia. In 4 other patients, there was only water intensity in the subcutis.

Conclusion.—Magnetic resonance imaging appears to be a promising means of identifying various forms of edematous disease.

▶ The unbelievable images obtained by MRI in edematous limbs have been previously noted (1). These authors make the interesting observation that lymphatic edema has MRI characteristics permitting differentiation from venous edema. The actual differential rests with the presence or absence of a trabecular structure in the subcutaneous tissue, which the author believes

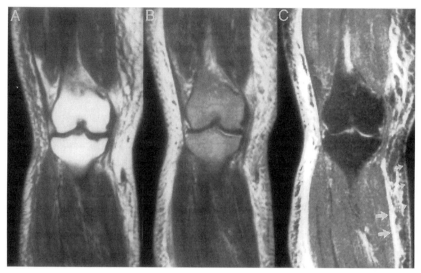

Fig 3–16.—Lymphatic edema of the right lower limb after treatment for uterine cervical cancer. Subcutaneous trabecular structures are shown with low signal intensity on the T1-weighted image (A) and high signal intensity on the T2-weighted image (B). Short inversion time inversion recovery (STIR) image (C) shows a greater signal intensity of trabecular structures, and it also shows high signal bands along cutaneous (curved arrows) and fascial (straight arrows) surface. (Courtesy of Fujii K: MR imaging of edematous limbs in lymphatic and nonlymphatic edema. Acta Radiol 35:262–269, 1994.)

indicates dilated collateral lymphatic channels. I suspect that in the future we will obtain MR images in extremity edema to assist us in differential diagnosis.

Reference

1. 1994 YEAR BOOK OF VASCULAR SURGERY, p 451.

Detection and Quantitation of Calcific Atherosclerosis By Ultrafast Computed Tomography in Children and Young Adults With Homozygous Familial Hypercholesterolemia
Hoeg JM, Feuerstein IM, Tucker EE (National Heart, Lung, and Blood Inst, National Inst of Health, Bethesda, Md; Warren G Magnuson Clinical Ctr, Bethesda, Md; The Uniformed Services Univ of the Health Sciences, Bethesda, Md; et al)
Arterioscler Thromb 14:1066–1074, 1994   145-96-3–32

Objective.—Ultrafast CT was used in an attempt to detect calcific lesions of coronary atherosclerosis in 11 consecutive children and young adults who were homozygous for familial hypercholesterolemia (FH). Their baseline total plasma cholesterol levels ranged from 488 to 1,277 mg/dL.

Method.—The heart and thoracic aorta were examined by ultrafast CT using the 100-msec high-resolution mode. No intravenous contrast material was used. Standard quantification methods were used to score the coronary arteries and aorta for calcification.

Results.—Ultrafast CT scanning detected calcific atherosclerosis in all 9 subjects who were older than 12 years of age, including all who had angina. Angiography demonstrated significant stenotic lesions in 7 of the 11 individuals examined. Computed tomography was more sensitive than angiography in detecting lesions in the aortic root and coronary ostia; these are the initial sites of disease in those homozygous for FH. The volume of calcification correlated with the degree and duration of hyper-cholesterolemia as well as with the presence of angina. All 7 patients with angina, but only 1 of 4 who were asymptomatic, had a volume score exceeding 150 cu mm.

Conclusions.—Deposits of calcium phosphate are frequently detected by ultrafast CT in young individuals who are homozygous for FH. They are more common in the aorta than in the coronary arteries, and they correlate with the presence of angiographic stenoses.

▶ The new ultrafast CT scans are amazing. They apparently have a 100-msec acquisition time, 3-mm slice thickness, and 1 mm in plane spatial resolution. Because of these remarkable characteristics, it is possible to quickly detect and quantitate coronary artery calcific deposits. In this fascinating study, the authors examined 11 patients, 3–37 years of age, who were homozygous for hypercholesterolemia. Each patient had a very high serum level of cholesterol. The fast CT scan detected calcific atherosclerosis of the coronary artery in all 9 patients older than 12 years. Increasingly, a number of authors are concluding that the detection of coronary calcification is an excellent marker for both coronary and peripheral atherosclerotic disease. As I noted in the 1995 YEAR BOOK (1), I suspect that ultrafast CT will become an important tool for future epidemiologic studies.

Reference

1. 1995 YEAR BOOK OF VASCULAR SURGERY, p 124.

Serial Magnetic Resonance Imaging of Experimental Atherosclerosis Detects Lesion Fine Structure, Progression and Complications *in vivo*
Skinner MP, Yuan C, Mitsumori L, Hayes CE, Raines EW, Nelson JA, Ross R
(Univ of Washington, Seattle)
Nature Med 1:69–73, 1995   145-96-3–33

Background.—Accurate, noninvasive imaging of atherosclerotic lesions and following their progress in vivo have proved difficult.

Objective.—An advanced MRI technique has been developed with which to noninvasively and serially image advanced atherosclerotic lesions in the abdominal aorta of rabbits given an atherogenic diet.

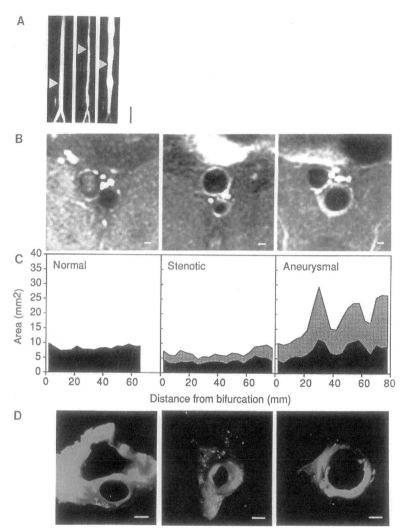

Fig 3–17.—Magnetic resonance imaging of normal, stenotic, and aneurysmal vessels. Abdominal aortas from 2 rabbits containing advanced lesions of atherosclerosis were imaged 14 months after injury and initiation of atherosclerotic diet and were compared with the abdominal aorta of an equivalent-sized control, fed a normal diet. In each panel, the same normal aorta is shown on the **left**, a diseased and stenotic aorta is shown in the **middle**, and a diseased and aneurysmal aorta is shown on the **right**. **A**, magnetic resonance TOF (time-of-flight) angiography of a ventral view (2D TOF, flip angle = 40 degrees; TR = 46 msec, TE = 4.6 msec, FOV = 12 cm, matrix = 256 × 128). *Vertical bar* = 1 cm. *Arrowheads* indicate the sites from which the axial views and sections were obtained in B and D. **B**, axial views of PDW images acquired with fat suppression. Two-dimensional fast spin echo (TE = 6,000 msec, TE = 24 msec, FOV = 9 cm, matrix = 256 × 256/echo train length = 8). The sites from which these images were taken are denoted by *arrows* in the TOF images. *Bar* represents 1 mm. **C**, lumen and wall measurements. The lumen and wall were outlined for each axial section for the length of the abdominal aorta. The area was calculated from the number of pixels in each area (1 pixel = .124 mm²). The distance of each section (at its midpoint) from the bifurcation is shown on the x axis, and areas (mm²) for lumen (*black*) and wall (*hatched*) are shown on the y axis. **D**, dissection microscopy of perfusion fixed arteries. Sections were referenced to the bifurcation and correspond with the images shown in **B**. (Courtesy of Skinner MP, Yuan C, Mitsumori L, et al: Serial magnetic resonance imaging of experimental atherosclerosis detects lesion fine structure, progression and complications *in vivo. Nature Med* 1:69–73, 1995.)

Method.—Images were acquired using a phased-array volume coil, and the arteries subsequently were evaluated ex vivo to correlate the imaging findings with the histologic characteristics of the plaque.

Results.—The images made it possible to detect progressive disease that increased the lesion mass and decreased the arterial lumen. Intralesional alterations also were detected. The images correlated with the histologic appearances of the fibrous cap, necrotic core, and fissures (Fig 3–17).

Conclusions.—The ability to image atherosclerotic plaques noninvasively should prove useful in assessing various therapeutic interventions. In particular, it will be useful to identify lipid-rich plaques, which are considered more prone to complications than more stable plaques composed of fibrous connective tissue.

▶ Research regarding the detailed characterization of atherosclerotic plaques hopefully leading to the prediction of unstable plaques has centered on the use of intravascular ultrasound and MRI. These authors have concluded that MRI has considerable potential in plaque morphological studies.

Raynaud's Phenomenon and Cold Stress Testing: A New Approach
Naidu S, Baskerville PA, Goss DE, Roberts VC (King's College Hosp, London and East Dulwich Grove, England)
Eur J Vasc Surg 8:567–573, 1994   145-96-3–34

Background.—Raynaud's attacks are ascribed to the so-called "critical closing" phenomenon when the digital arteries undergo spasm and close in response to progressive cooling. A number of methods have demonstrated this change, but none has provided a rapid and reproducible means of testing for Raynaud's phenomenon (RP).

Methods.—The digital arteries were imaged in real time using a high-frequency ultrasound technique in conjunction with cold challenge testing. The hand was immersed in water at 10° C for 5 minutes, after which the middle finger again was imaged using a 20-MHz transducer probe. Forty patients with primary RP and 20 with secondary RP were examined, along with 22 normal individuals with no history of cold sensitivity.

Results.—Digital artery diameter decreased by 92.4% on average after cold challenge in the patients with RP and by 8.7% in normal subjects. If a 45% decrease in arterial diameter was taken as the cutoff point, the test was 96.6% sensitive and 100% specific for identifying RP.

Conclusion.—Ultrasonic monitoring of digital artery diameter during cold challenge holds promise for confirming a clinical diagnosis of RP and also for evaluating treatment.

▶ There is a need for an objective reproducible test for the diagnosis of RP. Throughout the years, we have found the digital hypothermic perfusion test described by Nielsen and Lassen (1) to be at least 90% accurate and highly useful. These authors propose direct visualization of the digital arteries using high-frequency ultrasound. Although I suspect that their test is quite accurate, I see no advantage over the Nielsen test, which works very well. Inasmuch as the Nielsen test has now been standardized by more than 15 years of clinical use, I will stick with that one.

Reference

1. Nielsen SL, Lassen NA: Cold sensitivity of the digital arteries evaluated by measurement of digital blood pressure after local cooling. *J Applied Physiol* 43:907–910, 1977.

Effects of Saline, Mannitol, and Furosemide on Acute Decreases in Renal Function Induced By Radiocontrast Agents
Solomon R, Werner C, Mann D, D'Elia J, Silva P (New England Deaconess Hospital, Boston; Joslin Diabetes Ctr, Boston; Harvard Medical School, Boston)
N Engl J Med 331:1416–1420, 1994   145-96-3–35

Background.—Actue radiocontrast-induced reductions in renal function are an important cause of nosocomial renal insufficiency. Various prophylactic approaches have been recommended, such as saline hydration and the administration of mannitol or furosemide, to decrease the risk for this complication of the administration of a radiocontrast agent. However, no randomized studies have directly compared these approaches.

Methods.—Seventy-eight patients with chronic renal insufficiency having cardiac angiography were prospectively studied. By random assignment, the patients received 0.45% saline alone for 12 hours before and 12 hours after angiography, saline plus mannitol, or saline plus furosemide. Mannitol and furosemide were administered immediately before angiography. An acute radiocontrast-induced reduction in renal function was defined as an increase in the baseline serum creatinine level of at least 0.5 mg/dL within 48 hours of radiocontrast injection.

Findings.—In 26% of the patients, the serum creatinine level increased at least 0.5 mg/dL after angiography. Eleven percent of the 28 patients in the saline group had a similar increase in the serum creatinine level compared with 28% of the 25 patients in the mannitol group and 40% of the 25 patients in the furosemide group. The mean increase in the serum creatinine level 48 hours after angiography was significantly higher in patients given furosemide than in those given saline (Fig 3–18).

Conclusions.—In patients with chronic renal insufficiency with or without diabetes mellitus, the best way to prevent acute reductions in renal function was through hydration with 0.45% saline for 12 hours before and 12 hours after the administration of radiocontrast agents. Neither mannitol nor furosemide added to this hydration protocol improved outcomes.

▶ This interesting, prospective, randomized study examined patients with moderate preexisting renal failure who were undergoing cardiac angiography and were randomized to receive treatment with saline alone, saline plus

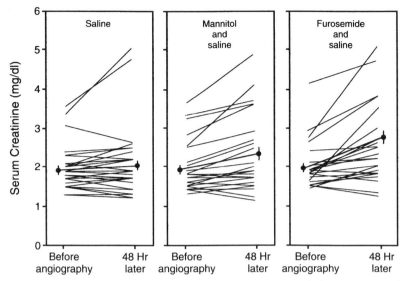

Fig 3–18.—Serum creatinine levels immediately before the administration of radiocontrast agent (after 12 hours of hydration) and 48 hours later in patients with chronic renal insufficiency. The mean ± SE for each treatment group is indicated by the heavy lines and circles. The increase in serum creatinine levels was significantly greater in the furosemide group than in the saline group ($P < .01$ by t-test). To convert values for the serum level of creatinine to µmol/L, multiply by 88.4. (Courtesy of Solomon R, Werner C, (Reprinted by permission of Solomon R, Werner C, Mann D, et al: Effects of saline, mannitol, and furosemide on acute decreases in renal function induced by radiocontrast agents. *N Engl J Med* 331:1416–1420, 1994. Copyright 1994, Massachusetts Medical Society.)

mannitol, or saline plus furosemide to minimize contrast nephrotoxicity. It is interesting that hydration with saline alone provided better renal protection than treatment with saline plus either mannitol or furosemide. The authors did not investigate the role of dopamine in providing renal protection in this population (1). On balance, I am willing to accept their conclusions that treatment with saline alone is not only as good as, but probably is better than, saline plus any other agent.

Reference

1. 1994 YEAR BOOK OF VASCULAR SURGERY, p 116.

4 Nonatherosclerotic Conditions

Buerger's Disease

Thrombolysis and Angioplasty for Acute Lower Limb Ischemia in Buerger's Disease

Hodgson TJ, Gaines PA, Beard JD (Royal Hallamshire Hosp, Sheffield, England)
Cardiovasc Intervent Radiol 17:333–335, 1994   145-96-4-1

Introduction.—Buerger's disease frequently is managed conservatively, but acute limb ischemia may develop and lead to amputation, unless salvage measures are urgently undertaken.

Case Report.—Man, 24, a smoker, had had paresthesias in his foot for 8 months and had recently noted an anesthetic great toe. Emergency angiography showed the

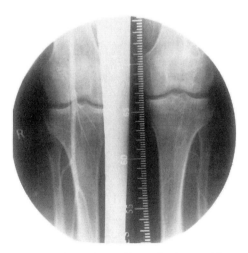

Fig 4–1.—Initial angiogram revealing occlusion of left popliteal artery with a small amount of anterior tibial artery filling. Normal popliteal artery and trifurcation on the **right.** (Courtesy of Hodgson TJ, Gaines PA, Beard JD: Thrombolysis and angioplasty for acute lower limb ischemia in Buerger's disease. [Figure 1] *Cardiovasc Intervent Radiol* 17:333–335, 1994. Reprinted by permission of Springer-Verlag.)

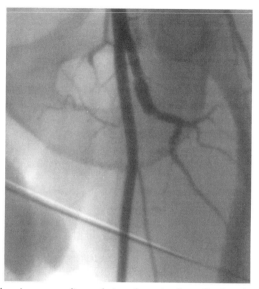

Fig 4–2.—Initial angiogram revealing occlusion of a major descending branch of the left profunda femoris artery. (Courtesy of Hodgson TJ, Gaines PA, Beard JD: Thrombolysis and angioplasty for acute lower limb ischemia in Buerger's disease. [Figure 2] *Cardiovasc Intervent Radiol* 17:333–335, 1994. Reprinted by permission of Springer-Verlag.)

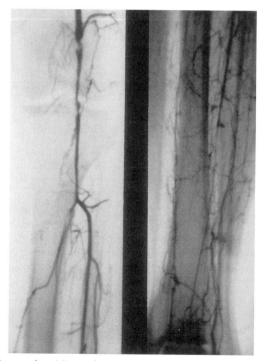

Fig 4–3.—Angiogram after 12 hours of streptokinase, revealing a long popliteal artery stenosis with improved flow into the calf. (Courtesy of Hodgson TJ, Gaines PA, Beard JD: Thrombolysis and angioplasty for acute lower limb ischemia in Buerger's disease. [Figure 3] *Cardiovasc Intervent Radiol* 17:333–335, 1994. Reprinted by permission of Springer-Verlag.)

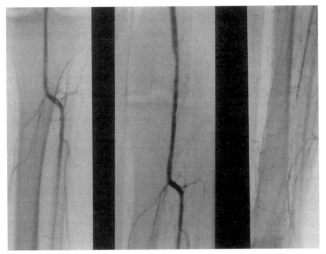

Fig 4–4.—Angiogram after popliteal and anterior tibial artery angioplasty. (Courtesy of Hodgson TJ, Gaines PA, Beard JD: Thrombolysis and angioplasty for acute lower limb ischemia in Buerger's disease. [Figure 4] *Cardiovasc Intervent Radiol* 17:333–335, 1994. Reprinted by permission of Springer-Verlag.)

left popliteal artery to be totally occluded; the anterior tibial artery was slightly filled in the calf (Fig 4–1). A major descending branch of the deep femoral artery was absent (Fig 4–2). Streptokinase and heparin were infused into the thrombosed vessel 8 hours later. Most of the thrombus resolved, revealing a long popliteal artery stenosis. Multiple collateral vessels were present in the calf (Fig 4–3). Angioplasty using balloons of varying diameter relieved the popliteal artery stenosis, but the anterior tibial artery stenosis changed little (Fig 4–4). The foot improved clinically. Pain and paresthesias had totally resolved 48 hours after angioplasty. The patient stopped smoking and, after 2 years, both feet remained free of pain and there was no claudication.

Conclusion.—This case shows the value of aggressive thrombolysis and angioplasty when a patient with Buerger's disease has acute limb ischemia develop.

▶ I selected this paper for its novelty. We have treated a rather large number of patients with Buerger's disease here at Oregon Health Sciences Center, but we have been able to achieve durable vascular repair in very few. This interesting case report showing prolonged benefit at 24 months is noteworthy. I should point out that "Spikey" Gaines is probably the most aggressive interventional radiologist in England. I am quite unclear as to how generalizable results, such as those reported in this article, may be; however, based on this report alone, I will give consideration to this form of therapy in the future.

Plantar or Dorsalis Pedis Artery Bypass in Buerger's Disease

Sasajima T, Kubo Y, Izumi Y, Inaba M, Goh K (Asahikawa Med College, Japan)
Ann Vasc Surg 8:248–257, 1994   145-96-4-2

Background.—Buerger's disease (thromboangiitis obliterans) most often begins with painful ischemic ulceration on 1 toe, usually developing after injury. Typically, there are cycles of healing and recurrent ulceration. The disorder tends to resist conservative measures when multiple segments at the level of the ankle are occluded.

Patients.—Thirteen patients with this form of Buerger's disease underwent 15 below-ankle bypass procedures. Ten of the bypasses were for intractable toe ulcers that caused severe pain, and 5 were for either ischemic changes that threatened the foot or disabling foot claudication. The average age of these patients was 46 years; 4 were female. Six of the 13 had undergone sympathectomy previously. In all cases, the 3 main crural arteries or both tibial arteries were occluded at the level of the ankle.

Methods.—The medial and lateral plantar arteries were readily distinguished on the preoperative angiogram (Fig 4–5). Only clearly outlined

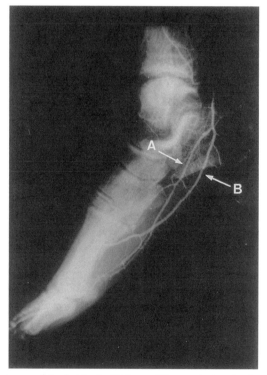

Fig 4–5.—Arteriogram of the foot in the 30-degree oblique projection showing the medial plantar artery (A) and the lateral plantar artery (B). (Courtesy of Sasajima T, Kubo Y, Izumi Y, et al: Plantar or dorsalis pedis artery bypass in Buerger's disease. *Ann Vasc Surg* 8:248–257, 1994.)

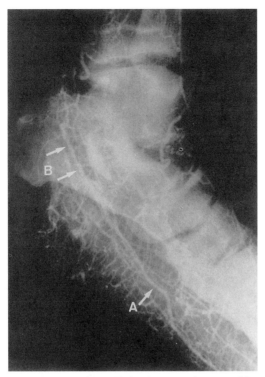

Fig 4–6.—Preoperative arteriogram of man, 48, showing a normal segment of the medial plantar artery (A) and a patent but diseased segment (B). The latter segment had edematous intimal thickening with periarterial adhesions at operation. (Courtesy of Sasajima T, Kubo Y, Izumi Y, et al: Plantar or dorsalis pedis artery bypass in Buerger's disease. *Ann Vasc Surg* 8:248–257, 1994.)

arterial segments (Fig 4–6) were used for the anastomoses. Ten bypasses were to the medial or lateral plantar arteries, 2 were to the common plantar artery, and 3 were to the dorsalis pedis artery.

Results.—The 3 early graft failures were ascribed to thrombosis at the cross-clamping site, anastomosis to a diseased segment, and arterial spasm. All 3 graft failures that occurred more than 3 months after surgery resulted from progressive disease in patients who continued smoking. In those who stopped smoking, all grafts remained patent and functioned adequately.

Conclusion.—A bypass to the arteries of the foot, either plantar vessels or the dorsalis pedis artery, can provide excellent long-term symptomatic relief to patients with medically refractory Buerger's disease who are willing to stop smoking.

▶ See the comment after Abstract 145-96-4–1. We have not been able to achieve good results with arterial bypass in Buerger's disease. These investigators performed a small number of bypasses below the ankle for patients with Buerger's disease, obtaining a gratifying intermediate-term patency of 60%. Unfortunately, their life-table, which is based on short-term follow-up and small patient numbers, is only valid through the 12-month period because of high standard error. One, of course, may legitimately wonder whether patients with Buerger's disease in Japan are the same as those we see in America. I simply do not know. My pessimism concerning the durability of arterial bypass in patients with Buerger's disease is not altered by this article. We do have to conclude, however, that some patients do seem to get intermediate-term benefit. I wonder, however, whether the angioplasty described in Abstract 145-96-4–1 may not be the better option.

Marfan Syndrome

Surgical Management of Aortic Dissection in Patients with the Marfan Syndrome
Smith JA, Fann JI, Miller C, Moore KA, DeAnda A Jr, Mitchell RS, Stinson EB, Oyer PE, Reitz BA, Shumway NE (Stanford Univ School of Medicine, Calif)
Circulation 90:II235–II242, 1994   145-96-4–3

Background.—Patients with Marfan syndrome are at risk of a number of significant cardiovascular complications, one of the most lethal of which is aortic dissection.

Patients.—Forty of 360 patients operated on for aortic dissection in the years 1963–1992 had Marfan syndrome. The patients, whose average age was 35 years, included 16 with acute type A, 2 with acute type B, 18 with chronic type A, and 4 with chronic type B dissections. The aortic arch was involved by dissection in 29 patients. Thirteen patients had acute aortic valve insufficiency preoperatively and, in 3 cases, the aorta had ruptured into the pericardial space. Peripheral pulses were lost in 9 patients. In a majority of cases, the primary intimal tear was located in the ascending aorta.

Treatment.—Twenty-two patients had the ascending aorta and aortic valve replaced, with or without reimplantation of the coronary artery. In 5 other patients, only the ascending aorta was replaced. Nine patients had replacement of the descending thoracic aorta.

Results.—Operative mortality was 10%. Fifteen late deaths occurred during a total of 216 patient-years of follow-up (average, 5.4 years), 7 of them resulting from late aortic sequelae. Actuarial survival was 71% at 5 years, 54% at 10 years, and 22% at 15 years (Fig 4–7). Fourteen patients required 20 late operations on the aorta.

Conclusion.—More aggressive medical treatment and earlier surgery, as well as closer postoperative surveillance by serial imaging of the entire aorta, may improve the outlook for patients with aortic dissection complicating Marfan syndrome.

▶ The group at Stanford University School of Medicine, led by Dr. Craig Miller, has had significant experience in the treatment of aortic dissection in patients with Marfan syndrome. During the course of many years, they had an operative mortality rate of only 10% with these difficult patients. The

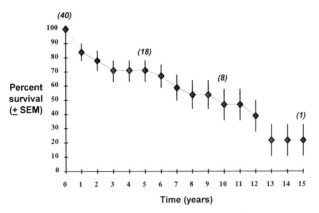

Fig 4–7.—Actuarial survival for all patients including early deaths in the hospital. The *error bars* represent 1 SEM. The *numbers in parentheses* represent the numbers of patients at risk at each interval. (Courtesy of Smith JA, Fann JI, Miller C, et al: Surgical management of aortic dissection in patients with the Marfan syndrome. *Circulation* 90:II235–II242, 1994.)

long-term actuarial survival was 71%, 54%, and 22% at 5, 10, and 15 years. A number of patients required additional aortic operations. This is a well-described clinical report of aortic surgery in a difficult patient group.

Marfan Syndrome: The Variability and Outcome of Operative Management
Coselli JS, LeMaire SA, Büket S (Baylor College of Medicine, Houston; Methodist Hosp, Houston)
J Vasc Surg 21:432–443, 1995   145-96-4–4

Objective.—The outcome of surgery for Marfan syndrome was examined in 69 patients who had a total of 79 operations in the years 1989–1994.

Methods.—The operations included 28 composite valve graft replacements and 29 graft replacements of the thoracoabdominal aorta (Fig 4–8). The patients had previously had 57 procedures on the aorta. Forty-two patients required more than 1 operation, and nearly one fourth of the patients had 3 or more procedures.

Results.—A single hospital death occurred, for a 30-day survival rate of 98.7%; the long-term survival rate was 96.2%. Only 1 of 38 patients undergoing replacement of the distal aorta (2.6%) became paraplegic. No patient had a stroke after surgery using profound hypothermic circulatory arrest.

Conclusions.—Surgery on the aorta prolongs the survival of patients with Marfan syndrome and causes little morbidity, but multiple operations often are necessary. Lifelong cardiovascular surveillance is necessary to detect recurrent disease or new lesions.

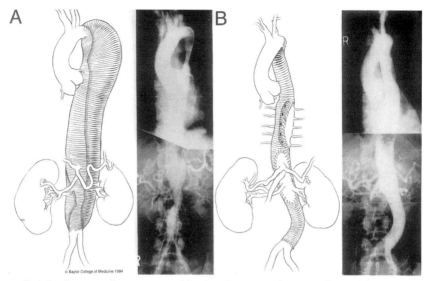

Fig 4–8.—**A,** preoperative aortogram and drawing of a patient with extensive thoracoabdominal aortic aneurysm (Crawford type II) caused by chronic DeBakey type III dissection. **B,** postoperative aortogram and drawing of a patient after thoracoabdominal aortic aneurysm replacement. (Courtesy of Coselli JS, LeMaire SA, Büket S: Marfan syndrome: The variability and outcome of operative management. *J Vasc Surg* 21:432–443, 1995.)

▶ This article presents another large patient group. The authors report extremely good surgical results—interestingly, with minimal neurologic impairment in these difficult patients. The operative mortality rate of 1.3% in the past 5 years appears unprecedented. This article is accompanied by the absolutely classic Baylor medical illustrations, the likes of which I have never seen from any other institution.

Composite Graft Repair of Marfan Aneurysm of the Ascending Aorta: Results in 150 Patients
Gott VL, Cameron DE, Pyeritz RE, Gillinov AM, Greene PS, Stone CD, Alejo DE, McKusick VA (Johns Hopkins Med Institutions, Baltimore, Md)
J Card Surg 9:482–489, 1994
145-96-4–5

Introduction.—Between 1976 and 1994, 150 consecutive patients with Marfan syndrome underwent composite graft repair of an ascending aorta aneurysm. Twenty-six patients had preoperative dissection of the ascending aorta, with a mean diameter of 7.8 cm; 7 patients had aortic diameters of 6.5 cm or less.

Technique.—The Bentall technique was used with several modifications, including the elimination of the "blood tight" aneurysm wrap and the increasing use of coronary artery buttons in patients with low-lying coronary ostia. Twenty-four patients had mitral valve procedures.

Outcome.—There were no deaths among the 138 patients who underwent elective composite graft repair or among the 24 patients who had mitral procedures. One early death occurred among the 12 patients who underwent urgent operation; this patient arrived at the hospital with a rupturing aneurysm. Among the 149 survivors, 14 (9%) late deaths occurred, for an actuarial survival rate of 93% at 1 year, 92% at 5 years, 81% at 10 years, and 73% at 14 years. Multivariate analysis identified New York Heart Association class III or IV and male sex as significant independent predictors of mortality. Late complications directly related to the composite graft were gratifyingly low and included coronary dehiscence in 2 (1%) patients and thromboembolic events in 3 (2%). Eight (5%) patients had endocarditis: 2 responded to antibiotics, 3 died before widespread availability of cryopreserved homografts, and 3 treated with antibiotics and homograft root replacement had no evidence of recurrent infection. Eight patients required a subsequent procedure on the distal unoperated aorta, and all survived.

Summary.—The Bentall operative technique provides excellent early and long-term results in patients with Marfan aneurysm of the ascending aorta. Composite graft repair is mandated when the aneurysm reaches 5.5–6 cm, even in asymptomatic patients. With a family history of dissection, operative intervention should occur when the aneurysm reaches 5 cm in diameter. Endocarditis remains an important late complication, and root re-replacement with a cryopreserved aortic homograft root has become the treatment of choice when antibiotic therapy fails.

► Abstracts 145-96-4–3 through 145-96-4–5 present a remarkable group of patients who had aortic surgery in association with Marfan syndrome. The extremely low operative mortalities are noted, especially among the elective patients. The actuarial survival in the patients without dissection was quite good. These patients underwent surgery using the composite graft valve-containing prosthesis. My conclusion from these 3 papers is that, in experienced centers, the outcome of aortic surgery in patients with Marfan disease has improved markedly. I reluctantly congratulate the thoracic surgeons on their accomplishment in this difficult area.

Progression of Aortic Dilatation and the Benefit of Long-Term β-Adrenergic Blockade in Marfan's Syndrome
Shores J, Berger KR, Murphy EA, Pyeritz RE (Johns Hopkins Univ, Baltimore, Md)
N Engl J Med 330:1335–1341, 1994   145-96-4–6

Background.—Progressive enlargement of the aortic root is the most serious clinical feature of Marfan syndrome. In untreated patients, the associated aortic dissection and regurgitation shorten life expectancy by as much as one third. Halpern et al. suggested that β-adrenergic blockade might have the effect of protecting the aortic root by reducing the impulse (rate of pressure change) of left ventricular ejection and the heart rate.

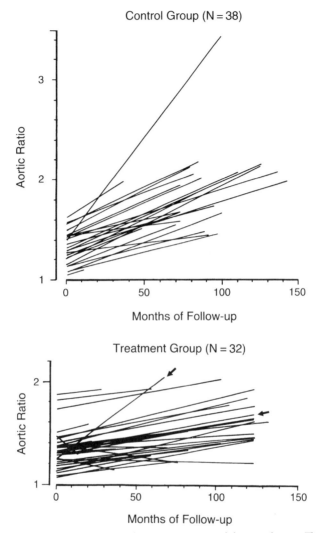

Fig 4–9.—Changes in the aortic ratio in the treatment group and the control group. The aortic ratio is the ratio of the diameter of the aorta measured in a patient to the diameter expected in a subject with the same body surface area and age. The ratio in each patient is presented as a fitted regression line. The data points are not shown, but the length of each line indicates the length of follow-up. One patient in the control group had an exceptional aortic ratio (more than 3.4) at 100 months. Two patients in the treatment group (*arrows*) did not comply with propranolol therapy. (Reprinted by permission of Shores J, Berger KR, Murphy EA, et al: Progression of aortic dilatation and the benefit of long-term β-adrenergic blockade in Marfan's syndrome. *N Engl J Med* 330:1335–1341, 1994. Copyright 1994, Massachusetts Medical Society.)

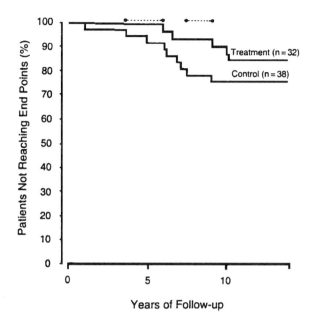

Fig 4–10.—Kaplan-Meier survival analysis based on the clinical end points in the study (death, congestive heart failure, or aortic regurgitation, aortic dissection, or cardiovascular surgery). The *dashed lines* indicate the periods when the 90% confidence limits for the difference between the curves did not include zero. The curves diverge the most in the middle years but do not intersect at any point. (Reprinted by permission of Shores J, Berger KR, Murphy EA, et al: Progression of aortic dilatation and the benefit of β-adrenergic blockade in Marfan's syndrome. *N Engl J Med* 330:1335–1341, 1994. Copyright 1994, Massachusetts Medical Society.)

Study Plan.—In a randomized, open-label study, the use of propranolol was evaluated in adult and adolescent patients with classic Marfan syndrome. Thirty-two patients were given propranolol in an initial dose of 10 mg 4 times daily, and the dose was increased until either the heart rate remained less than 100 beats per minute during exercise or the systolic time interval, corrected for heart rate, rose 30%. Thirty-eight other patients of similar age and cardiovascular characteristics were untreated. The patients were followed up clinically for about 10 years on average, and the dimensions of their aortic root were monitored by M-mode echocardiography.

Results.—The mean dose of propranolol was 212 mg daily and the mean serum drug level on optimal dosing was 135 ng/mL. Figure 4–9 shows the regression lines for the aortic ratio in each patient during the study. The rate of dilatation of the aortic root was significantly less in propranolol-treated patients than in the control group. Nine control patients and only 3 who actually took their prescribed drug reached a clinical end point: death, congestive heart failure, aortic regurgitation, aortic dissection, or cardiovascular surgery. The survival of patients who did not reach a clinical end point is shown in Figure 4–10. Two of the control patients died, and postmortem examinations showed no aortic dissection or obvious cause of death. Only 1 patient had a third-degree atrioventricular block and required a dose reduction.

Discussion.—Beta-adrenergic blockade effectively slows the development of aortic root dilatation in some patients with Marfan syndrome. It may be advantageous to use a β_1-selective agent such as atenolol, which has a longer therapeutic half-life and fewer side effects than propranolol.

▶ It has been speculated for years that propranolol may protect the aortic root from dilatation in patients with Marfan syndrome by reducing the rate of pressure change within the cardiac cycle. These authors report a prospective, randomized trial of propranolol in 70 patients with Marfan syndrome. They were followed up for an average of 9.3 years in the control group and 10.7 years in the treatment group. Prophylactic β-adrenergic blockade was effective in slowing the rate of aortic dilatation and diminishing the development of aortic complications in patients with Marfan syndrome. The authors note that the drug atenolol may actually be more effective, but this was not available when this study began. Thus, available evidence supports the use of prophylactic β-blockade in young patients with Marfan syndrome.

Quantitative Differences in Biosynthesis and Extracellular Deposition of Fibrillin in Cultured Fibroblasts Distinguish Five Groups of Marfan Syndrome Patients and Suggest Distinct Pathogenetic Mechanisms
Aoyama T, Francke U, Dietz HC, Furthmayr H (Stanford Univ, Calif; Johns Hopkins Univ, Baltimore, Md)
J Clin Invest 94:130–137, 1994   145-96-4–7

Introduction.—In patients with Marfan syndrome (MFS), elastic and nonelastic tissues from significantly affected organs show abundant microfibrils. Skin and cultured fibroblasts from these patients show a dramatic decrease in the number of microfibrils. The results of pulse-chase studies of [^{35}S]cysteine-labeled fibrillin performed on fibroblast strains from patients with MFS were reported.

Methods and Findings.—Fifty-five patients with MFS—including 13 with identified mutations of the fibrillin-1 gene—and 10 controls were studied. Five groups of patients could be distinguished by quantitation of soluble intracellular and insoluble extracellular fibrillin. The 8 patients in group I and the 19 patients in group II synthesized reduced amounts of normal-sized fibrillin. The 6 patients in group III, the 18 patients in group IV, and the 4 patients in group V showed normal fibrillin synthesis. On measurement of extracellular fibrillin deposition, patients in groups I and III deposited 35% to 70% of control values; those in groups II and IV deposited less than 35%; and those in group V deposited more than 70%.

The group I protein phenotype was found in a patient with a deletion mutant with a low transcript level from the mutant allele and in 7 additional patients. In this group, MFS resulted from a reduction in microfibrils associated with a null allele, an unstable transcript, or an altered fibrillin product that was synthesized in low amounts. For the patients in groups II and IV, who represented 68% of the patients with MFS, a dominant negative effect appeared to be the main pathogenetic mechanism. The mutant allele in these fibroblasts makes products that appear to interfere with microfibril formation. The group II phenotype was characterized by insertion, deletion, and exon skipping mutations that result in smaller fibrillin products. One of the group II cell culture media showed a truncated, 60-kD form of fibrillin with specific fibrillin antibodies. Of the 9 known missense mutations that gave rise to abnormal fibrillin molecules of normal size, 7 were in group IV.

Conclusions.—Distinct groups of patients with MFS are suggested by differences in the synthesis and extracellular deposition of collagen. In addition to being a useful diagnostic tool, this classification may provide a useful basis for studying the relationship between the clinical phenotype and underlying pathogenesis of MFS.

▶ It was recognized several years ago that MFS is causally related to mutations in the fibrillin gene on chromosome 15 (1). These investigators, using extremely sophisticated techniques, have identified 5 different groups of fibrillin abnormalities in patients with MFS. It appears that the fibrillin abnormalities may be either a reduction in fibrillin synthesis or a distinct abnormality in the fibrillin molecule, depending on the exact genetic abnormality present. I am pleased to note that there are some people out there who can understand this complicated material.

Reference

1. 1993 YEAR BOOK OF VASCULAR SURGERY, p 141.

Arteritis

Thoracic Aortic Aneurysm and Rupture in Giant Cell Arteritis: A Descriptive Study of 41 Cases
Evans JM, Bowles CA, Bjornsson J, Mullany CJ, Hunder GG (Mayo Clinic and Med School, Rochester, Minn)
Arthritis Rheum 37:1539–1547, 1994   145-96-4–8

Background.—Giant-cell arteritis (GCA), a common form of vasculitis, is associated with a broad range of symptoms and findings. The features and outcomes of patients with GCA and aneurysms or rupture of the thoracic aorta were examined.

Methods.—A computerized indexing system was used to identify patients with GCA treated during a 40-year period. The presence of thoracic aortic aneurysms (TAA) with or without aortic valve insufficiency was established by findings on radiographs. CT scans, ultrasound studies of the thorax, angiograms of the aorta, and postmortem evaluation.

Clinical Features at Diagnosis of Giant-Cell Arteritis in 41 Patients With Giant-Cell Arteritis and Involvement of the Thoracic Aorta

Feature	No. of patients
Age at onset, years	
Median	67
Range	52–88
Sex, M/F	10/31
History of hypertension (>140/90 mm Hg)	14
Duration of symptoms prior to diagnosis, months	
Median	2
Range	0–118
Malaise	29
Weight loss	15
Fever	14
Headaches	25
Polymyalgia rheumatica	22
Jaw claudication	14
Tender or swollen temporal artery	25
Visual disturbance	9

(Courtesy of Evans JM, Bowles CA, Bjornsson J, et al: Thoracic aortic aneurysm and rupture in giant cell arteritis: A descriptive study of 41 cases. *Arthritis Rheum* 37:1539–1547, 1994.)

Findings.—Thirty-one women and 10 men with GCA had TAA and/or rupture. Features of GCA at or before diagnosis are listed in the table. In 3 patients, TAA developed before GCA was diagnosed. In 5, aortic findings were noted near the time of diagnosis and in 33, after the diagnosis. Acute aortic dissection occurred in 16 patients, causing the deaths of 8 patients. Nineteen patients also had aortic valve insufficiency resulting from aortic root dilation. Congestive heart failure developed in 15 of these patients. A total of 21 operations were done in 18 patients for TAA resection and/or aortic valve replacement or repair. In 10 patients, aortitis was documented histologically.

Conclusions.—Thoracic aortic complications in patients with GCA are associated with serious outcomes that may be fatal. Such complications have been under-recognized. Physicians need to be alert to the development of these complications at any time in the course of GCA, which may occur many years after the usual symptoms have subsided.

▶ We normally associate GCA with occlusive disease of the brachiocephalic circulation or, more rarely, with abdominal aortic coarctation. However, this condition most assuredly can cause TAA. This retrospective study described 41 patients with GCA associated with TAA, rupture of the thoracic aorta, or both. Three fourths of the patients were women. The clinical findings are noted. The clinician must be aware of the possibility of TAA when encountering a patient with GCA. Interestingly, GCA is substantially a disease of old age. The median age of the patients studied was 67 years.

Takayasu Arteritis

Kerr GS, Hallahan CW, Giordano J, Leavitt RY, Fauci AS, Rottem M, Hoffman GS (National Inst of Allergy and Infectious Disease, Bethesda, Md; George Washington Univ, Washington, DC)
Ann Intern Med 120:919–929, 1994   145-96-4–9

Objective.—The clinical features, angiographic findings, and response to treatment of patients with Takayasu's arteritis were evaluated prospectively.

Patients.—Between 1970 and 1990, 58 women and 2 men with Takayasu's arteritis were seen at the National Institutes of Health. The disease occurred far more often in Asians compared with other racial groups. The patients were followed up prospectively for a median of 5.3 years.

Clinical Features.—The median age at disease onset was 25 years (range, 7–64 years). Juveniles had a delay in diagnosis that was nearly 4 times that of adults. Systemic symptoms occurred in only 33% of patients at the onset of disease and in another 10% during the course of the disease. The

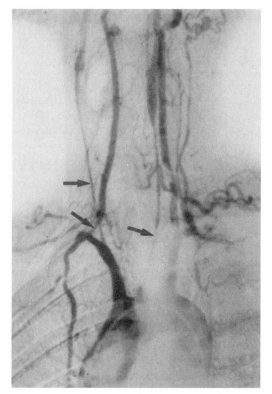

Fig 4–11.—Angiogram showing critical stenoses. Long segments of critical stenoses (> 70%) (*arrow*) of both common carotid arteries, the subclavian artery, and the proximal right vertebral arteries. (Courtesy of Kerr GS, Hallahan CW, Giordano J, et al: Takayasu arteritis. *Ann Intern Med* 120:919–929, 1994.)

clinical course ranged from asymptomatic to catastrophic with stroke. Vascular ischemic symptoms were the hallmark of the disease (Fig 4–11) and were seen as a bruit in 80%, particularly in the carotid vessels. Stenotic lesions were 3.6-fold more common than aneurysms, and 68% of the patients had extensive vascular disease. Hypertension was less common and was often associated with renal artery stenosis. Other findings included inflammatory bowel disease, erythema nodosum, and sarcoidosis. The erythrocyte sedimentation rate was an unreliable marker of disease course.

Treatment/Outcome.—Forty-eight patients received glucocorticoids alone or in combination with a cytotoxic agent for active disease. Remission was achieved in 60% of the patients treated with glucocorticoids alone, and the addition of cytotoxic agents induced remission in 40% of steroid-resistant patients. However, about half of those who achieved remission later relapsed. Twenty percent of patients had a monophasic disease that did not require therapy. Thirty patients underwent 79 vascular procedures (table). Although clinically significant palliation occurred, usually after angioplasty or bypass of severely stenotic vessels, complications, including restenosis, were common. Arterial biopsy specimens from clinically inactive patients showed active vasculitis in 44% of patients. Only 9 of 34 patients were not functionally affected by their disease on long-term follow-up, but mortality as a result of Takayasu's arteritis was low (2%).

Vascular Procedures and Complications Among 60 Patients With Takayasu's Arteritis

Procedure	Site of Procedure	Patients	Procedures	Procedures Complicated	Complications/ Number of Patients*
		n		%	*n/n*
Bypass		23	50	30	15/9
	Common carotid		12		
	Subclavian or axillary (or both)		10		
	Iliofemoral		7		
	Renal		7		
	Coronary		6		
Angioplasty		11	20	45	9/6
	Subclavian		8		
	Renal		7		
	Iliofemoral		4		
	Thoracic aorta		1		
Aneurysm repair	Aorta	3	3	0	0/3
Aortic valve replacement		2	2		1/1
Iliofemoral thrombectomy		2	2	0	0/2
Iliofemoral endarterectomy		1	1		1/1
Nephrectomy		1	1		
Total for all procedures		30	79		

Note: 30 patients required 79 procedures (2.6 procedures/patient).
* Complications included restenosis, thrombosis, hemorrhage, infection, and aneurysm formation. Thirty-six percent of 39 procedures using synthetic grafts had complications, whereas 9% of 11 procedures using autologous grafts had complications.
(Courtesy of Kerr GS, Hallahan CW, Giordano J, et al: Takayasu arteritis. *Ann Intern Med* 120:919–929, 1994.)

Summary.—Takayasu's arteritis is rare in North America. It is heterogenous in presentation, progression, and response to therapy, with limited reliability of clinical, laboratory, and angiographic markers of disease activity. Most patients with Takayasu's arteritis require repeated and, at times, prolonged courses of therapy. In addition, most patients have substantial morbidity, but mortality is low.

▶ The research group at the National Institute of Allergy and Infectious Disease has the largest group of patients with fully characterized Takayasu's arteritis under active follow-up in the United States. This publication presents their overview of this large patient group that was followed up for many years. The overwhelming majority of their patients were Asian and female. Interestingly, surgical biopsy material from patients with clinically inactive disease showed active arteritis in 44%. The medical treatment of this disease was difficult. On balance, Takayasu's arteritis is a virulent, life-threatening disease that requires diligent medical attention. I consider this group from the NIH to be the most important source of information on Takayasu's arteritis in America.

Gallium Scintigraphy in the Diagnosis and Total Lymphoid Irradiation of Takayasu's Arteritis

Meyers KEC, Thomson PD, Beale PG, Morrison RCA, Kala UK, Jacobs DWC, Pantanowitz D, Lakier RH, Esser JD (Univ of the Witwatersrand, Johannesburg, South Africa)

S Afr Med J 84:685–688, 1994   145-96-4–10

Background.—Takayasu's arteritis (TA) causes substantial morbidity and mortality in children, mainly as a result of renovascular hypertension.

Patients.—Ten children with TA complicated by renovascular hypertension have been treated in the past 10 years. All had an increased sedimentation rate and a purified protein derivative reaction exceeding 15 mm.

Management and Outcome.—Gallium scintigraphy demonstrated sites of active vascular inflammation in 3 of 4 patients, which became negative after total lymphoid irradiation (TLI). The last 6 children regained a normal sedimentation rate after TLI, and all those with active inflammation had normal scintigraphic findings (Figs 4–12 and 4–13). Renal bypass grafting was followed by clotting in all 5 treated kidneys, but 6 of 11 kidneys managed by autografting or allografting were functional. All 4 patients managed conventionally with steroids, antituberculosis drugs, and/or cyclophosphamide died within 18 months of the diagnosis of TA. In contrast, 5 of the 6 patients treated with TLI were alive after 32–54 months of follow-up.

Conclusion.—Total lymphoid irradiation effectively counters vascular inflammation in TA. Combined with immunosuppressive therapy and autotransplantation for renal artery stenosis, younger patents with TA now have an improved outlook.

24 hours

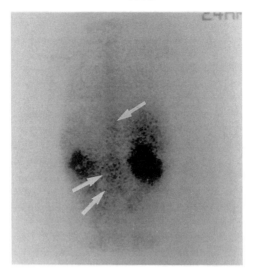

Posterior

Fig 4–12.—Gallium-67 citrate posterior planar view of patient 8 pre–total lymphoid irradiation at 24 hours. Uptake (*arrows*) is demonstrated in the region of the descending thoracic abdominal aorta and the common iliac arteries. (Courtesy of Meyers KEC, Thomson PD, Beale PG, et al: Gallium scintigraphy in the diagnosis and total lymphoid irradiation of Takayasu's arteritis. *S Afr Med J* 84:685–688, 1994.)

48 hours

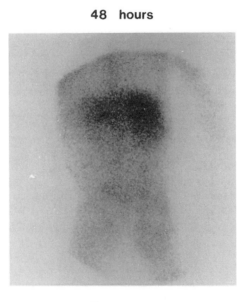

Posterior

Fig 4–13.—Gallium-67 citrate posterior planar view of patient 8 post–total lymphoid irradiation at 48 hours. All evidence of increased aortic uptake has disappeared. (Courtesy of Meyers KEC, Thomson PD, Beale PG, et al: Gallium scintigraphy in the diagnosis and total lymphoid irradiation of Takayasu's arteritis, *S Afr Med J* 84:685–688, 1994.)

▶ This article describes the use of gallium scans in children with TA. The gallium apparently is taken up by the inflammatory cells in the areas of active arteritis, allowing localization of disease. Interestingly, the researchers used lymphoid irradiation in a number of these patients, following an immuno-suppressive low-dose irradiation schedule similar to that used in some centers in preparation for renal transplantation. They believed they achieved good clinical improvement in a number of patients. The use of gallium scanning to actively localize areas of arteritis, although interesting, does not, at present, appear important in clinical decision-making.

Arterial Reconstruction for Non-Specific Arteritis (Takayasu's Disease): Medium to Long Term Results
Robbs JV, Abdool-Carrim ATO, Kadwa AM (Univ of Natal, Republic of South Africa)
Eur J Vasc Surg 8:401–407, 1994   145-96-4-11

Background.—The value of reconstructive arterial surgery for Takayasu's arteritis remains uncertain. Patients with this disorder commonly die of stroke, ruptured aneurysm, complications of renovascular hypertension, or renal failure.

Patients.—The results of arterial reconstruction were reviewed in 134 patients who were referred to a vascular service over 11 years, 81 of whom were considered suitable for operation. The patients were 3 to 45 years of age (average, 29.5 years). Twenty-eight patients had disease limited to the aortic arch (type I); 41 had involvement of the descending aorta (type II); 6 had both arch and aortic disease (type III); 2 had associated cardiac lesions (type IV); and 4 had isolated peripheral vascular lesions (type V). Seventy percent of the lesions were aneurysmal in nature. Operative management is summarized in the table.

Results.—Operative mortality was 3.6% in patients with type I involvement and 4% in those with types II to IV disease. The latter deaths

Operative Management

Type O (*n* = 28)	
Aortic arch reconstruction	12
Interposition graft	14
Subclavian-subclavian bypass	1
Ligation I.C.A.	1
Type II, III, IV (*n* = 49)	
Thoracoabdominal aortic replacement + bypass	26
Aortoiliac aneurysm replacement	18
Nephrectomy	2
Aortobiofemoral bypass	1
Iliorenal bypass	1
Type V (*n* = 4)	
Interposition graft	4

(Courtesy of Robbs JV, Abdool-Carrim ATO, Kadwa AM: Arterial reconstruction for non-specific arteritis [Takayasu's disease]: Medium to long term results. *Eur J Vasc Surg* 8:401–407, 1994.)

occurred after surgery for ruptured aneurysm. No electively operated patient died. On follow-up for up to 11 years after surgery, 5% of the patients had progressive and ultimately fatal disease, and another 9% had progression but survived. Three of the surviving patients had further surgery. Renovascular hypertension improved or resolved in 19 of the 22 patients affected.

Conclusion.—Reconstructive surgery is reasonably safe and helps prevent life-threatening complications in patients with symptomatic Takayasu's arteritis and those with aneurysms.

▶ Takayasu's arteritis must be endemic in South Africa. Of the 81 patients undergoing surgery in this series, 70% of the lesions were operated on for aneurysmal degeneration. The overall operative mortality was 4%, and there were no deaths after elective surgery. This is, by far, the largest modern surgical report regarding Takayasu's arteritis of which I am aware. The principles of surgery generally include the use of bypass grafts instead of endarterectomies, taking care to originate and terminate grafts in grossly normal arteries. I am impressed by this large experience.

Analysis of Steroid Related Complications and Mortality in Temporal Arteritis: A 15-Year Survey of 43 Patients
Nesher G, Sonnenblick M, Friedlander Y (The Hebrew Univ, Jerusalem)
J Rheumatol 21:1283–1286, 1994   145-96-4–12

Introduction.—Corticosteroids (CS) are the preferred treatment of temporal arteritis (TA), but they may—as may the disease itself—lead to severe, even fatal complications.

Patients and Treatment.—Steroid-related complications were studied in 43 consecutive patients who received a diagnosis of TA at a single center in Israel in 1978–1992. The disease was histologically confirmed in all but 4 instances. The patients, 28 women and 15 men with a mean age of 75.5 years, were followed up for a mean of 3 years. All patients received prednisone in starting doses of 30 mg–80 mg daily. Patients with ocular involvement began treatment with 60 mg–80 mg daily.

Results.—Major CS-related side effects developed in 58% of the patients, with the most common being fracture, infection, and a complex of diabetes, congestive heart failure, and hypertension (table). Three-fourths of the patients who were 75 years of age or older at the time TA was diagnosed had CS-related side effects compared with 37% of younger patients. Side effects also were dose-related. Seven deaths, including 5 caused by respiratory infection, probably were related to prednisone therapy. The overall standardized mortality ratio was 2.1, mainly reflecting an excess of deaths from severe infection in the first year of illness.

Conclusion.—Patients with TA are at risk of serious CS-related complications. Treatment should be individualized, taking the patient's age, the severity of disease, and co-existing medical conditions into account.

Prevalence of Major Corticosteroid-Related Complications in
43 Patients With Temporal Arteritis

CS Related Complication	Patients (*n*)	Duration of Therapy Until Complication (mean ± SD)
Fractures	15	12 ± 11months
Infections	9	6 ± 5 months
DM, CHF, hypertension	8	3 ± 2 weeks
Depression/psychosis	3	4 ± 2 weeks
Bleeding peptic ulcers	2	4 ± 3 months
AVN of hip joint	2	19 ± 6 months

Abbreviations: AVN, avascular necrosis; *CHF*, congestive heart failure; *DM*, diabetes mellitus.
(Courtesy of Nesher G, Sonnenblick M, Friedlander Y: Analysis of steroid related complications and mortality in temporal arteritis: A 15-year survey of 43 patients. *J Rheumatol* 21:1283–1286, 1994.)

▶ The conclusion appears inescapable: old people receiving high-dose steroids do not do well. Twenty-five of 43 consecutive patients treated with high-dose prednisone had major steroid complications develop, including fractures and severe infection. Seven of 19 deaths occurring during the study appeared to be related to steroid treatment. Perhaps much lower doses of steroids, with the addition of cytotoxic agents, would have been preferable. See the comment after Abstract 145-96-4–13.

Treatment of Glucocorticoid-Resistant or Relapsing Takayasu Arteritis With Methotrexate

Hoffman GS, Leavitt RY, Kerr GS, Rottem M, Sneller MC, Fauci AS (National Inst of Allergy and Infectious Diseases, Bethesda, Md; Cleveland Clinic Found, Ohio)
Arthritis Rheum 37:578–582, 1994   145-96-4–13

Background.—Perhaps half of all patients with Takayasu's arteritis respond to glucocorticoid treatment. Those who are resistant may respond to the addition of daily cyclophosphamide administered in low dosages, but significant toxic effects are a possibility and in some patients, the disease continues to progress.

Methods.—The efficacy of methotrexate (MTX) was examined in an open-label study of 16 patients with Takayasu's arteritis. These patients had multifocal angiographic lesions and had failed to respond to daily glucocorticoid treatment for at least 1 month or had relapsed. Oral MTX was added to the current steroid regimen in a dose of approximately .3 mg/kg per week, not exceeding 15 mg per week at the outset. The average maintenance dose was 17.1 mg. The average follow-up was nearly 3 years.

Results.—Thirteen of the 16 patients (81%) entered remission, but 7 patients relapsed as glucocorticoid therapy was tapered. Resumption of steroid therapy again resulted in remission, and 3 of these patients have been able to stop using steroid. In all, 8 patients have remained in remission for 18 months on average, 4 of them without requiring either steroid or MTX. Three patients continued to progress despite combined treatment.

Conclusion.—The addition of a weekly low dose of MTX to glucocorticoid therapy is an effective treatment approach in patients whose disease is resistant to steroid treatment alone.

▶ Patients with Takayasu's arteritis appear to require high doses of steroids, which typically are difficult to taper or withdraw. These authors believe the addition of MTX to the treatment regimen assists in the induction of remission and reduces the need for ongoing glucocorticoid therapy. Vascular surgeons should be aware of this.

Miscellaneous

Midaortic Syndrome and Hypertension in Childhood
O'Neill JA Jr, Berkowitz H, Fellows KJ, Harmon CM (Children's Hosp of Philadelphia)
J Pediatr Surg 30:164–172, 1995   145-96-4-14

Background.—The midaortic syndrome is a type of fibromuscular hyperplasia, of unknown cause, that produces narrowing of the abdominal aorta and its renal and visceral branches. The symptoms depend on the degree and site of vascular narrowing.

Patients.—Among 45 patients operated on for marked renovascular hypertension, the cases of 17 who were found to have midaortic syndrome were reviewed. The patients were 5 months to 15 years of age; the average age was 10 years. The clinical features included malignant hypertension, congestive heart failure, oliguric renal failure, and claudication. Intestinal angina was not seen, even in patients with involvement of the celiac or superior mesenteric artery or both.

Treatment and Outcome.—Balloon angioplasty, done in 2 patients, did not achieve lasting effects. One patient underwent primary nephrectomy. Twelve of the other patients underwent aorto-aortic bypass graft surgery, with bilateral renal artery bypasses in 9 of them and unilateral renal bypass in 3. Four patients had only bilateral renal bypasses. Most patients had narrowed visceral arteries; however, excellent collateral vessels were the rule, and no patient has required visceral arterial reconstruction. During a mean follow-up of 4 years, 12 patients have been cured of hypertension, and 5 have improved. Claudication, heart failure, and renal failure all were relieved. The reinforced saphenous veins used for renal artery bypass have not showed aneurysmal degeneration.

Recommendations.—Children who are hypertensive with midaortic syndrome are best managed by aggressive single-stage vascular reconstruction. Patch aortoplasty with either autogenous artery or a prosthesis is useful when the narrowed aortic segment is short, but bypass has proved easier when extensive involvement is present. Woven Dacron aorto-aortic bypass grafts have been used, making them long enough to allow for growth and placing them behind the left kidney. Vein grafts are reinforced with Dacron net.

▶ All 17 patients reported in this article were symptomatic with complaints of hypertension, congestive heart failure, or oliguric renal failure. Leg claudication was a minor complaint. Elevated blood pressure was present in all patients. Generally, the author preferred Dacron aorto-aortic grafts with associated renal bypasses, with the vein reinforced by Dacron. The results generally appear to be quite satisfactory. I disagree with the authors' assessment that this condition represents fibromuscular dysplasia. I find myself in general disagreement with his preference for aorto-aortic Dacron bypasses. Dr. James Stanley makes an impassioned plea for use of autogenous tissue whenever possible, and I believe he is correct.

Vascular Complications in Ehlers-Danlos Syndrome
Mattar SG, Kumar AG, Lumsden AB (Emory Univ, Atlanta, Ga)
Am Surg 60:827–831, 1994   145-96-4-15

Background.—Type IV Ehlers-Danlos syndrome (EDS), the arterial or ecchymotic form, results from defective type III collagen and often produces vascular complications. These include multiple aneurysms and the spontaneous rupture or dissection of large and small arteries. The operative management of these patients has proved to be hazardous and often ineffective.

Three Cases.—Man, 63, who was known to have EDS, had severe pain develop acutely in his back and chest and had CT findings of pericardial and mediastinal fluid consistent with a hemorrhage. An iliac artery aneurysm also was noted. The mediastinal hematoma resolved with conservative management. Boy, 11 years, had rupture of an aortic pseudoaneurysm (Fig 4–14) and died intraoperatively when the aorta was partially transected by clamps. Woman, 24, who was previously shown to have multiple abdominal aneurysms and an internal carotid aneurysm, had a pulsatile abdominal mass and aortographic evidence of multiple renal artery aneurysms on both sides (Fig 4–15). The infrarenal aorta and both internal iliac arteries also bore aneurysms. The patient did well after removal of the aortic aneurysm and exclusion of the internal iliac artery aneurysms.

Conclusion.—The fragility of arterial vessels in patients with type IV EDS creates a serious operative risk, but mortality from hemorrhage in unoperated patients is even greater.

▶ Type IV EDS is associated with a defect in type III collagen synthesis. This is the variant of EDS associated with extremely fragile arteries, multiple aneurysms, spontaneous rupture, and arterial dissections. The authors of this article present several case reports that demonstrate the difficulties in dealing with these patients. Vascular surgery is possible but extremely

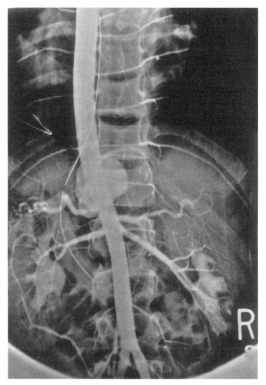

Fig 4–14.—Aortogram revealing a pseudoaneurysm in the suprarenal aorta. (Courtesy of Mattar SG, Kumar AG, Lumsden AB: Vascular complications in Ehlers-Danlos Syndrome. *Am Surg* 60:827–831, 1994.)

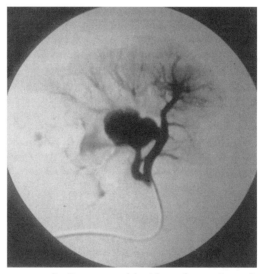

Fig 4–15.—Aortogram revealing 2 aneurysms of the right renal artery, 5 cm × 8 cm and 6 cm × 3 cm in size, giving the appearance of a single bilobed aneurysm. (Courtesy of Mattar SG, Kumar AG, Lumsden AB: Vascular complications in Ehlers-Danlos syndrome. *Am Surg* 60:827–831, 1994.)

hazardous, and the outcome is unpredictable. In an especially memorable patient with EDS type IV, whom we have dealt with here, 7 aneurysms have been currently diagnosed and treated. To date, all but 1 of the operative repairs have required ligation because of recurrent aneurysm formation. Interestingly, this patient's ruptured aorta has been successfully treated to date with an endovascular graft placed directly across the defect. Please do not mention this, because it may tarnish my image as one who is uniformly opposed to endovascular therapy.

Vascular Involvement in Behçet's Disease: 8-Year Audit
Kuzu MA, Özaslan C, Köksoy C, Gürler A (Univ of Ankara, Turkey)
World J Surg 18:948–954, 1994   145-96-4-16

Background.—Behçet's disease is a multisystem disorder, the hallmarks of which are recurrent ulceration of the oral cavity and genitals and relapsing iritis. In addition, both arteries and veins may be involved, resulting in arterial and venous occlusions, aneurysm formation, and the development of varices. From 7% to 29% of cases have been reported to have vascular involvement.

Objective.—The frequency of vascular disease was determined in 1,200 patients with Behçet's disease seen from 1983 to 1992.

Findings.—Venous manifestations were present in 14.4% of patients and arterial involvement in 1.6% (table). Venous thrombosis was by far the most common venous manifestation of Behçet's disease. Twenty-two patients had superior or inferior vena cava syndrome, and 5 had varices. Arterial aneurysms most frequently involved the femoral artery. Three patients had arterial occlusions.

Conclusion.—Behçet's disease should be considered when a young adult patient with either venous or arterial abnormalities is seen by a vascular surgeon.

▶ Patients with Behçet's disease are prone to arterial and venous thrombosis as well as aneurysm formation. This remarkable paper describes the follow-up of 1,200 patients with this condition from Turkey. Without ques-

Details of Patients With Vascular Involvement		
Parameter	Venous involvement	Arterial involvement
No. of patients	173* (14.4%)	19* (1.6%)
No. of cases	181	22
Age (years)	33 (17–170)	35 (22–60)
Duration of Behçet's disease (years)	6 (1–5)	5 (1–16)
Male/female	142/31	17/2

Results are expressed as the median and range.
* Some patients had more than 1-system involvement.
(Courtesy of Kuzu MA, Özaslan C, Köksoy C, et al: Vascular involvement in Behçet's disease: 8-Year audit. *World J Surg* 18:948–954, 1994. Copyright 1994, Springer-Verlag.)

tion, the most frequent vascular event in these patients was venous thrombosis, which occurred in 15%. Arterial thrombosis was uncommon, and aneurysm formation was rare. Although this paper presents no new insights into this disease, it does give a good account of the relative frequency with which various vascular abnormalities are present and, as such, is an important epidemiologic paper.

Intermittent Claudication Due to Spinal Stenosis in a Vascular Surgical Practice
Stansby G, Evans G, Shieff C, Hamilton G (Royal Free Hosp School of Medicine, London)
J R Coll Surg Edinb 39:83–85, 1994   145-96-4–17

Introduction.—Patients with intermittent claudication experience a delayed limping that is not present with the first steps. This complaint is usually associated with occlusive arterial disease, but it may be associated with spinal canal stenosis. In a retrospective study, the frequency and nature of intermittent claudication caused by spinal stenosis was assessed.

Methods.—The records of 271 patients referred to a vascular surgeon over 26 months with intermittent claudication were reviewed. The patients were assessed clinically and were evaluated to establish or exclude the diagnosis of vascular claudication.

Results.—In 21 of the 271 patients (87%), spinal claudication was confirmed with CT or CT myelography. There were no statistically significant differences between the patients with and without spinal stenosis with respect to gender or age. However, there were significantly fewer smokers among the patients with spinal claudication. The presenting complaints in the spinal claudication group included sensory symptoms such as numbness or paresthesias in 62%, back pain in 38%, and leg pain when walking in 67%. These symptoms were bilateral in 71% of the patients. Reduced Doppler pressures were noted in 29%.

Discussion.—There was an 8% incidence of intermittent claudication because of spinal stenosis in this population. Both spinal and vascular claudication occurred primarily in elderly patients. Although patients may have congenital spinal canal stenosis, symptoms usually do not occur without the addition of acquired degenerative disease. Sensory symptoms or back pain, or both, in addition to the cramping leg pain suggest the possibility of spinal canal stenosis, even though these patients will not usually have neurologic abnormalities. However, both vascular disease and spinal stenosis may occur concurrently, thereby complicating diagnosis.

▶ In 1 vascular consultant's practice, an unbelievable 8% of patients referred for claudication ultimately had spinal stenosis diagnosed. I think we have seen 1 such patient in our most recent 1,000 claudicants. This is really an epidemiologic paper, attempting to give the relative frequency with which this uncommon condition occurs. The prevalence cited in this article is dramatically greater than what we see. It must be noted that spinal stenosis is not the only cause of neurogenic claudication. Any lesion of the cauda equina may produce the condition. Some of the less common lesions include tumor, hemangioma, etc. The finding of an atypical claudication history with a prolonged recovery time, especially if associated with relief when bending forward at the waist, and a normal arterial examination, including normal ankle pressure recovery after treadmill, must lead to consideration for an imaging study of the lumbar spine. This is another classic condition that shows up far more often on board examinations than in the clinic.

Interferon-Alpha-2a for the Treatment of Complex Hemangiomas of Infancy and Childhood
Ricketts RR, Hatley RM, Corden BJ, Sabio H, Howell CG (Emory Univ, Atlanta, Ga; Med College of Georgia, Atlanta)
Ann Surg 219:605–614, 1994   145-96-4–18

Background.—Hemangiomas, the most frequent tumors in infants and children, most often grow rapidly until the infant is aged 6–8 months and then stabilize and begin to involute in the second year of life. Complete resolution occurs in 90% of all cases by age 10 years. Hemangiomas that do not follow this course may threaten vital organs and extremities and are associated with a 20% to 50% mortality. Typically, aggressive treatment has included high-dose steroids, arterial ligation, or surgical resection. Each of these treatments may present serious risks to, or may be ineffective with, some individuals. The results of treating 5 patients with complex hemangiomas with interferon-α2a were reviewed.

Patients and Methods.—The 4 infants and 1 child were aged 4 weeks to 28 months. Three patients were male and 2 were female. Three were white and 2 were black. All had complex hemangiomas. Two of these patients had received prior therapy, 1 with compression, and 1 with prednisone plus blood product replacement therapy. Interferon-α2a was administered subcutaneously at a beginning dose of 1 million units m^2/day over 1 week. The dose was then advanced over 1 week to 3 million units/m^2/day. Therapy was continued for 5–11 months based on the response of the lesion to treatment.

Result.—Three of the 5 patients had total or near total regression (Fig 4–16), 1 had partial regression, and 1 had stabilization after 6 months of treatment but no regression. In this patient, the lesion was ablated with 3 KTP laser treatments. A severe consumptive coagulopathy resolved immediately after the initiation of therapy in 1 patient. All patients have grown and developed normally and there have been no recurrences after a mean follow-up of 9.25 months. Minor, transient side effects occurred in 2 patients.

Conclusions.—These findings are in agreement with those of other studies supporting the effectiveness of interferon-α2a in treating complex

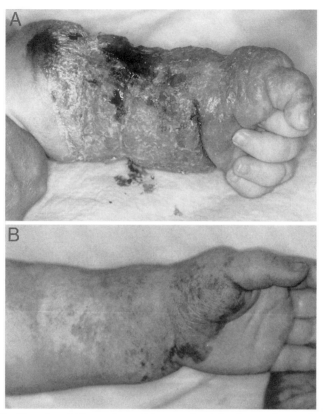

Fig 4-16.—Circumferential hemangioma of the arm of an infant boy, aged 6 months, before (**A**) therapy and after (**B**) completion of therapy with interferon-α2a. (Courtesy of Ricketts RR, Hatley RM, Corden BJ, et al: Interferon-α-2a for the treatment of complex hemangiomas of infancy and childhood. *Ann Surg* 219:605–614, 1994.)

hemangiomas. It is recommended that interferon-α2a be considered as the first-line agent in the treatment of complex hemangiomas of infants and children.

▶ See also the comment after Abstract 145-96-1–49. Since the first report of the use of interferon-α2a for the treatment of hemangioma in 1989, this treatment has attracted a great deal of attention. It is known that steroids are occasionally successful in these patients, and it is noted in the comment after Abstract 145-96-1–49 that antiangiogenesis factor is also being considered. The obvious reason all of these medical therapies are undergoing active investigation is because there is no good surgery for this condition. I am sure we will hear more about this interesting subject in the future.

Aspirin Use and the Risk for Colorectal Cancer and Adenoma in Male Health Professionals

Giovannucci E, Rimm EB, Stampfer MJ, Colditz GA, Ascherio A, Willett WC (Harvard Med School, Boston; Brigham and Women's Hosp, Boston; Harvard School of Public Health, Boston)
Ann Intern Med 121:241–246, 1994   145-96-4–19

Objective.—The evidence to date that nonsteroidal anti-inflammatory drugs reduce the risk of colorectal cancer, and possibly other gastrointestinal tumors, remains inconclusive. This purported association was examined in a prospective cohort study.

Methods.—A total of 47,900 male health professionals throughout the United States, who were aged 40–75 years, responded to a questionnaire mailed to them in 1986. Nearly 60% of those eligible were dentists and 20% were veterinarians. Optometrists, osteopaths, podiatrists, and pharmacists formed the rest of the cohort. Questionnaires concerning cancer and the use of aspirin were again sent in 1988 and 1990.

Findings.—There were 251 new diagnoses of colorectal cancer during the study. The regular use of aspirin at least twice a week was associated with a total relative risk (RR) for colorectal cancer of .68. The RR of metastatic or fatal colorectal cancer was .51. These risk estimates were observed after controlling for age, history of polyps, previous endoscopy, parental history of colorectal cancer, smoking, body mass, level of physical activity, and the intake of red meat, alcohol, and vitamin E. Men who were regular users of aspirin in 1986 continued to have a lower risk of colorectal cancer when followed up to 1992, regardless of subsequent aspirin use (table). When those who had endoscopy for fecal blood were excluded, men who used aspirin were at lower risk of being diagnosed as having a colorectal adenoma.

Conclusion.—Men who use aspirin regularly over the long term may be at substantially lower risk for colorectal cancer. Further work is needed to determine the effective dose of aspirin and how long it must be used.

▶ I though this article was sufficiently interesting to include in the YEAR BOOK, although I did not really know where to place it. I think it is fascinating

Relative Risk for Colorectal Cancer in Subsequent Periods, by Aspirin Use in 1986

Aspirin Use in 1986	Follow-up		
	1986 to 1987	1988 to 1989	1990 to 1992
Total colorectal cancer Age-adjusted RR (95% CI)	0.78 (0.46 to 1.32)	0.72 (0.51 to 1.02)	0.67 (0.41 to 1.08)
Advanced colorectal cancer* Age-adjusted RR (95% CI)	0.50 (0.21 to 1.22)	0.50 (0.27 to 0.91)	0.43 (0.18 to 1.04)
Fatal colorectal cancer Age-adjusted RR (95% CI)	0.42 (0.15 to 1.18)	0.57 (0.24 to 1.37)	0.18 (0.03 to 1.00)

* Patients with advanced cancers are those with metastases at diagnosis plus fatal cases.
(Courtesy of Giovannucci E, Rimm EB, Stampfer MJ, et al: Aspirin use and the risk for colorectal cancer and adenoma in male health professionals. *Ann Intern Med* 121:241–246, 1994.)

to note that the regular use of simple aspirin (2 times per week or less) is associated with a clearly decreased risk for colorectal cancer. In the absence of aspirin allergy or upper gastrointestinal bleeding, it seems that we should strongly consider regular use of aspirin both for ourselves and our patients. The low dose of 80 mg given once daily appears adequate.

Call Mosby Document Express at **1 (800) 55-MOSBY** to obtain copies of the original source documents of articles featured or referenced in the YEAR BOOK series.

5 Perioperative Considerations

Coronary Disease

Surgical Therapy for Coronary Artery Disease Among Patients With Combined Coronary Artery and Peripheral Vascular Disease

Rihal CS, Eagle KA, Mickel MC, Foster ED, Sopko G, Gersh BJ (Mayo Clinic and Mayo Found, Rochester, Minn; Massachusetts General Hosp, Boston; Univ of Washington, Seattle; et al)

Circulation 91:46–53, 1995   145-96-5–1

Study Population.—A retrospective cohort analysis was done based on 1,834 patients in the Coronary Artery Surgery Study registry who had both coronary artery disease, with at least 1 operable vessel, and clinically diagnosed peripheral vascular or cerebrovascular disease. Of the patients, 80% were men; the mean patient, age was 56 years. Coronary bypass surgery was nonrandomly done in 986 patients, whereas 848 patients were managed medically. None of the former patients had previous cardiac surgery.

Results.—The perioperative mortality rate was 4.2%. Of 1,100 deaths occurring during an average follow-up of 10.4 years, 80% were from cardiovascular causes. The survival rates at 4–16 years were significantly higher in the surgical group (Fig 5–1). On multivariate analysis, the type of treatment was independently predictive of survival. Benefit of surgery was limited to patients with triple-vessel coronary artery disease and was inversely correlated with the preoperative ejection fraction. Significantly more patients who had surgery lived without myocardial infarction.

Conclusion.—Coronary revascularization improves the long-term outcome in patients who have both coronary artery disease and peripheral vascular disease.

▶ What we have here, dear reader, is a classic example of post hoc analysis. The patients with peripheral vascular disease in the Coronary Artery Surgery Study have been retrospectively analyzed according to whether they underwent coronary bypass. Keep in mind that this was not a prospective end point of the study and that these patients were not stratified for peripheral vascular disease during randomization. The authors claim to find increased

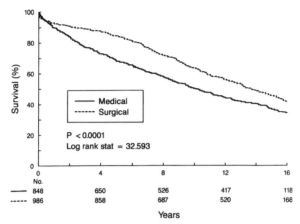

Fig 5–1.—Kaplan-Meier estimated probability of survival among 1,834 patients with peripheral vascular disease enrolled in the Coronary Artery Surgery Study registry. The survival curve is adjusted for the number of diseased coronary arteries. (Courtesy of Rihal CS, Eagle KA, Mickel MC, et al: Surgical therapy for coronary artery disease among patients with combined coronary artery and peripheral vascular disease. *Circulation* 91:46–53, 1995. Reproduced with permission. *Circulation.* Copyright 1995, American Heart Association.)

survival in the coronary bypass cohort within this group of patients with vascular disease. It is important to note that post hoc analysis can only be used as a hypothesis-seeking—never, never a hypothesis-proving—exercise. In return for this clear demonstration of a lack of understanding of the basic tenets of clinical research, I award these authors the prestigious Camel Dung Award.

A Randomized Trial Comparing Coronary Angioplasty With Coronary Bypass Surgery
King SB III, for the Emory Angioplasty Versus Surgery Trial (EAST) (Emory Univ, Atlanta, Ga)
N Engl J Med 331:1044–1050, 1994   145-96-5-2

Objective.—A comparison of the clinical outcome after percutaneous transluminal coronary angioplasty (PTCA) with that after coronary artery bypass grafting (CABG) in patients with multivessel coronary disease was made in a 3-year prospective, randomized trial. The Emory Angioplasty Versus Surgery Trial was a single-center study that enrolled patients being referred for the first time for coronary revascularization.

Study Population.—Of 5,118 patients screened for inclusion in the trial, 842 were eligible and 392 agreed to participate. Of these, 194 patients were assigned to CABG and 198 to PTCA. Baseline characteristics were comparable in the 2 groups. Forty percent of all participants had triple-vessel coronary artery disease; 80% had Canadian Cardiovascular Society class III or class IV angina. Mean ejection fraction was 61%.

Results.—Angioplasty reduced stenosis by 20% or more and left less than 50% residual stenosis in 88% of treated vessels, and all treated

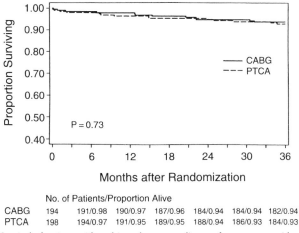

No. of Patients/Proportion Alive

CABG	194	191/0.98	190/0.97	187/0.96	184/0.94	184/0.94	182/0.94
PTCA	198	194/0.97	191/0.95	189/0.95	188/0.94	186/0.93	184/0.93

Fig 5-2.—Survival of patients with multivessel coronary disease after treatment with coronary artery bypass grafting (*CABG*) or percutaneous transluminal coronary angioplasty (*PTCA*). The number of patients at risk and the estimated probability of surival are shown below the figure for each 6-month interval. (Reprinted by permission of King SB III, for the Emory Angioplasty Versus Surgery Trial (EAST): A randomized trial comparing coronary angioplasty with coronary bypass surgery. *N Engl J Med* 331:1044-1050, 1994. Copyright 1994, Massachusetts Medical Society.)

arteries were dilated in 77% of patients. One patient died in relation to bypass surgery, and 10% of patients in the CABG group had a Q-wave infarction. Mortality in the PTCA group also was 1%, and 3% of patients had myocardial infarction. Deaths from all causes were comparably frequent in the 2 treatment groups (Fig 5-2). Only 1 patient in the CABG

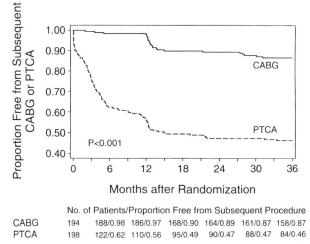

No. of Patients/Proportion Free from Subsequent Procedure

CABG	194	188/0.98	186/0.97	168/0.90	164/0.89	161/0.87	158/0.87
PTCA	198	122/0.62	110/0.56	95/0.49	90/0.47	88/0.47	84/0.46

Fig 5-3.—Proportion of patients remaining free from coronary artery bypass grafting (CABG) or percutaneous transluminal coronary angioplasty (PTCA) after the initial revascularization procedure. The number of patients at risk and the estimated probability of survival are shown below the figure for each specified 6-month period. (Reprinted by permission of King SB III, for the Emory Angioplasty Versus Surgery Trial (EAST): A randomized trial comparing coronary angioplasty with coronary bypass surgery. *N Engl J Med* 331:1044-1050, 1994. Copyright 1994, Massachusetts Medical Society.)

group required further surgery, but PTCA patients required 42 operations during 3 years of follow-up (Fig 5–3). At 3 years, 75% of CABG patients and 51% of those in the PTCA group had revascularization of 80% or more index segments. Cardiac function was comparable in the 2 groups, and there were no differences in activity level or work status.

Conclusion.—The choice between CABG and PTCA for multivessel coronary artery disease should be based on the patient's preference and on the possible need for subsequent procedures.

▶ These authors have the laudable intent of objectively comparing coronary angioplasty with coronary bypass surgery. In many ways, this may be like attempting to compare nephropexy to hysteropexy. They conclude that in a prospectively randomized series, the CABG group and the PTCA group generally behave about the same, although the PTCA group required more touch-up procedures, as one may predict. My present opinion is that coronary angioplasty is a fairly good procedure for patients who do not need very much, but it has a limited duration of action. Coronary bypass appears better, but I wonder by how much? See also the comment after Abstract 145-96-5–3.

A Randomized Study of Coronary Angioplasty Compared With Bypass Surgery in Patients With Symptomatic Multivessel Coronary Disease
Hamm CW, for the German Angioplasty Bypass Surgery Investigation (Univ Hosp Eppendorf, Hamburg, Germany; Klinikum Bogenhausen, Munich; Univ of Mainz, Germany)
N Engl J Med 331:1037–1043, 1994   145-96-5–3

Introduction.—Coronary artery bypass grafting (CABG) has become standard therapy for symptomatic patients with multivessel coronary artery disease. Percutaneous transluminal coronary angioplasty (PTCA), which is standard for symptomatic patients with single-vessel disease, also has been extended to selected patients with multivessel disease. The two alternatives were compared in a randomized study of patients with multivessel disease who required complete revascularization.

Methods.—Of 8,981 patients with multivessel coronary artery disease at 8 centers screened for inclusion in the German Angioplasty Bypass Surgery Investigation, 359 were randomized to undergo CABG or PTCA. All patients needed complete revascularization of at least 2 major vessels supplying different regions of the myocardium, and all procedures were judged clinically necessary and technically feasible. The patients received the routine surgical or angioplastic care at their hospital; decisions made during the procedures and throughout follow-up were left to the discretion of the treating physicians. The outcomes of the 2 groups were compared 1 year after the procedures.

Results.—The CABG group underwent grafting of an average of 2.2 vessels, and the PTCA group had dilation of an average of 1.9 vessels. The median hospitalization was 19 days with CABG vs. 5 days with PTCA.

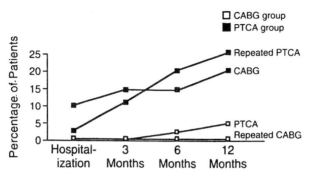

Fig 5–4.—Rate of further interventions (coronary artery bypass grafting [*CABG*] or percutaneous transluminal coronary angioplasty [*PTCA*] in the 2 treatment groups during the initial hospitalization and 3, 6, and 12 months later. (Reprinted with permission of Hamm CW, for the German Angioplasty Bypass Surgery Investigation: A randomized study of coronary angioplasty compared with bypass surgery in patients with multivessel coronary artery disease. *N Engl J Med* 331:1037–1043, 1994. Copyright 1994, Massachusetts Medical Society.)

The procedure was associated with Q-wave myocardial infarction in 8% of the CABG group vs. 2% of the PTCA group. There was no significant difference in inhospital mortality: 2.5% with CABG and 1% with PTCA. Discharge assessments showed freedom from angina in 93% of the CABG group vs. 82% of the PTCA group.

In the year after the procedure, 44% of the PTCA group required further interventions: repeat PTCA in 23%, CABG in 18%, and both in 3%. In contrast, only 6% of the CABG group required repeat procedures: repeat CABG in 1% and PTCA in 5% (Fig 5–4). One-year follow-up assessments showed freedom from angina in 74% of the CABG group and 71% of the PTCA group. Both groups had comparable improvements in exercise capacity, although significantly more patients in the CABG group (22%) did not require antianginal medications compared with PTCA group (12%).

Conclusions.—For properly selected patients with symptomatic multivessel coronary artery disease, CABG and PTCA yield approximately equal improvements in angina after 1 year of follow-up. However, patients undergoing PTCA are more likely to require further interventions and antianginal medications to achieve the same outcome as those undergoing CABG. On the other hand, patients undergoing CABG are more likely to have an acute myocardial infarction during the procedure. The findings will be useful in clinical decision-making; the results will be assessed again at 5 and 10 years' follow-up.

▶ See the comment after Abstract 145-96-5-2. In this rather small prospective, randomized series, angioplasty and CABG again resulted in equivalent improvement in angina after 1 year. Again, the PTCA patients were more likely to require additional interventions than were the CABG patients.

Effect of Coronary Artery Bypass Graft Surgery on Survival: Overview of 10-Year Results From Randomised Trials by the Coronary Artery Bypass Graft Surgery Trialists Collaboration

Yusuf S, Zucker D, Peduzzi P, Fisher LD, Takaro T, Kennedy JW, Davis K, Killip T, Passamani E, Norris R, Morris C, Mathur V, Varnauskas E, Chalmers TC (National Heart, Lung, and Blood Inst, Bethesda, Md; McMaster Univ, Hamilton, Ontario, Canada; Hebrew Univ, Jerusalem; et al)
Lancet 344:563–570, 1994   145-96-5-4

Objective.—Mortality data were reviewed from 7 randomized trials comparing initial coronary artery bypass graft (CABG) surgery with medical treatment in patients with stable coronary heart disease. In these patients, angina by itself did not make surgery necessary, and there was no history of myocardial infarction.

Study Population.—In the years 1972–1984, a total of 1,324 patients were randomized to undergo CABG surgery and 1,325 to receive medical treatment initially.

Results.—One fourth of the patients initially assigned to medical care had undergone CABG surgery at 5 years, one third after 7 years, and 41% at 10 years. All but 6% of the patients assigned to surgery in fact underwent surgery. Patients who had surgery had significantly lower mortality than those given medical treatment at all intervals (Fig 5–5). Patients with left main coronary artery disease and those at the highest risk, both clinically and angiographically, benefited most from CABG surgery.

▶ The only reason for performing extensive coronary testing in patients preparing to undergo vascular surgery is that you must believe that the discovery and treatment of significant coronary disease will either reduce

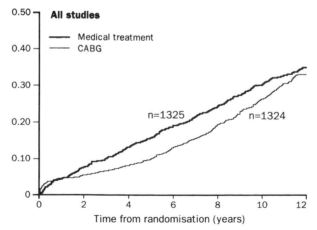

Fig 5–5.—Survival curve for the overall population. (Courtesy of Yusef S, Zucker D, Peduzzi P, et al: Effect of coronary artery bypass graft surgery on survival: Overview of 10-year results from randomised trials by the coronary artery bypass graft surgery trialists collaboration. *Lancet* 3444:563–570, 1994. Copyright 1994, The Lancet Ltd.)

the mortality associated with the subsequent vascular procedure or prolong life. Unfortunately, it does not reduce mortality, as convincingly shown in many studies, including our own (1). Prolongation of life is a very sticky topic. You can see my opinion of the data presented by the group in the comment after Abstract 145-96-5-1. This particular paper is a bit better in that survival was an identified end point of the studies and a number of studies were analyzed using the meta-analysis technique. These studies, however, are compromised by having been done in the 1970s, the presence of 41% crossover to surgery of the medical limb, and the fact that almost all the patients were relatively young males.

Whether any of these data are relevant to the vascular surgery population is highly speculative. Nonetheless, these authors found about a 5% improvement in survival at each analytic point up to 10 years, with most of the benefit being in patients with left main disease or multivessel disease. For the reasons listed, these data are suspect, and the benefits, if present at all, are minimal. I continue to be unimpressed by the objective benefits of extensive routine preoperative coronary evaluation in vascular patients.

Incidentally, it is interesting to note that what these preoperative studies detect is high-grade coronary stenosis. What we think kills people with fatal myocardial infarction is mid-range stenosis associated with an unstable plaque that ruptures and causes thrombosis. Therefore, what these studies are detecting is probably not what really is killing people with coronary disease. Nonetheless, the entire field has provided employment for generations of cardiologists and cardiac surgeons. Why should I stand in the way of economic progress?

Reference

1. Taylor LM, et al: The incidence of perioperative myocardial infarction in general vascular surgery. *J Vasc Surg* 15:52–61, 1992.

Left Ventricular Dysfunction During Infrarenal Abdominal Aortic Aneurysm Repair
Gillespie DL, Connelly GP, Arkoff HM, Dempsey AL, Hilkert RJ, Menzoian JO
(Boston Univ)
Am J Surg 168:144–147, 1994   145-96-5-5

Background.—In patients undergoing surgical repair of an abdominal aortic aneurysm (AAA), pulmonary artery occlusion pressure (PAOP) may underestimate the resuscitative volumes needed before the aortic cross-clamp is released. The pressure-volume relationships associated with the repair of an AAA were examined.

Methods.—The study included 22 patients who were undergoing AAA repair. All had simultaneous monitoring of PAOP with a pulmonary artery catheter (PAC) and estimated left ventricular diastolic volume with the use of two-dimensional transesophageal echocardiography (TEE). Both the

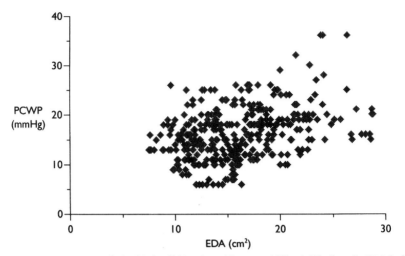

Fig 5–6.—Pressure-area relationship for all 22 patients. (Courtesy of Gillespie DL, Connelly GP, Arkoff HM, et al: Left ventricular dysfunction during infrarenal abdominal aortic aneurysm repair. *Am J Surg* 168:144–147, 1994. Reprinted with permission from *American Journal of Surgery.*)

PAC and TEE data were collected before, during, and after aortic occlusion. The TEE cross-sectional images were made at the midpapillary level.

Results.—Overall, there was a weak correlation between the PAOP and the left ventricular end-diastolic area (LVEDA) (Fig 5–6). There was a wide variation in LVEDA at a given PAOP value, even for individual patients. As the operation proceeded, the correlation between PAOP and LVEDA weakened further. It was strongest before aortic cross-clamping, weaker during cross-clamping, and weaker still after unclamping.

Conclusions.—In patients undergoing AAA, the correlation between PAOP and LVEDA is not strong. The strength of this correlation decreases during surgery, especially after release of the aortic cross-clamp. This may result from changes in LV compliance. Valuable help in guiding volume resuscitation during AAA repair may be obtained through TEE monitoring.

▶ These authors raise the interesting question of whether we should continue to use pulmonary artery wedge pressure to guide fluid resuscitation during infrarenal aortic surgery. They find that TEE-determined LVEDA varies widely for a given pulmonary artery pressure. The 2 correlate even worse during aortic clamping and unclamping. The authors recommend TEE as a valuable adjunct in guiding volume resuscitation in patients undergoing AAA repair. I find this an interesting area of research, but I am not sure of its relevance. We have not recognized any particular difficulties in fluid management during aneurysm surgery. Although we may be overlooking a great many potential problems, they have not evolved into actual difficulties. It frightens me to give anesthesiologists yet 1 more gadget to play with and bill for when they should be paying attention to the patient.

Late Survival After Perioperative Myocardial Infarction Complicating Vascular Surgery

Yeager RA, Moneta GL, Edwards JM, Taylor LM Jr, McConnell DB, Porter JM (Oregon Health Sciences Univ, Portland; Portland Veterans Affairs Med Ctr, Ore)

J Vasc Surg 20:598–606, 1994   145-96-5–6

Background.—In patients undergoing vascular surgery, perioperative myocardial infarction (PMI) is a serious and potentially fatal complication. However, there are few data on the long-term outcomes of patients who survive PMI. Cardiac outcomes and survival in peripheral vascular surgery patients with symptomatic and asymptomatic nonfatal PMI were studied prospectively.

Methods.—From 1989 to 1992, all vascular surgery patients were monitored for PMI by using serial creatine kinase and myocardial band isoenzyme measures and ECG. Those PMIs associated with chest pain, arrhythmia, congestive heart failure, or hypotension were categorized as symptomatic, whereas those detected by biochemical measurements or ECG only were categorized as asymptomatic. When PMI occurred, the patients were monitored prospectively. The late survival of patients with and without PMI was compared.

Results.—Forty-seven of the 1,561 major peripheral vascular procedures performed were associated with PMIs, for an incidence of 3%. There were 11 fatal and 31 nonfatal PMIs; 5 other patients with PMI died of non–heart-related causes during their operation. Eight of the 31 patients with nonfatal PMIs were identified solely on the basis of creatine kinase and myocardial band isoenzyme elevation. The mean follow-up was 28 months. During this time, patients with nonfatal PMI had higher rates of subsequent myocardial infarction and coronary artery revascularization. However, there were no significant differences in survival: 1-year survival was 80% for patients with and 90% for those without PMI, and the 4-year survival rate was 51% and 60%, respectively (Fig 5–7). The clinical course of patients with "chemical" PMI was similar to that of controls.

Conclusions.—The risk of subsequent adverse cardiac events and coronary artery revascularization is increased for peripheral vascular surgery patients who have a nonfatal PMI. However, survival at 1 and 4 years is similar for patients with and without PMI. When the PMI is asymptomatic (detected by biochemical measurements only) the outcome is similar to that of patients without PMI. Such "chemical" PMIs may thus be of little clinical significance.

▶ In this study, our group's Dr. Yeager asks the haunting question, "What happens to vascular surgery patients who have the misfortune to suffer a PMI?" Eleven of 47 patients who had a PMI died, for a mortality rate of 23%, which is considerably less than the 50% frequently quoted for PMI. During follow-up for a mean of almost 28 months, there was a higher incidence of both subsequent myocardial infarction and coronary artery bypass among

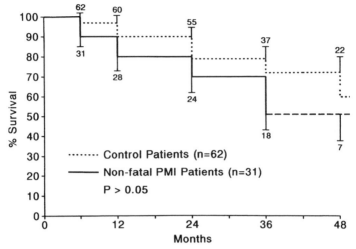

Fig 5–7.—Long-term survival of patients with perioperative myocardial infarction (*PMI*), compared with control patients, as determined by life-table analysis. (*Courtesy of Yeager RA, Moneta GL, Edwards JM, et al: Late survival after perioperative myocardial infarction complicating vascular surgery.* J Vasc Surg 20:598–606, 1994.)

the patients with nonfatal PMI compared with controls; however, survival was not different. The lack of a survival difference through 4 years is interesting and continues to indicate to us the absence of any pressing need for extensive preoperative coronary evaluation in vascular surgery patients.

Is There Detrimental Gender Bias in Preoperative Cardiac Management of Patients Undergoing Vascular Surgery?

Hutchinson LA, Pasternack PF, Baumann FG, Grossi EA, Riles TS, Lamparello PJ, Giangola G, Adelman M, Imparato AM (New York Univ)
Circulation 90:II220–II223, 1994   145-96-5–7

Background.—Past studies have raised the possibility that gender-driven differences in the assessment and management of patients with coronary artery disease may help explain the higher hospital mortality rates recorded in women having angioplasty, coronary atherectomy, and coronary bypass surgery.

Methods.—This possibility was examined by reviewing the management and outcome of 350 men and 128 women who had peripheral vascular surgery and were monitored perioperatively for myocardial ischemia.

Results.—The men and women were similar in age at the time of surgery and had comparably frequent and lengthy episodes of silent myocardial ischemia. Nevertheless, significantly fewer women than men had undergone coronary bypass surgery (6% vs. 17%). Perioperative infarction occurred in 4% of each group. Actuarial analysis showed that, 2 years

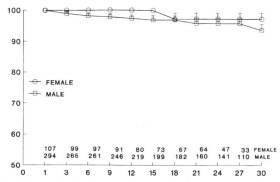

Fig 5–8.—Actuarial rates of survival, expressed as months after operation and percentage of patients, from late cardiac death for male and female patients who underwent peripheral vascular surgery. (Courtesy of Hutchinson LA, Pasternack PF, Baumann FG, et al: Is there detrimental gender bias in preoperative cardiac management of patients undergoing vascular surgery? *Circulation* 90:II220–II223, 1994. Reproduced with permission. *Circulation.* Copyright 1994, American Heart Association)

postoperatively, 80% of women and 72% of men had escaped late cardiac death (Fig 5–8) and nonfatal cardiac-related events (Fig 5–9).

Conclusion.—Although sex bias in preoperative cardiac management may not have compromised the long-term cardiac outcome in these women, even better results might have been achieved had more of them undergone cardiac revascularization.

▶ Here it is again ladies and gentlemen, that rare politically correct article. As I have previously stated, if you can find any suspicion of sex bias in a patient cohort, you have a guarantee of automatic publication. Is there really a sex bias in the preoperative cardiac management of patients undergoing vascular surgery? My response to the haunting question asked by the

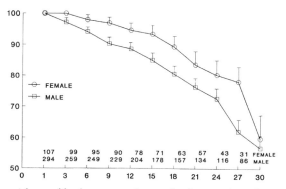

Fig 5–9.—Actuarial rates of freedom, expressed as months after operation and percentage of patients, from late cardiac-related adverse events other than late cardiac death for male and female patients who underwent peripheral vascular surgery. (Courtesy of Hutchinson LA, Pasternack PF, Baumann FG, et al: Is there detrimental gender bias in preoperative cardiac management of patients undergoing vascular surgery? *Circulation* 90:II220–II223, 1994. Reproduced with permission. *Circulation.* Copyright 1994, American Heart Association.)

authors is the same as that of the bright-eyed young man who, when asked the difference between ignorance and apathy, promptly answered "I don't know and I don't care."

Effects of Captopril on Ischemic Events After Myocardial Infarction: Results of the Survival and Ventricular Enlargement Trial
Rutherford JD, on behalf of the SAVE Investigators (Univ of Texas Southwestern Med Ctr, Dallas)
Circulation 90:1731–1738, 1994   145-96-5–8

Background.—Survivors of myocardial infarction (MI) are at increased risk of nonfatal and fatal ischemic events. In the Survival and Ventricular Enlargement (SAVE) trial, recurrent MI was the most prominent predictor of a poor outcome; it increased the risk of death sevenfold.

Methods.—Predictors of recurrent MI were sought in a series of 2,231 patients who survived the acute phase of MI and a nuclide ventricular ejection fraction of 40% or less, and who were randomly assigned to receive captopril therapy or placebo. They were followed up for an average of 42 months.

Results.—Recurrent MI was relatively likely to occur in patients who had had an MI or who were functionally disabled before the index infarction and in those with higher systolic blood pressure. The baseline left ventricular ejection fraction was not a significant predictive factor. Captopril therapy reduced the risk of recurrent MI by one fourth and the risk of dying after recurrent MI by nearly one third (table). Patients assigned to receive captopril also were less likely to require revascularization, but the rate of unstable angina was unaffected. The overall risk of major ischemic events was reduced by 14% in captopril-treated patients.

Conclusion.—Long-term captopril therapy should help prevent recurrent MI, even in patients whose left ventricular function is relatively well preserved. It also appears to reduce the need for cardiac revascularization.

Effect of Captopril on Ischemic and Morbid Events

No. With Event (%)

Event	Captopril ($n = 1115$)	Placebo ($n = 1116$)	Risk Reduction, % (95% CI)	P
Clinical MI	133 (12)	170 (15)	25 (5–40)	0.015
Clinical MI followed by death	56	80	32 (4–51)	0.029
Fatal MI (died within 10 days of MI)	32	43	28 (⁻14–54)	0.159
Revascularization	154 (14)	195 (17)	24 (6–39)	0.010
Hospitalization for unstable angina	135 (12)	133 (12)	0 (⁻26–22)	0.930
Any of above	327 (29)	363 (33)	14 (0–26)	0.047

Abbreviations: CI, confidence interval; *MI*, myocardial infarction.
(Courtesy of Rutherford JD, on behalf of the SAVE Investigators: Effects of captopril on ischemic events after myocardial infarction: Results of the Survival and Ventricular Enlargement Trial. *Circulation* 90:1731–1738, 1994. Reproduced with permission. *Circulation*. Copyright 1994, American Heart Association.)

► The SAVE trial has shown that survivors of MI with left ventricular dysfunction derive survival benefit from the long-term administration of the angiotensin-converting enzyme (ACE) inhibitor captopril. The purpose of this study was to determine the predictors of recurrent MI in study participants and to examine the effect of captopril on myocardial ischemic events. The authors' conclusions include the interesting observations that recurrence of MI was independent of left ventricular ejection fraction, and that the need for cardiac revascularization was reduced in patients receiving long-term captopril. Although the mechanisms of benefit are not worked out with ' precision, there seems to be little doubt that ACE inhibitors are beneficial after MI.

The Effect of Peripheral Vascular Disease on In-Hospital Mortality Rates With Coronary Artery Bypass Surgery
Birkmeyer JD, for the Northern New England Cardiovascular Disease Study Group (Dartmouth-Hitchcock Med Ctr, Lebanon, NH; Med Ctr Hosp of Vermont, Burlington; Maine Med Ctr, Portland; et al)
J Vasc Surg 21:445–452, 1995   145-96-5–9

Introduction.—Considerable evidence suggests that patients with peripheral vascular disease (PVD) who undergo coronary artery bypass grafting (CABG) have an elevated perioperative mortality rate compared with patients without PVD. This association was addressed by a regional cohort study of patients who had CABG.

Methods.—Demographic, historical, and clinical data were obtained prospectively for 3,003 consecutive patients who had CABG in northern New England during a period of nearly 3 years. Medical records were reviewed retrospectively to confirm comorbidities, including PVD. The causes of inhospital deaths were recorded prospectively. Logistic regression analysis was used to calculate the influence of PVD on inhospital mortality, while adjusting for potential confounders.

Results.—Of 3,003 patients who had CABG, 796 patients (26.5%) had PVD and 2,207 patients (73.5%) did not (table). Carotid bruit was the most common indicator of PVD, followed by a history of claudication and absent pedal pulses. Patients with PVD tended to be older and were more likely to be women than patients without PVD. Patients with subclinical PVD were particularly likely to be women. Patients with PVD were also more likely to have co-morbidity, especially diabetes in those with lower extremity occlusive disease, and indicators of more severe heart disease. Poorer left ventricular function was modestly significant in patients with PVD, and there was more advanced coronary disease in this group. Compared with patients without PVD, patients with PVD had an inhospital mortality rate that was 2.4-fold higher.

Patients who had CABG before a scheduled peripheral vascular procedure had the highest mortality rate (25%). Multivariate analysis adjusting for age, sex, body surface area, ejection fraction, left ventricular end-

Prevalance of PVD and Death in 3,003 Patients Undergoing CABG

	Prevalence		In-hospital deaths	
	n	%	*n*	%
No PVD	2207	73.5	70	3.2
PVD overall	796	26.5	61	7.7
CABG before planned vascular surgery	20	0.7	5	25.0
History of CVA	105	3.5	8	7.6
History of TIA	98	3.3	5	5.1
Prior carotid endarterectomy	108	3.6	8	7.4
Carotid stenosis				
By history alone	28	0.9	1	3.6
Known ≥50% by imaging study	78	2.6	6	7.7
Carotid bruit	334	11.1	27	8.1
History of claudication	238	7.9	19	8.0
Prior lower extremity revascularization	82	2.7	7	43.7
Prior amputation (nontraumatic)	16	0.5	7	43.7
Lower extremity arterial ulcer	13	0.4	1	7.7
Absent pedal pulses				
Unilaterally	103	3.4	7	6.8
Bilaterally	180	6.0	26	14.4
Abdominal aortic aneurysm				
Surgically repaired	26	0.9	3	11.5
Not repaired	31	1.0	2	6.5

Abbreviations: CABG, coronary artery bypass grafting; PVD, peripheral vascular disease.
(Courtesy of Birkmeyer JD, for the Northern New England Cardiovascular Disease Study Group: The effect of peripheral vascular disease on in-hospital mortality rates with coronary artery bypass surgery. *J Vasc Surg* 21:445–452, 1995.)

diastolic pressure, surgical priority, prior CABG, and co-morbidity score revealed that PVD was a significant independent risk factor for inhospital mortality, attributed mainly to the increased risk of lower extremity occlusive disease, which doubled the risk of death. The most common cause of death was cardiac failure in patients with PVD; fatal dysrhythmias were also significantly more common in this group.

Discussion.—The presence of PVD was a substantial independent risk factor for inhospital death after CABG, mainly because of lower extremity occlusive disease. Prophylactic CABG for patients expected to have major peripheral vascular surgery may not improve short-term survival. More study is required to determine the long-term effects of CABG in patients with PVD and to investigate the mechanisms affecting the association between PVD and increased inhospital death in patients who have CABG.

▶ This article concludes that mortality after CABG is increased in patients with PVD and that vascular disease is an independent predictor of CABG mortality. This is a very large study involving several centers and a regional cohort of more than 3,000 patients. I think I already knew its conclusion. Although it is reassuring to have my bias confirmed, isn't it intuitive that patients with diffuse rather than focal occlusive disease are not going to do as well after surgery? Perhaps the most interesting part of this study is the observation that patients with lower extremity disease had an increased risk, whereas those with carotid stenosis did not. That is a little puzzling. Hopefully these authors will continue to put this important database to good use.—W. Abbott, M.D.

▶ Increased CABG mortality in vascular patients is another good reason for staying off the routine coronary screening bandwagon.—J.M. Porter, M.D.

Does Routine Stress-Thallium Cardiac Scanning Reduce Postoperative Cardiac Complications?
Seeger JM, Rosenthal GR, Self SB, Flynn TC, Limacher MC, Harward TRS (Univ of Florida, Gainesville)
Ann Surg 219:654–663, 1994   145-96-5–10

Background.—In patients who require aortic reconstruction but have myocardial ischemia, initial cardiac revascularization may limit the risk of cardiac complications after surgery on the aorta, but this has not been documented. These patients may be identified by stress-thallium myocardial scintigraphy.

Methods.—Stress-thallium myocardial perfusion imaging was performed before operation in 146 patients who required reconstructive surgery on the aorta. Coronary angiography was done when indicated. The outcome was compared with that of 172 similar patients who did not have scintigraphic assessment before surgery.

Results.—Coronary angiography was performed in 41% of the study group, and 11.6% of patients underwent cardiac revascularization. In contrast, only 15% of the comparison patients had coronary angiography and 4% underwent revascularization. Serious cardiac events were more prevalent in patients with fixed perfusion defects on stress-thalium scanning (table), but neither cardiac complications nor cardiac deaths were significantly less frequent than in patients who were not scanned before aortic reconstruction. The only factors that significantly predicted postoperative cardiac events were advanced age and the occurrence of intraoperative complications.

Conclusion.—Significant coronary artery disease is quite prevalent in patients who require aortic reconstruction, but initial coronary bypass surgery does not reduce either the short-term or long-term cardiac mortality.

▶ This nonrandomized study compares the postoperative performance of 146 aortic patients undergoing preoperative stress-thallium cardiac scanning with 172 similar patients without stress-thallium scanning. It is fascinating

Correlation Between Cardiac Events and Stress Thalium Defects

	All Cardiac Events	Serious Cardiac Events
Redistribution ($n = 70$)	22.9%	8.6%
Fixed defect ($n = 25$)	36.0%*	28.0%*
Normal ($n = 49$)	14.3%	6.1%

* Significantly different from both redistribution and normal groups ($P < 0.05$ by exact contingency table analysis).
(Courtesy of Seeger JM, Rosenthal GR, Self SB, et al: Does routine stress-thallium cardiac scanning reduce postoperative cardiac complications? *Ann Surg* 219:654–663, 1994.)

that 41% of the patients undergoing stress-thallium testing underwent coronary arteriography, and 11.6% underwent cardiac revascularization. Cardiac mortality, complications, and long-term mortality were similar in both groups. The authors conclude, appropriately, that prophylactic preoperative cardiac intervention in patients undergoing vascular surgery does not reduce operative or long-term mortality. Dr. Seeger takes the clear position that the risk and expense of routine stress-thallium testing and subsequent cardiac revascularization cannot be justified. Hurrah! He got it right.

Coronary Artery Disease Is Highly Prevalent Among Patients With Premature Peripheral Vascular Disease
Valentine RJ, Grayburn PA, Eichhorn EJ, Myers SI, Clagett GP (Dallas VA Med Ctr; Univ of Texas Southwestern Med Ctr, Dallas)
J Vasc Surg 19:668–674, 1994   145-96-5–11

Background.—The early development of peripheral atherosclerosis in a young adult is very debilitating. A majority of deaths in this population are ascribed to myocardial infarction, but the prevalence of associated coronary artery disease (CAD) in patients with premature peripheral vascular disease remains uncertain.

Methods.—The coronary arteries were evaluated in 59 consecutive male veterans in whom peripheral vascular disease developed in the lower extremity before the age of 45 years. Coronary angiography was done when exercise stress testing was not feasible or when the results were abnormal.

Results.—Forty-three of the 59 patients (71%) were found to have a 50% or greater narrowing of a major coronary artery. Myocardial infarction had occurred in 11 of 17 patients with single-vessel CAD; 3 of 4 with 2-vessel disease; and 18 of 22 with triple-vessel or more extensive disease. Nineteen of the patients with extensive CAD and 4 with single- or 2-vessel disease had undergone either coronary bypass graft surgery or percutaneous transluminal coronary angioplasty. Five patients died during the study, 4 of myocardial infarction and 1 of stroke.

Conclusion.—Young adult males with peripheral vascular disease frequently have CAD develop as well and are at substantial risk of complications.

▶ In recent years, a number of interesting papers by Dr. Valentine and his associates have focused on the patterns and outcomes of arterial occlusive disease in young patients. In 59 consecutive male military veterans younger than 45 years of age with symptomatic peripheral vascular disease, 71% had significant coronary lesions by arteriography. The authors correctly conclude that premature peripheral atherosclerosis is associated with a high prevalence of coronary disease. The authors then make the unsupported, gratuitous recommendation that correction of such disease is highly desirable to minimize subsequent cardiac complications. Unfortunately, no data underly this profound recommendation. Let's face it, available data indicate coronary artery bypass surgery really does not accomplish very much.

**Characteristics of Patients at Risk for Perioperative Myocardial Infarc-
tion After Infrainguinal Bypass Surgery: An Exploratory Study**
Gillespie DL, LaMorte WW, Josephs LG, Schneider T, Floch NR, Menzoian
JO (Boston Univ)
Ann Vasc Surg 9:155–162, 1995   145-96-5–12

Background.—Many patients who undergo infrainguinal bypass surgery have diffuse atherosclerosis, and perioperative myocardial infarction
(MI) is the cause of more than 50% of the operative deaths. A preoperative
cardiac risk evaluation is therefore essential before infrainguinal bypass
surgery, but it is questionable whether all patients need an extensive
cardiac workup. The clinical characteristics that might help in selecting
patients for more extensive cardiac evaluation were sought in an exploratory study.

Methods.—The case-control study included 22 patients with perioperative MI after elective infrainguinal bypass surgery and 191 controls without apparent perioperative MI. In addition to such recognized risk factors
as a history of angina or MI, the association of perioperative MI with the
results of common preoperative laboratory tests, preoperative use of certain medications, and such intraoperative factors as duration of surgery or
type of anesthesia were examined.

Results.—The factors associated with perioperative MI included a history of angina, prior MI, or coronary artery disease; the need for certain
cardiac drugs; higher white blood cell (WBC) counts; ST-segment depression; left bundle-branch block; and long duration of surgery. The independent factors on multiple logistic regression analysis were preoperative
antiarrhythmic medications (odds ratio [OR], 26.4), nitrates (OR, 8.4),
calcium channel blockers (OR, 5.5), and aspirin (OR, 6.8), as well as
ST-segment depression (OR, 11.8), WBC count (OR, 1.27), and duration
of surgery (OR, 2.2/hr).

Conclusions.—In addition to the previously recognized risk factors, the
risk of perioperative MI in patients undergoing infrainguinal bypass surgery was linked to certain cardiac medications, greater WBC counts, and
longer duration of surgery. If incorporated into the routine preoperative
risk assessment, these variables could help in identifying patients who need
more extensive preoperative cardiac evaluation.

▶ Papers such as this one do not help me. I suspect we would all be better
off if multiple logistic regression analysis had never been discovered. Nonetheless, we are informed that a variety of variables predict perioperative MI
in patients undergoing infrainguinal bypass surgery. Some of these variables
include preoperative antiarrhythmic drugs, nitrates, calcium channel blockers, aspirin, ST-segment depression, WBC elevation, and duration of surgery.
The only 1 of these that possibly interests me is duration of surgery. In
recent years, we have consistently used multiple operating teams whenever
practical, which includes virtually every patient with leg bypass, every patient with axillofemoral bypass, and certain patients with aortofemoral by-

pass. Our average operating time is slightly under 2 hours, based almost totally on the use of multiple operating teams. I do believe that short duration of surgery is preferable to long duration of surgery, a conclusion strengthened by advancing age and diminished bladder capacity.

Hypothermia

Hypothermia During Elective Abdominal Aortic Aneurysm Repair: The High Price of Avoidable Morbidity
Bush HL Jr, Hydo LJ, Fischer E, Fantini GA, Silane MF, Barie PS (Cornell Univ, New York)
J Vasc Surg 21:392–402, 1995   145-96-5–13

Background.—Hypothermia is a common occurrence during abdominal aortic aneurysm (AAA) repair. Although hypothermia could help protect tissue during the relative ischemia caused by aortic cross-clamping, it may also be associated with adverse effects involving decreased oxygen delivery at the microcirculatory level. The effects of intraoperative hypothermia on morbidity and mortality after elective abdominal aortic reconstruction were evaluated in a retrospective study.

Methods.—The review included 262 patients undergoing elective AAA repair. Data on core temperature, age, Acute Physiology and Chronic Health Evaluation (APACHE) II and III scores, fluid resuscitation, and perioperative organ dysfunction were collected prospectively. Hypothermia was defined as a temperature of less than 34.5°C.

Results.—The hypothermic and nonhypothermic patients had comparable preoperative risk factors, except that women had a higher risk of hypothermia. In the postoperative period, the APACHE scores were significantly higher in the hypothermia group. Patients with hypothermia who died had significantly longer rewarming times, suggesting that marked hypoperfusion was present. Requirements for fluids, transfusion, vasopressors, and inotropic drugs were all greater in the hypothermic patients. Organ dysfunction occurred in 53% of the hypothermic patients vs. 29% of the nonhypothermic patients. Mortality was 12% vs. 2%. The mean length of stay in the ICU was 9 days for the hypothermic patients vs. 5 days for the nonhypothermic patients, and the mean hospital stay was 24 vs. 15 days, respectively. The only significant predictor of intraoperative hypothermia on multivariate analysis was female sex. Once initial hypothermia had developed, it was a significant predictor of prolonged hypothermia and of organ failure. Death was significantly predicated by organ failure and acute myocardial infarction.

Conclusions.—The occurrence of hypothermia after AAA repair is associated with various physiologic abnormalities and with increased morbidity and mortality. Although there are many possible interacting etiologic factors in patients undergoing aortic surgery, maintenance of body temperature is one that can and should be controlled.

► We avoid hypothermia in our vascular patients, because our operating room air conditioner usually does not work. Just what is the role of hypothermia in clinical surgery? These investigators conclude that in patients undergoing infrarenal aortic aneurysm repairs, hypothermia is clearly detrimental. Patients with hypothermia had greater fluid and transfusion requirements, a greater need for vasopressors and ionotropes, and a significantly higher incidence of organ dysfunction and death. These authors recommend, correctly, that we should make every effort to avoid hypothermia during surgery. The obvious expedients of a warm room, heating blanket, and warmed intravenous fluids come to mind. If your routine postoperative aortic patients have a core temperature below 34°C, you should pay close attention to this information.

Normothermia Versus Hypothermia During Cardiopulmonary Bypass: A Randomized, Controlled Trial
Tönz M, Mihaljevic T, von Segesser LK, Schmid ER, Joller-Jemelka HI, Pei P, Turina MI (Univ Hosp, Zurich, Switzerland)
Ann Thorac Surg 59:137–143, 1995   145-96-5–14

Background.—There is some evidence linking the systemic inflammatory reaction that occurs during cardiopulmonary bypass (CPB) with the systemic perfusion temperature during bypass. Normothermic CPB has become increasingly popular because of the renewed interest in normothermic myocardial protection. The effects of perfusion temperature on the systemic effects of CPB were evaluated in a prospective, randomized study.

Methods.—Thirty patients undergoing elective coronary artery bypass grafting were randomized to receive either normothermic or hypothermic CPB. Temperatures were 36°C in the warm group and 28°C in the cold group. Before, during, and after CPB, the investigators made serial hemodynamic measurements and took blood samples.

Results.—The 2 groups were not significantly different in their need for vasopressors, their urinary output, or their fluid balance during CPB. Despite the lack of difference in vasoactive drug administration, systemic vascular resistance during the early postoperative period was significantly lower in the normothermic group: 880 vs. 1,060 dyne·s·cm^{-5}. Cardiac index was higher in the normothermic group, 3.6 vs. 2.9 L ·min^{-1}·m^{-2}. Patients receiving hypothermic CPB had significantly greater median blood loss—370 vs. 490 mL/m^2 of body surface area—leading to the need for more transfusions of erythrocytes and fresh frozen plasma. Patients in both groups had elevated plasma levels of tumor necrosis factor and soluble tumor necrosis factor during and after CPB.

Conclusions.—In patients undergoing CPB, the temperature of CPB appears to have an important effect on postoperative hemodynamic status and blood loss. No additional adverse systemic effects are noted with normothermic CPB. For selected patients, normothermic CPB appears to be a favorable alternative to hypothermic CPB.

▶ This article is included because it supports the conclusion reached in Abstract 145-96-5–13. The authors of this prospective randomized trial compared hypothermic CPB to normothermic CPB, making multiple appropriate measurements. They, too, find significant benefits in favor of normothermic bypass. We are forced to conclude that hypothermia for almost any type of surgery is losing its attractiveness.

Miscellaneous Topics

The Ankle-Brachial Index as a Predictor of Survival in Patients With Peripheral Vascular Disease
McDermott MM, Feinglass J, Slavensky R, Pearce WH (Northwestern Univ, Chicago)
J Gen Intern Med 9:445–449, 1994   145-96-5–15

Background.—Patients with peripheral vascular disease frequently have advanced atherosclerotic disease in other vascular beds. Patients with an abnormal ankle-brachial index (ABI) reportedly have mortality rates up to 5 times higher than those without atherosclerotic disease in the lower extremity.

Methods.—The ABI was evaluated as a predictor of survival in a retrospective series of 422 patients who had an ABI less than 0.92 when first seen in 1987 and who were followed up through 1991.

Results.—The cumulative probability of survival at 52 months was 69% for patients whose ABIs ranged from 0.5 to 0.91; 62% for those with ABIs of 0.31 to 0.49; and 47% when the ABI was 0.3 or less (Fig 5–10). The relative risk of dying for patients with an ABI of 0.3 or less, compared with those whose ABIs were 0.5 to 0.91, was 1.8. Survival also was compromised by age older than 65 years; congestive heart failure; and a diagnosis of cancer, renal failure, or chronic pulmonary disease.

Conclusion.—The ABI is a reliable means of predicting survival in patients with peripheral vascular disease. Further work will show whether patients with low ABIs will benefit from a workup for coronary or cerebrovascular atherosclerosis or measures to modify coronary risk factors.

▶ It is always a relief to note internists belatedly discovering the wheel. The authors conclude, remarkably, that the ABI in patients with peripheral vascular disease actually correlates with patient survival. That this observation was noted and published by vascular surgeons a decade ago seems to have escaped these authors. For this oversight, I award them an honorable mention Camel Dung Award.

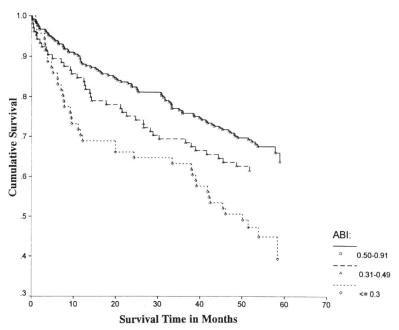

Survival Time in Months

Fig 5–10.—Survival stratified by ankle–brachial index (*ABI*). (Courtesy of McDermott MM, Feinglass J, Slavensky R, et al: The ankle-brachial index as a predictor of survival in patients with peripheral vascular disease. *J Gen Intern Med* 9:445–449, 1994.)

Systemic Hypertension Induced by Aortic Cross-Clamping: Detrimental Effects of Direct Smooth Muscle Relaxation Compared With Ganglionic Blockade

Moursi MM, Facktor MA, Zelenock GB, D'Alecy LG (Univ of Michigan, Ann Arbor)

J Vasc Surg 19:707–716, 1994   145-96-5–16

Background.—When the infrarenal aorta is cross-clamped in the course of vascular reconstruction, systemic hypertension frequently develops above the clamp. Much of the morbidity and some of the deaths associated with cross-clamping are related to hypertension, prompting numerous pharmacologic attempts to minimize the effects of clamp-related hypertension.

Methods.—The efficacy of nitroprusside (NP) and trimethaphan camsylate (TC) was examined in dogs in which aortas were cross-clamped for 90 minutes. Antihypertensive treatment was given for 30 minutes, starting after 30 minutes of cross-clamping.

Results.—The mean arterial pressure increased from 80 mm Hg to 140 mm Hg when the aortic clamp was applied. The pressure returned to preclamp levels in TC-treated animals, but decreased by only about 50% in those given NP, despite the use of substantial doses. The mean (and

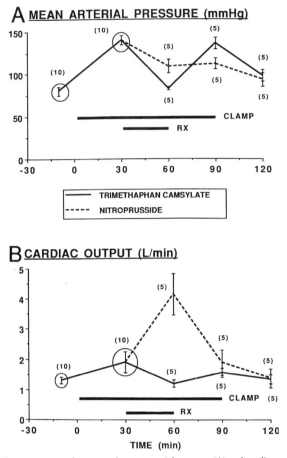

Fig 5–11.—The time course of suprarenal mean arterial pressure (A) and cardiac output (B) before, during, and after application of the infrarenal aortic cross-clamp. Treatment with trimethaphan camsylate (TC) was more effective antihypertensive medication than treatment with NP. Ninety-minute cross-clamp time and 30 minutes of intraoperative drug therapy are indicated as *solid horizontal bars*. Both groups (*n* = 10) are pooled for the preclamp and period A periods and are represented by circles. B shows a dramatic and significant increase in cardiac output in the nitroprusside group. The TC group experienced no significant cardiac output changes. The sample sizes are shown in parentheses. (Courtesy of Moursi MM, Facktor MA, Zelenock GB, et al: Systemic hypertension induced by aortic cross-clamping: Detrimental effects of direct smooth muscle relaxation compared with ganglionic blockade. *J Vasc Surg* 19:707–716, 1994.)

standard error of the mean) values for suprarenal blood pressure for the TC and NP groups are shown in Figure 5–11. Cardiac output increased by 115% in the NP-treated animals, and the cardiac minute work doubled as a result. In the TC group, the cardiac output decreased by 36%.

Conclusion.—The ganglionic blocker TC is preferable to NP in countering the systemic hypertension induced by aortic cross-clamping.

▶ It is always refreshing to see deeply held beliefs challenged. These authors point out that the use of NP to relieve hypertension above an aortic clamp is associated with an increase in cardiac work and cardiac energy requirements, which may be detrimental. In this study, the use of a ganglionic blocker appeared to achieve the same level of superclamp pressure reduction without imposing extra metabolic demands on the heart. The authors suggest that perhaps we should be using the ganglionic blocker clinically. I shall have to think about this.

General Practitioner Referral of Patients With Symptoms of Peripheral Vascular Disease
Michaels JA, Galland RB (Royal Berkshire Hosp, Reading, England)
J R Coll Surg Edinb 39:103–105, 1994   145-96-5-17

Objective.—Because general practitioners are known to vary widely in their referral practices, a questionnaire survey was planned to learn the circumstances prompting them to refer patients with peripheral vascular disease to a district general hospital in England.

Method.—A single-page questionnaire was sent to 100 general practitioners asking about their referral practices for patients with claudication, ischemic rest pain, or an abdominal aortic aneurysm. Replies were received from 77% of those queried.

Results.—More than half of the respondents would not refer a patient, aged 70 years, who had claudication at a half mile, or a patient aged 80 years, having claudication at 100 meters (table). Nearly 45% of the respondents would not refer a patient, aged 80 years, who had a palpable abdominal aneurysm.

Implications.—Many elderly patients who have symptoms of claudication or an asymptomatic abdominal aortic aneurysm are not referred. The remedy, in part, lies in making clinicians more aware of the less invasive treatments now available and of the benefits of aneurysm surgery.

▶ I really did not know where to put this article, so I put it in this section, but at the end. Even though this curious article is not really concerned with traditional vascular surgery, it does address the important issue of referral patterns, a topic with which we are all going to be increasingly concerned in the brave new world of HMOs and managed care. This study indicates a sobering lack of information among general practitioners about peripheral vascular disease.

Although this survey was conducted in England, I am convinced that similar circumstances exist in the United States. For reasons unknown to me, we have selected the least qualified group of doctors in the country (family practitioners) to serve as gatekeepers and case managers for pa-

Number and Type of General Practitioner Referrals for Patients With Various Symptoms of Peripheral Vascular Disease (Percentage of Those Responding)

Type of patient/symptoms	No referral	Routine referral	Urgent referral	Emergency admission
60-year-old with claudication at half a mile	11 (14.5)	59 (77.6)	6 (7.9)	0
70-year-old with claudication at half a mile	40 (52.6)	36 (47.4)	0	0
80-year-old with claudication at half a mile	71 (93.4)	5 (6.58)	0	0
60-year-old with claudication at 100 m	3 (4.1)	36 (48.6)	35 (47.3)	0
70-year-old with claudication at 100 m	8 (10.8)	53 (71.6)	13 (17.6)	0
80-year-old with claudication at 100 m	45 (60.8)	27 (36.5)	2 (2.7)	0
Sudden onset claudication 5 days previously	1 (1.3)	5 (6.6)	63 (82.9)	7 (9.2)
Sudden onset claudication <24 h previously	0	3 (3.95)	23 (30.3)	50 (65.8)
Gradual onset rest pain	4 (5.4)	40 (54.1)	27 (36.5)	3 (4.1)
Sudden onset rest pain 5 days previously	0	1 (1.3)	54 (70.1)	22 (28.6)
Sudden onset rest pain <24 h previously	0	0	10 (13.2)	66 (86.8)
80-year-old with asymptomatic abdominal aneurysm	34 (44.2)	35 (45.5)	8 (10.4)	0
Painful abdominal aortic aneurysm	1 (1.3)	11 (14.5)	36 (47.4)	28 (36.8)

(Courtesy of Michaels JA, Galland RB: General practitioner referral of patients with symptoms of peripheral vascular disease. *J R Coll Surg Edin* 39:103–105, 1994. Reprinted with permission of Blackwell Science, Ltd.)

tients in the HMO future. If we do not have the ability to change this, we had better get busy educating general practitioners about peripheral vascular diseae. At our own institution, we are rarely asked to give any talks to the family practice residents about vascular disease. They know little and appear vacuously unconcerned.

6 Thoracic Aorta

Aortic Arch

Does Routine Use of Aortic Ultrasonography Decrease the Stroke Rate in Coronary Artery Bypass Surgery?
Duda AM, Letwin LB, Sutter FP, Goldman SM (Lankenau Hosp and Med Research Ctr, Wynnewood, Pa)
J Vasc Surg 21:98–109, 1995   145-96-6-1

Background.—Stroke is still a serious and costly complication of coronary artery bypass grafting (CABG). Embolization of unsuspected atheromatous material during manipulation of the ascending aorta is a major cause of stroke in the immediate postoperative period.

Methods.—The value of routine intraoperative surface ultrasound scanning in preventing strokes was examined in 195 consecutive patients who had CABG. A normal aorta is seen in Figure 6–1. Abnormal ultrasound findings (Fig 6–2) prompted changes in surgical technique. The outcome was compared with that in 164 earlier patients in whom the aorta was evaluated only by inspection and palpation.

Results.—Significant disease was detected in 3 of the earlier patients (2%). In 2 cases, hypothermic fibrillatory arrest was used without cross-clamping of the aorta, and the left ventricle was vented. One patient had a single cross-clamp placed. Five controls (3%) had a stroke, and 6 (3.6%) died. Stroke directly contributed to one of the deaths. Of the subsequent patients, 20 had moderate and 7 had severe ultrasound abnormalities. In 14 patients, hypothermic fibrillatory arrest was substituted for cross-clamping, and the left ventricle was vented. In 3 patients, the aortic cannulation site was changed or a single cross-clamp was used. In 2 other cases, the placement of proximal anastomoses or all arterial grafts was altered. The mortality rate was 2.6%; there were no strokes.

Conclusion.—The risk of stroke after CABG may be limited by intraoperative ultrasound study of the ascending aorta and by making appropriate changes in the operative technique.

▶ The aortic arch is an increasingly recognized source of atheroembolic debris that can cause symptomatic cerebral and peripheral embolism (1). Cardiac surgeons have belatedly come to the conclusion that manipulation of the ascending aorta during cannulation for CABG surgery is a major cause of

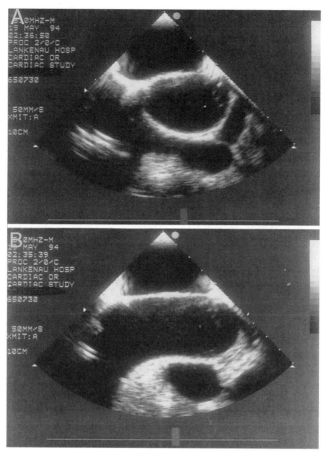

Fig 6–1.—Normal ascending aorta, which requires no change in operative technique, is shown: transverse (A) and longitudinal (B) views. (Courtesy of Duda AM, Letwin LB, Sutter FP, et al: Does routine use of aortic ultrasonography decrease the stroke rate in coronary artery bypass surgery? *J Vasc Surg* 21:98–109, 1995.)

embolization, frequently producing symptoms in the immediate postoperative period. These investigators examined the routine use of intraoperative surface aortic ultrasonography to guide the conduct of CABG surgery. Twenty-seven of 168 patients in the experimental group had significant aortic arch atherosclerotic involvement, which was considered severe in 7, leading to modification of surgical technique in 19 patients. No strokes occurred in this group compared with 5 strokes in a near-term historical control group. This is important information, suggesting that aortic arch atherosclerosis may be the cause of a significant percentage of strokes that occur in conjunction with coronary artery bypass grafting.

Reference

1. 1993 YEAR BOOK OF VASCULAR SURGERY, p 163.

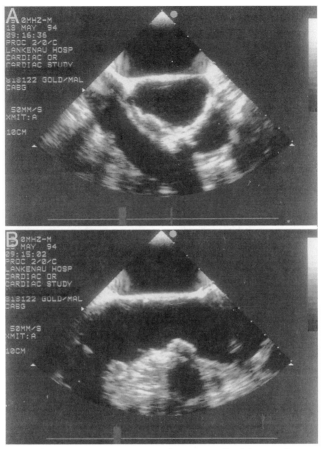

Fig 6–2.—Severe disease involving the anterior and posterior walls of the ascending aorta and arch is shown in transverse (**A**) and longitudinal (**B**) views. (Courtesy of Duda AM, Letwin LB, Sutter FP, et al: Does routine use of aortic ultrasonography decrease the stroke rate in coronary artery bypass surgery? *J Vasc Surg* 21:98–109, 1995.)

Atherosclerotic Disease of the Aortic Arch and the Risk of Ischemic Stroke
Amarenco P, Cohen A, Tzourio C, Bertrand B, Hommel M, Besson G, Chauvel C, Touboul P-J, Bousser M-G (Université Pierre et Marie Curie, Paris; Recherches Epidémiologiques en Neurologie et Psychopathologie, Villejuif, France; Centre Hospitalier Universitaire de Grenoble, France)
N Engl J Med 331:1474–1479, 1994   145-96-6–2

Background.—Atherosclerotic disease of the aortic arch may be a source of cerebral emboli. The risk of ischemic stroke associated with atherosclerotic disease of the aortic arch was quantified.

Methods.—Two hundred fifty patients were enrolled in a prospective case-control study of the frequency and thickness of atherosclerotic plaques in the ascending aorta and proximal arch. All these patients were hospitalized with ischemic stroke. Transesophageal echocardiography was performed in the patients and in an equal number of controls; all were older than age 60 years.

Findings.—Fourteen percent of the patients and 2% of the controls had atherosclerotic plaques of 4 mm or greater in thickness. The odds ratio for ischemic stroke among patients with such plaques was 9.1 after adjusting for atherosclerotic risk factors. Among the 78 patients with brain infarcts with no obvious cause, 28.2% had plaques of 4 mm or greater in thickness. Among the 172 patients with infarcts of known possible or likely causes, this proportion was 8.1%. Plaques of 4 mm or greater in the aortic arch were unrelated to the presence of atrial fibrillation or stenosis of the extracranial internal carotid artery, whereas plaques with thicknesses of 1–3.9 mm were often associated with carotid stenosis of 70% or more.

Conclusion.—There appears to be a strong, independent relationship between atherosclerotic disease of the aortic arch and the risk of ischemic stroke. This relationship was especially strong when plaques were thick. As a result, atherosclerotic disease of the aortic arch should be considered a risk factor for ischemic stroke and a possible source of cerebral emboli.

▶ In a study similar to that reported in Abstract 145-96-6–1, these investigators used transesophageal echocardiography to examine the ascending aorta and proximal arch in 250 consecutive hospitalized stroke patients older than age 60 years, and the findings were compared with those in control patients. Significant arch atherosclerosis was found in 14.4% of patients vs. 2% of controls. The authors found a strong independent association between atherosclerotic aortic arch disease and the risk of stroke, which was especially strong with thick plaques. Taken together, Abstracts 145-96-6–1 and 145-96-6–2 indicate a significant increase in the recognition of the importance of aortic arch atherosclerotic disease by the nonvascular surgical community.

TEE-Trauma

Transesophageal Echocardiography in the Diagnosis of Traumatic Rupture of the Aorta
Smith MD, Cassidy JM, Souther S, Morris EJ, Sapin PM, Johnson SB, Kearney PA (Univ of Kentucky, Lexington; Veterans Affairs Med Ctr, Lexington, KY)
N Engl J Med 332:356–362, 1995   145-96-6–3

Background.—Standard chest radiography is useful in the initial screening of traumatic rupture of the aorta. However, diagnosis requires confirmation by aortography, CT, or MRI before surgical repair. The safety and efficacy of transesophageal echocardiography in patients with suspected acute traumatic injury to the thoracic aorta were assesssed prospectively.

Study Methods.—Transesophageal echocardiography of the aorta was attempted in 101 patients with possible traumatic rupture of the aorta. Echocardiography and aortography were performed sequentially in each patient.

Findings.—Transesophageal echocardiography was completed successfully in 93 patients. It could not be completed in 7 because of lack of cooperation and in 1 because of maxillofacial trauma. The test was done with no complications, despite a high mean injury-severity score. The mean time required for the test was 29 minutes. Eleven of the 93 studies showed aortic rupture near the isthmus, which was confirmed by aortography, surgery, or autopsy (Fig 6–3). As a result, transesophageal echocardiography had a sensitivity of 100% and a specificity of 98% for the detection of aortic injury (Fig 6–4). One false positive result occurred on echocardiography.

Conclusion.—Transesophageal echocardiography is a very sensitive, specific method for detecting injury to the thoracic aorta. It can be done safely

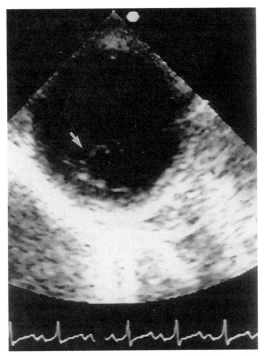

Fig 6–3.—Horizontal-plane transesophageal echocardiogram of a patient with confirmed aortic rupture. A thin, highly mobile linear flap (*arrow*) was evident at the cross-sectional level of the aortic isthmus. (Reprinted by permission of Smith MD, Cassidy JM, Souther S, et al: Transesophageal echocardiography in the diagnosis of traumatic rupture of the aorta. *N Engl J Med* 332:356–362, 1995. Copyright 1995, Massachusetts Medical Society.)

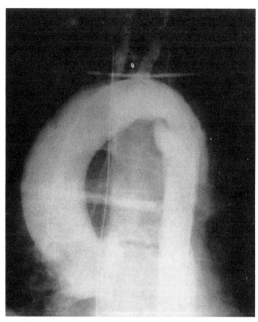

Fig 6–4.—Aortogram (anteroposterior view) of a patient with a positive transesophageal echocardiogram. The aortic contour is disrupted in the descending aorta just below the arch. This appearance and site of injury are typical of patients with deceleration injuries of the aorta. (Reprinted by permission of Smith MD, Cassidy JM, Souther S, et al: Transesophageal echocardiography in the diagnosis of traumatic rupture of the aorta. *N Engl J Med* 332:356–362, 1995. Copyright 1995, Massachusetts Medical Society.)

and rapidly in critically injured patients who have a possible traumatic rupture of the aorta. The results compare favorably with aortography.

▶ This interesting study compared the use of transesophageal echocardiography (TEE) with aortography in the diagnosis of traumatic rupture of the thoracic aorta in 101 patients. Transesophageal echocardiography was actually accomplished in 93 of 101 patients, whereas aortography was accomplished in all. Remarkably, TEE, which was performed in an average time of 29 minutes, showed a sensitivity of 100% and a specificity of 98%, with 1 false positive study. The authors appropriately conclude that TEE is a highly accurate method of detecting injury to the thoracic aorta. It may actually be more accurate than aortography.

Further Experience with Transesophageal Echocardiography in the Evaluation of Thoracic Aortic Injury
Buckmaster MJ, Kearney PA, Johnson SB, Smith MD, Sapin PM (Univ of Kentucky, Lexington, Ky)
J Trauma 37:989–995, 1994   145-96-6–4

Objective.—The role of transesophageal echocardiography (TEE) in diagnosing thoracic aortic injuries was examined in a prospective series of

160 patients who had blunt injury of the thoracic aorta. The TEE was performed in 121 patients, most often on the basis of the chest radiographic findings alone. Thirty-nine patients had aortography.

Results.—The TEE correctly identified 14 aortic injuries (Fig 6–5). Five injuries were confirmed by aortography, 7 at surgical exploration, and 2 at autopsy. In 2 other cases, the TEE findings suggested injury in patients who had aortic injuries, but the findings were not diagnostic. With these exceptions, TEE findings were 100% sensitive and specific for aortic injury. By contrast, aortography was 99% specific but had a sensitivity of only 73%.

Conclusion.—Aortography may no longer be the "gold standard" for diagnosing blunt injuries of the thoracic aorta. The TEE is an accurate bedside method of detecting these injuries. Several patients have undergone surgery after TEE alone. Aortography may be done when the TEE findings are equivocal, TEE cannot be tolerated or is contraindicated, or other vascular injuries are suspected.

▶ The same authors, with the addition of a new author named Buckmaster, have now extended their observation period from 24 to 33 months and the number of patients observed from 101 to 160; however, their results have remained the same. They continued to find TEE to be as good as or better than aortography in the diagnosis of thoracic aortic injury. To the authors, for polluting the literature with almost identical publications, I present the Camel Dung Award.

In defense of the *New England Journal of Medicine*, however, I notice the authors did not refer to their previous paper in the one they published in the journal. I am hardly surprised. I suppose this reinforces the old adage: "If you have good data, there's no sense in limiting it to a single publication." I note with pleasure the recent, although belated, vituperative editorial in the *New England Journal of Medicine* directed against the authors of this article for their duplicate publication (1).

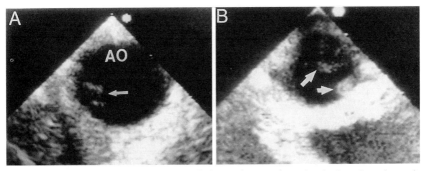

Fig 6–5.—Characteristic ultrasonographic findings of aortic disruption in 2 patients (*arrows*). (Courtesy of Buckmaster MJ, Kearney PA, Johnson SB, et al: Further experience with transesophageal echocardiography in the evaluation of thoracic aortic injury. *J Trauma* 37:989–985, 1994.)

Reference

  1. Editorial. *N Engl J Med* 333:449–450, 1995.

Thoracic Aneurysm

Graft Replacement of the Descending Thoracic Aorta: Results of "Open" Distal Anastomosis

Scheinin SA, Cooley DA (Texas Heart Inst, Houston)
Ann Thorac Surg 58:19–23, 1994   145-96-6–5

Background.—The availability of rapid autotransfusion has made it feasible to repair aneurysms of the descending thoracic or thoracoabdominal aorta by an "open" technique, in which a single cross-clamp is placed proximal to the aneurysm to exsanguinate the lower body.

Series.—The risk of cord injury was examined in 71 consecutive patients (50 men and 21 women) with an average of 63 years who had this operation. Seventy-six percent of the patients were symptomatic, and 86% were hypertensive. Medial degeneration was the diagnosis in 63% of cases and aortic dissection in 22.5%. Five patients were admitted with a ruptured aorta.

Management and Outcome.—Thirty-one patients had the entire descending thoracic aorta replaced. The thoracoabdominal aorta was replaced in 21 cases, and a segment of descending thoracic aorta was replaced in 19. The distal ischemic time averaged 22 minutes. An average of 2,099 mL of blood was returned by autotransfusion. Eight patients (11%) died within 30 days of operation of multiple organ failure, ischemic heart disease, or bleeding. Six patients (8.5%) had spinal cord dysfunction; 4 had paraparesis, and 2 had paraplegia. Four patients required dialysis because of renal insufficiency.

Conclusion.—If the intercostal and lumbar arteries can drain freely while the aorta is occluded, the CSF and central venous pressures are more readily controlled. Exsanguination of the lower body permits the distal anastomosis to be constructed during a brief period of ischemia.

▶ Dr. Cooley has hit upon the notion that thoracic aortic aneurysms can be more safely resected by performing the distal anastomosis in an open fashion with cell saver and limited distal aorta dissection. In this article he reports on 71 consecutive patients with an 11% mortality, an 8.5% incidence of spinal cord dysfunction, and a 5.6% incidence of renal failure. Although this is an interesting technique, these results are not the stuff that dreams are made of. I notice he had reported the first 31 patients previously (1); the results have improved slightly since the earlier publication. See Abstract 145-96-6–6 for a repeat discussion of the same patient group.

Reference

  1. 1994 YEAR BOOK OF VASCULAR SURGERY, p 186.

Further Experience With Exsanguination for Descending Thoracic Aneurysms

Cooley DA (Texas Heart Inst, Houston)

J Cardiovasc Surg 9:625–630, 1994   145-96-6–6

Background.—When a descending thoracic aortic aneurysm is resected and replaced by a graft, aortic cross-clamping may lead to ischemic injury of the spinal cord. Limiting the cross-clamp time to less than 30 minutes is the most effective way of preventing cord injury. Continuous autotransfusion makes it possible to decompress the distal aorta by means of back-bleeding through the distal aorta and the segmental spinal arteries.

Methods.—A single aortic cross-clamp is applied proximal to the lesion and an "open" distal anastomosis is performed, limiting dissection of the distal aorta (Fig 6–6). Most often, the proximal cross-clamp was placed between the left common carotid and left subclavian arteries or just distal to the left subclavian artery.

Patients.—This technique was used in 71 consecutive patients with aortic aneurysms. The entire descending thoracic aorta was involved in 31 cases, the thoracoabdominal aorta in 21, the proximal descending thoracic aorta in 15, and the distal descending thoracic aorta in 4. Nearly two thirds of the aneurysms were secondary to medial degeneration or atherosclerosis. Dissection was present in 16 cases. Three fourths of the patients were symptomatic; in 5 cases, the aneurysm had ruptured.

Results.—The average ischemic interval was 22.4 minutes, and an average of 2,099 mL of autologous blood was salvaged during the procedure. Eight patients (11.3%) died early in the postoperative period. Six surviving patients (8.5%) had spinal cord dysfunction, 2 of them after recovery from anesthesia. Cerebrospinal fluid pressures increased initially during cross-clamping, but then they declined when the aneurysm was opened and the abdominal aorta was decompressed. Four patients (5.6%) had renal failure.

Conclusion.—The exsanguination technique is now used on all patients requiring resection of a descending thoracic or thoracoabdominal aortic aneurysm.

▶ Just in case you didn't see the preceding article (Abstract 145-96-6–5), which described 71 patients and was published in the *Annals of Thoracic Surgery*, a report on the same 71 patients has now been published in the *Journal of Cardiovascular Surgery.* Happily, I am able to report that the results are the same. Dare I present Dr. Cooley the prestigious Camel Dung Award for this a remarkable example of triple publication? With this rarely encountered triple, Cooley demonstrates preservation of a remarkably active interest in publication apparently undiminished by advancing years.

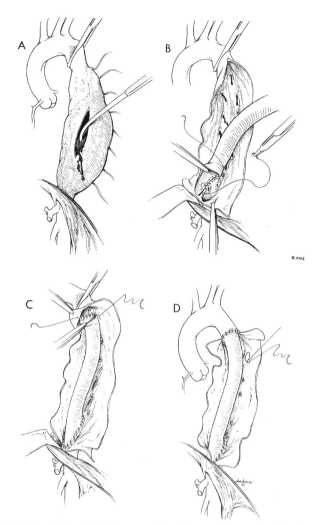

Fig 6–6.—Technique of "open" distal anastomosis used to repair aneurysms of the descending aorta. The distal anastomosis is performed without an aortic cross-clamp. (Reprinted with permission from the Society of Thoracic Surgeons [*The Annals of Thoracic Surgery*, 1992, vol 54, pp 932–936].)

Reversal of Delayed-Onset Paraplegia After Thoracic Aortic Surgery With Cerebrospinal Fluid Drainage

Hill AB, Kalman PG, Johnston KW, Vosu HA (Univ of Toronto)
J Vasc Surg 20:315–317, 1994   145-96-6–7

Background.—Two patients had delayed paraplegia develop after undergoing repair of a type I thoracoabdominal aneurysm; they responded to postoperative CSF drainage. Drainage was not begun preoperatively in these patients because of the need for urgent repair.

Patients.—Woman, 53, had a known aneurysm that had recently expanded. Surgery became urgent when severe chest pain persisted despite treatment for hypertension. The clamp time was 32 minutes. Complete paraplegia was present 18 hours postoperatively. A CSF catheter was inserted, and 250 mL of CSF was drained in 24 hours to maintain a pressure of 10 mm Hg. The paralysis completely resolved in the next 24 hours. Man, 75, with a ruptured aneurysm had severe paralysis of the left leg and weakness of the right leg develop 24 hours after repair, which had entailed clamping for 30 minutes. A CSF catheter drained 110 mL of fluid in 24 hours, and normal function returned in both legs.

Conclusion.—Postoperative CSF drainage can improve circulation in the spinal cord and relieve neurologic deficits in patients who have CSF hypertension develop after surgery on the thoracic aorta. Routine drainage is recommended.

▶ This is a clear demonstration of reversal of what appeared to be a severe neurologic defect after thoracoabdominal aneurysm repair by the delayed initiation of spinal fluid drainage. It suggests that such an approach be considered—if CSF drainage is not already being performed—in every patient who has delayed-onset paraplegia develop.

Neurologic Deficit in Patients at High Risk With Thoracoabdominal Aortic Aneurysms: The Role of Cerebral Spinal Fluid Drainage and Distal Aortic Perfusion
Safi HJ, Bartoli S, Hess KR, Shenaq SS, Viets JR, Butt GR, Scheinbaum R, Doerr HK, Maulsby R, Rivera VM (Baylor College of Medicine, Houston, Tex)
J Vasc Surg 20:434–443, 1994   145-96-6–8

Background.—Neurologic deficit is a potentially devastating complication of thoracoabdominal aortic aneurysm (TAAA) surgery. The use of perioperative CSF drainage and distal aortic perfusion to prevent postoperative neurologic deficit in patients with high-risk TAAAs was prospectively evaluated.

Methods.—The analysis included 45 consecutive patients with high-risk TAAAs: 14 with type I and 31 with type II (Fig 6–7.) There were 36 men and 9 women, with a median age of 63 years. Dissection had occurred in 53% of patients, and 38% had had a previous proximal aortic replacement. Perioperative CSF drainage and distal aortic perfusion were performed in all patients. For distal aortic perfusion, a Pruitt catheter was used to perfuse the celiac axis, superior mesenteric, and renal arteries if possible (Fig 6–8). The aorta was clamped for a median of 42 minutes, and the intercostal artery was reattached in 78% of patients. The results were compared with those of a previous series of 112 patients who had a type I or III TAAA.

Results.—The perioperative survival rate was 96%. Two patients each had an early and late neurologic deficit, for a total incidence of 9%. By contrast, the incidence of neurologic deficit for the historical controls was

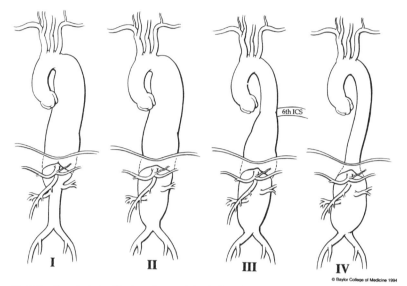

Fig 6–7.—Crawford classification, thoracoabdominal aortic aneurysm (TAAA) types I-IV. (Courtesy of Safi HJ, Bartoli S, Hess KR, et al: Neurologic deficit in patients at high risk with thoracoabdominal aortic aneurysms: The role of cerebral spinal fluid drainage and distal aortic perfusion. *J Vasc Surg* 20:434–443, 1994.)

31%. None of the patients with type I TAAAs who underwent CSF drainage had a neurologic deficit compared with 21% of those with type I TAAAs in the comparison group. For patients with type II TAAAs, the respective rates were 13% and 51%. Neurologic deficit occurred in 12% of patients with aortic dissection in the new series vs. 28% of those with aortic dissection in the comparison group. For patients without aortic dissection, the figures were 5% vs. 32%. Rates of neurologic deficit were 4% vs. 21% in patients with aortic clamp times of less than 45 minutes and 14% vs. 48% for those with longer clamp times.

Conclusion.—Perioperative CSF drainage and distal aortic perfusion can significantly reduce the occurrence of neurologic deficit in patients with high-risk TAAAs. This technique is recommended for patients with type I and II aneurysms and should be studied for use in patients with types III and IV aneurysms.

▶ Again, spinal fluid drainage is evaluated for its prophylactic benefit in the prevention of postoperative neurologic deficit in patients with thoracoabdominal aortic aneurysm resection. The 9% rate of paraplegia in the patients with spinal fluid drainage is distinctly superior to that of an historical control group with a rate of 31%. The authors conclude that both spinal fluid drainage and distal aortic perfusion are desirable in thoracoabdominal aortic aneurysm surgery. They must be correct, because this is our policy at Oregon Health Sciences University.

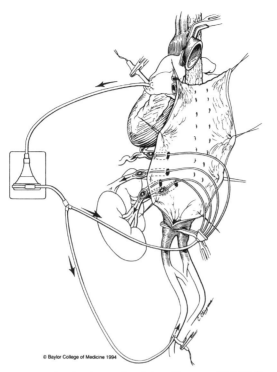

© Baylor College of Medicine 1994

Fig 6–8.—Left atrial to left feoral and visceral perfusion. (Courtesy of Safi HJ, Bartoli S, Hess KR, et al: Neurologic deficit in patients at high risk with thoracoabdominal aortic aneurysms: The role of cerebral spinal fluid drainage and distal aortic perfusion. *J Vasc Surg* 20:434–443, 1994.)

Influence of Segmental Arteries, Extent, and Atriofemoral Bypass on Postoperative Paraplegia After Thoracoabdominal Aortic Operations

Svensson LG, Hess KR, Coselli JS, Safi HJ (Lahey Clinic, Burlington, Mass; Baylor College of Medicine, Houston)
J Vasc Surg 20:255–262, 1994   145-96-6–9

Objective.—The risk factors for postoperative paraparesis and paraplegia were sought in a prospective series of 99 patients who underwent repair of a type I or type II thoracoabdominal aneurysm. In particular, the risk was related to the extent of the aneurysm, atriofemoral bypass, and whether patent segmental intercostal and lumbar arteries were reattached or oversewn.

Methods.—The patency of intercostal arteries from T3 to T12 and lumbar arteries from L1 to L4 was assessed by inspection during surgery. Motor function was graded daily for the first 5 days after surgery, and the worst score in the first postoperative month was used for analysis.

Results.—Thirty-one patients (32%) had a neurologic deficit develop within a month of surgery. In general, the risk of deficit could not be related to whether segmental vessels were reattached when patency was ignored. Nevertheless, 48% of patients who had 1 or more arteries at T11, T12, or L1 oversewn—frequently because they could not be reattached—had a deficit develop compared with 27% of those who had no patent arteries or had all patent vessels reattached. Sixty-three percent of the patients in whom all arteries at these levels were oversewn had a deficit develop. The risk of a deficit appeared to be less when patent arteries at other levels from T7 to L4 were reattached. Atriofemoral bypass correlated with a lesser risk of paralysis. Patients with more extensive aneurysms more often became paralyzed.

Conclusion.—Every attempt should be made to reattach patent segmental arteries at the time a thoracoabdominal aneurysm is resected, particularly those from T11 to L1. Where feasible, atriofemoral bypass appears to protect against neurologic complications.

▶ A remarkable 32% of patients in this series had a neurologic deficit postoperatively. The authors attempt to relate oversewing of segmental arteries at specific levels to neurologic outcome. Patients who had patent aortic branch arteries oversewn at the T11, T12, and L1 levels had a dramatic 48% neurologic deficit vs. 27% in patients who either did not have patent arteries at all or else had all patent arteries reattached. Spinal fluid drainage apparently was not used in these patients. On balance, this is a very high and disturbing incidence of neurologic deficit. It is noted that these patients underwent surgery over a number of years. Certainly, I suspect current results are markedly better.

Evolution of Surgical Techniques for Aneurysms of the Descending Thoracic Aorta: Twenty-Nine Years Experience With 659 Patients
Lawrie GM, Earle N, De Bakey ME (Baylor College of Medicine, Houston)
J Cardiovasc Surg 9:648–661, 1994   145-96-6–10

Series.—An aneurysm of the descending thoracic aorta was resected in 659 patients in the 4 decades from 1953 to 1993. Atherosclerotic disease was the predominant cause, and pain was the chief feature noted.

Results.—The perioperative mortality rate decreased from 24.2% in the first decade of the series to 14.03% in the years 1970–1993. Paraplegia developed in 4.1% of the patients, regardless of the time of surgery or the use of atriofemoral bypass. However, paraparesis, which occurred in 5.9% of all patients, was less frequent when atriofemoral bypass was used (table). Mortality from bleeding became more frequent later in the series, presumably because of systemic heparinization. Nearly half of all perioperative mortality and morbidity resulted from cardiac causes. The remainder was about equally divided among perioperative bleeding, pulmonary complications, and rupture of another aneurysmal segment. Cardiac causes were responsible for 30.6% of late deaths, and rupture of another aneurysm was responsible for 16.3%.

	Perioperative Results of Surgery			
	Date of Operation			
Factor	< 1965	1965–1970	> 1970	P
Perioperative mortality	57 (24.2%)	36 (18.1%)	32 (14.3%)	0.025
Paraplegia	9 (3.8%)	7 (3.5%)	11 (4.9%)	0.7
Paraparesis	2 (0.8%)	6 (3.0%)	31 (13.8%)	< 0.0001
Paraplegia/Paraparesis	11 (4.7%)	13 (6.5%)	42 (18.8%)	< 0.0001

(Reprinted by permission of Lawrie GM, Earle N, De Bakey ME: Evolution of surgical techniques for aneurysms of the descending thoracic aorta: Twenty-nine years experience with 659 patients. *J Cardiovasc Surg* 9:648–661, 1994.)

Implications.—A thorough preoperative assessment and evaluation of the entire aorta will help minimize complications and promote survival (Fig 6–9) when resecting descending thoracic aneurysms. If the clamp time is expected to exceed 30 minutes, the use of heparin-free circuits with centrifugal pumps should be considered. Regular, lifelong follow-up is essential.

▶ This is an interesting, lengthy, retrospective review of resection of descending thoracic aneurysms. The mortality rate of 14.3% is disturbing. Paraplegia and paraparesis occurred in 10% of the patients, and it was possibly reduced by the use of atriofemoral bypass. This is a moderately interesting, although not very exciting, retrospective review.

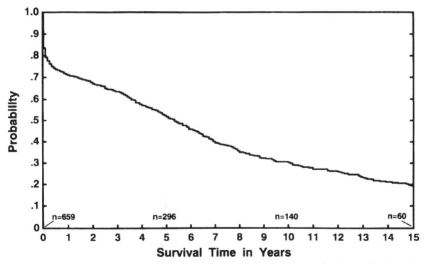

Fig 6–9.—Kaplan-Meier curve of survival probability for 659 patients after descending thoracic aneurysm resection. (Reprinted by permission of Lawrie GM, Earle N, De Bakey ME: Evolution of surgical techniques for aneurysms of the descending thoracic aorta: Twenty-nine years experience with 659 patients. *J Cardiovasc Surg* 9:648–661, 1994.)

Epidural Cooling for Regional Spinal Cord Hypothermia During Thoracoabdominal Aneurysm Repair
Davison JK, Cambria RP, Vierra DJ, Columbia MA, Koustas G (Harvard Medical School, Boston)
J Vasc Surg 20:304–310, 1994   145-96-6–11

Objective.—Because spinal cord injury remains an important problem in patients who require resection of a thoracic or thoracoabdominal aortic aneurysm, the efficacy of regional hypothermia was examined in 8 such patients.

Methods.—An epidural catheter was placed at the T11–12 level, and a thermistor catheter was placed in the subarachnoid space at the L3–4 level (Fig 6–10). Iced saline solution at 4°C was infused epidurally, about 30 minutes before planned aortic cross-clamping, until the CSF temperature decreased to about 25°C, and the infusion subsequently was adjusted to maintain this temperature until the aortic clamp was removed. The ther-

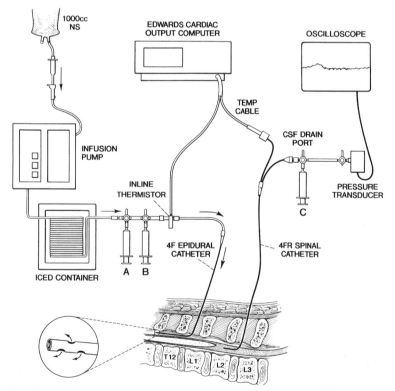

Fig 6–10.—Equipment setup for epidural cold infusion and measurement of CSF temperature and pressure. Syringe *A* for local anesthesia; syringe *B* for bolusing and removing infusate; syringe *C* for CSF drainage. (Courtesy of Davison JK, Cambria RP, Vierra DJ, et al: Epidural cooling for regional spinal cord hypothermia during thoracoabdominal aneurysm repair. *J Vasc Surg* 20:304–310, 1994.)

mistor catheter also served to monitor CSF pressure and allow drainage of fluid. A clamp-and-sew operative technique was used, with selective reattachment of the intercostal vessels.

Results.—The volume of iced saline infused ranged from 80 to 1,700 mL, and it averaged 489 mL, decreasing the mean CSF temperature to 26.9°C in 15–90 minutes (Fig 6–11). The CSF temperatures were maintained at 25.2°C to 27.6°C during aortic cross-clamping and returned to within 1°C of the body core temperature by the end of surgery. The mean CSF pressure increased, but it could be controlled by removing saline from the epidural space. No patient had a neurologic deficit postoperatively.

Conclusion.—Epidural cooling is an effective means of inducing hypothermia of the spinal cord during aortic cross-clamping for resection of an aneurysm of the thoracic or thoracoabdominal aorta.

▶ The authors present their initial experience with an innovative approach to achieving regional spinal cord hypothermia during thoracoabdominal aneurysm repair. This is based on experimental studies that have suggested regional hypothermia with a protective effect can be accomplished in animals during extensive aortic cross-clamping.

The authors were able to document the cooling effects of their epidural infusion system with a thermistor probe placed distally in the subarachnoid space. They noted some moderate increase in CSF pressure, although based

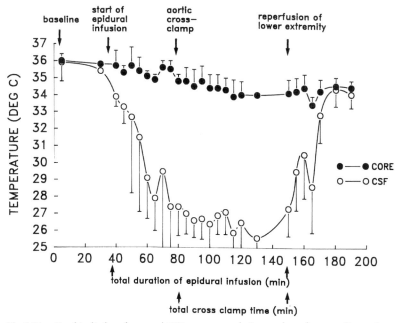

Fig 6–11.—Graphic display of core and CSF temperature during conduct of surgery. Data points are mean ± standard deviations from 8 patients. (Courtesy of Davison JK, Cambria RP, Vierra DJ, et al: Epidural cooling for regional spinal cord hypothermia during thoracoabdominal aneurysm repair. *J Vasc Surg* 20:304–310, 1994.)

on their clinical results, it did not have an untoward effect, and no patient had neurologic symptoms develop after extensive aortic replacement.

The method of repair of these aneurysms was the clamp-and-sew technique, which was originally described by Crawford; there were no attempts for extracorporeal support of the distal circulation, as recently reported by the Baylor group. It is likely that a combination of techniques will be the most effective approach in reducing the incidence of paraplegia. The experience reported in this article consists of only 8 patients; therefore, definitive statements regarding the effect of regional spinal cord hypothermia cannot be made. Perhaps consideration should be given to a drainage catheter to accompany the infusion technique so that low CSF pressures can be maintained during cooling, because this may further reduce the risk of spinal cord ischemia. This article has good documentation of the effects of regional spinal cord infusion of cold solution; it is an excellent contribution.—W. Quiñones-Baldrich, M.D.

Aneurysms of the Descending Thoracic Aorta: Three Hundred Sixty-Six Consecutive Cases Resected Without Paraplegia
Verdant A, Cossette R, Pagé A, Baillot R, Dontigny L, Pagé P (Univ of Montréal)
J Vasc Surg 21:385–391, 1995   145-96-6–12

Background.—The spinal cord is vulnerable to ischemia during surgery on the descending thoracic aorta. Cord injury has been described after cross-clamping for 18 minutes. Experience from more than 2 decades of use of the 9-mm Gott shunt (TDMAC-heparin shunt) for distal perfusion during aortic cross-clamping without systemic heparin was reported.

Methods.—A Dacron graft was used for aortic repair in 366 consecutive patients with an aneurysm between the left subclavian artery and the diaphragmatic crux. In 91.5% of the patients, no more than one third of the length of the aorta was resected. A Gott shunt was most often inserted into the ascending aorta, and it usually was inserted distally into the descending aorta.

Results.—Shunt flow, which was measured in 91 cases, ranged from 1,100 to 4,900 mL/min and averaged 2,526 mL/min. Distal pressure during shunting averaged 64.5 mm Hg. The aorta was cross-clamped from 8 minutes to 2 hours; the average time was 30 minutes. Hospital mortality was 12%; when ruptured aneurysms were excluded, it was 10%. No surviving patient had an immediate or delayed ischemic cord deficit. Nine patients had transient renal dysfunction, and 1 (.2%) had renal failure develop. There were 5 shunt-related deaths (1.3%), 2 caused by acute ascending aortic dissection and 3 by hemispheric stroke secondary to detached atherosclerotic debris.

Conclusion.—The Gott shunt is a highly reliable and relatively safe means of ensuring distal perfusion during aortic cross-clamping. Systemic heparin is not required. Paraplegia is effectively prevented when the extent of aortic resection and the cross-clamp time are minimized.

▶ Compare these results with those in Abstract 145-96-6–10. It is utterly amazing that no immediate or delayed ischemic spinal cord deficits were recognized in this entire cohort. The authors attribute these remarkable results to the use of the Gott shunt. Although I greatly admire the dramatic results reported in this article, I would be a bit concerned if I were going to be included in the next 100 patients who underwent surgery at this institution, because I suspect there is a high likelihood that their incidence of neurologic dysfunction is going to catch up with that of the rest of the world.

Technique for the Surgical Management of Mycotic Thoracoabdominal Aortic Aneurysms
Almdahl SM, Lie M, Vaage J, Dahl PE, Sørlie DG (Univ Hosp of Tromsø, Norway)
Eur J Surg 160:309–310, 1994   145-96-6–13

Background.—Mycotic aneurysms of the thoracoabdominal aorta are rare; fewer than 40 operatively treated patients have been reported. A problem is that no extra-anatomical route is available to maintain visceral perfusion. The consensus, based on very limited experience, is that an in situ Dacron graft should be implanted and the patient given antibiotics indefinitely.

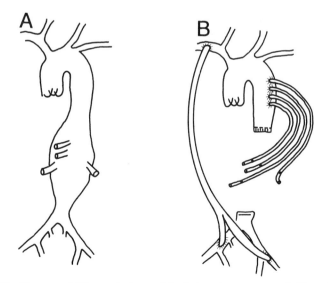

Fig 6–12.—Diagrams of (A) mycotic thoracoabdominal aortic aneurysm, and (B) condition after operation. (Courtesy of Almdahl SM, Lie M, Vaage J, et al: Technique for the surgical management of mycotic thoracoabdominal aortic aneurysms. *Eur J Surg* 160:309–310, 1994.)

Case Report.—Man, 46, was febrile when admitted with abdominal pain, and he had a tender epigastric mass. An emergency CT examination demonstrated pus surrounding a huge thoracoabdominal aneurysm. An 8-mm axillobifemoral bypass graft of reinforced polytetrafluoroethylene first was implanted using a right transthoracic approach to maintain perfusion of the lower body. A left thoracoretroperitoneal incision was then made to expose the thoracic aorta, and saphenous vein segments were taken from both thighs. After placement of an exclusion clamp on the descending thoracic aorta, 4 vein grafts were joined end-to-side to the thoracic aorta while continuous perfusion of the viscera and spine and avoidance of overload of the heart were provided by the bypass. Each of the grafts was joined to a visceral artery (Fig 6–12). The CSF pressure was reduced to less than 5 mm Hg. The aneurysmal segment was then removed along with inflamed retroperitoneal tissue. Dead space was filled with omentum. The patient was given antibiotic therapy for *staphylococcus aureus* infection, but systemic sepsis persisted. Multiple organ failure developed, and the patient died. No gross inflammation was evident in the area of surgery.

Conclusion.—Despite the outcome in this case, it appears worthwhile to consider using separate vein grafts and omental packing when repairing a mycotic thoracoabdominal aneurysm.

▶ This case report would have been more impressive had the patient survived. Nonetheless, we all encounter occasional patients with a thoracoabdominal repair who require graft excision because of ongoing severe sepsis. This technique—or some modification thereof—apppears to be about all we have available for these unfortunate patients.

7 Aortic Aneurysm

Small Aneurysm

The Cost-Effectiveness of Early Surgery Versus Watchful Waiting in the Management of Small Abdominal Aortic Aneurysms

Katz DA, Cronenwett JL (VA Med Ctr, White River Junction, Vt; Dartmouth-Hitchcock Med Ctr, Lebanon, NH)

J Vasc Surg 19:980–991, 1994   145-96-7–1

Background.—As surgery-related mortality rates decrease, surgical repair has been recommended for smaller and smaller abdominal aortic aneurysms (AAAs). There are 2 alternative strategies for managing AAAs measuring 4–5 cm in diameter: early repair, in which 4-cm AAAs are repaired at the time of diagnosis, and watchful waiting, in which ultrasound is done every 6 months to measure the size of the AAA and the aneurysm is repaired if it grows to 5 cm in diameter. Decision analysis techniques were used to compare the cost-effectiveness of these 2 approaches.

Methods.—For each strategy, the expected survival in quality-adjusted life-years (QALY) was calculated using a Markov decision tree model. Estimated probabilities of the various outcomes were derived from the literature. Using the costs of elective and emergency AAA repair at their hospital, the investigators calculated the additional cost per year of life saved with early surgery compared with watchful waiting. Cost-effectiveness ratios were expressed in dollars/QALY.

Results.—Expressed in 1992 dollars, the mean cost of elective AAA repair was $24,020, and that of emergency AAA repair was $43,208. The base-case analysis for this study concerned a man, 60, with a 4-cm AAA; the mortality rate of elective repair for such patients was 5%, and the annual rupture rate was 3.3%. In this analysis, early surgery improved survival by 0.34 QALY compared with watchful waiting. The associated incremental cost was $17,404/QALY. The cost-effectiveness of early AAA repair diminished with the increased mortality of elective surgery, the decreased risk of AAA rupture, and increased patient age. The factors that increased the cost-effectiveness of early repair were future increases in the risk of elective surgery, noncompliance with ultrasound monitoring, and increased threshold size for early repair (Fig 7–1).

Conclusion.—In appropriately selected patients, early surgery for 4-cm AAAs is a cost-effective management strategy. If $40,000/QALY is con-

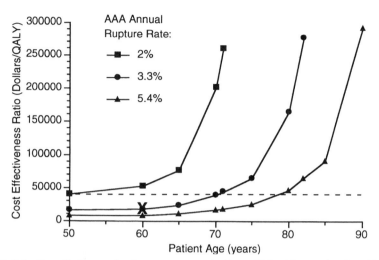

Fig 7–1.—Cost-effectiveness of early surgery compared with watchful waiting as a function of initial patient age for 3 different annual rupture rates for abdominal aortic aneurysms (*AAA*). The base-case analysis is indicated by the X. The *dotted line* indicates a cost-effectiveness ratio of $40,000/quality-adjusted life-years (*QALY*), below which health care interventions are generally considered cost-effective. (Courtesy of Katz DA, Cronenwett JL: The cost-effectiveness of early surgery versus watchful waiting in the management of small abdominal aortic aneurysms. *J Vasc Surg* 19:980–991, 1994).

sidered an "acceptable" cost-effectiveness ratio, early surgery appears to be suitable for patients as old as age 70 years, assuming an AAA rupture risk of at least 3% per year and an elective surgery-related mortality of no more than 5%. The cost-effectiveness data helped clarify the necessary trade-offs and ambiguities involved in managing patients with small AAAs; however, they do not replace the need for clinical judgment.

▶ Dr. Cronenwett and his associates embark on some unusual journeys from time to time. In this article, he and Dr. Katz use the politically correct language of the nouveau Washington bureaucrats to calculate the desirability of performing AAA surgery in terms of Markov decision analysis and QALY. With this arcane approach, early surgery on small 4-cm aneurysms improves survival by precisely 0.34 QALYs! I'll bet you did not know that. Interestingly, we also learn, that a QALY is worth precisely $40,000 to health care planners. Although I think this approach is utter hogwash, I appreciate Dr. Cronenwett's bringing it to our attention. Thank you, Jack.

Smoking and Growth Rate of Small Abdominal Aortic Aneurysms
MacSweeney STR, Ellis M, Worrell PC, Greenhalgh RM, Powell JT (Charing Cross and Westminster Med School, London)
Lancet 344:651–652, 1994   145-96-7-2

Background.—Smoking is a significant risk factor for abdominal aortic aneurysms. If it were possible to limit the rate at which small aneurysms grow, they might never reach the size at which surgical repair is considered.

Methods.—Aneurysm size was monitored by serial ultrasonography over 3 years in 43 patients with peripheral arterial disease, 33 men and 10 women 68–78 years of age. With 1 exception, the aneurysms initially measured less than 5 cm in diameter. One patient had a 6.3-cm aneurysm when first examined.

Results.—The aneurysms expanded at a median rate of 0.13 cm per year. The median rate was 0.16 cm per year for the 20 patients who currently smoked and 0.09 cm per year for current nonsmokers. An increased growth rate also was significantly correlated with the serum concentration of cotinine.

Conclusion.—Smokers with peripheral arterial disease who have a small abdominal aortic aneurysm would do well to stop smoking.

▶ This study of very few patients indicates that the growth rate of small aneurysms is slightly greater in those who smoke than in those who do not. Although statistical significance was achieved, I find the differences measured in one hundredths of a centimeter to be beyond the likely accuracy of ultrasonography, especially considering that a 3.5-MHz probe was required. I will reserve judgment.

A Statistical Analysis of the Growth of Small Abdominal Aortic Aneurysms

Grimshaw GM, Thompson JM, Hamer JD (Univ of Derby, England; Queen Elizabeth Hosp, Birmingham, England)
Eur J Vasc Surg 8:741–746, 1994   145-96-7–3

Background.—The issue of mass screening for abdominal aortic aneurysm to reduce mortality from unexpected rupture has engendered much interest. There is evidence that some patients with an abnormal aorta are not at high risk of rupture but nevertheless require monitoring.

Methods.—Ultrasound screening for abdominal aortic aneurysm was offered to 13,000 men 60–75 years of age, 76% of whom complied. Those whose initial aortic diameter measured 29–45 mm were offered serial ultrasonography.

Results.—The distribution of aortic diameters on initial screening is shown in Figure 7–2. The 302 individuals who had repeat studies included 93 who had more than 5 studies and an average of 7 during a mean of 32 months. Linear regression analysis of the rate of change of these aneurysms yielded an algorithm for aortic growth (Fig 7–3).

Conclusion.—Repeat ultrasound scanning at 2-year intervals appears to be adequate when the aortic diameter is less than 40 mm.

▶ Based on a complex analysis that is well beyond my ability to understand, these authors conclude that repeat scans for aneurysms that are less than 4 cm in diameter need only be performed once every 2 years, whereas for

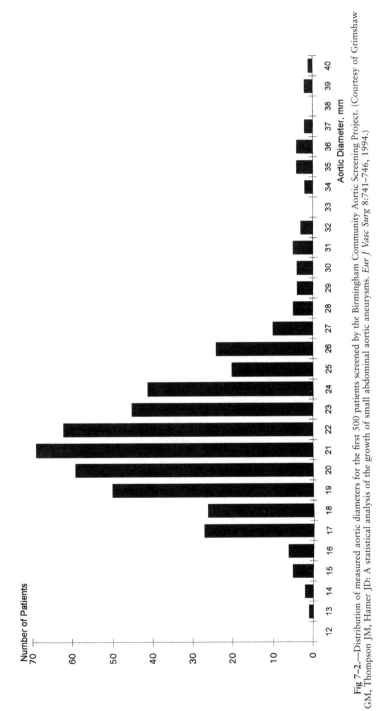

Fig 7–2.—Distribution of measured aortic diameters for the first 500 patients screened by the Birmingham Community Aortic Screening Project. (Courtesy of Grimshaw GM, Thompson JM, Hamer JD: A statistical analysis of the growth of small abdominal aortic aneurysms. *Eur J Vasc Surg* 8:741–746, 1994.)

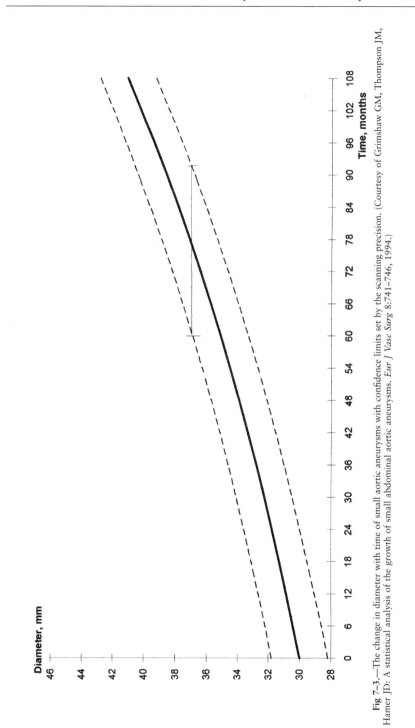

Fig 7–3.—The change in diameter with time of small aortic aneurysms with confidence limits set by the scanning precision. (Courtesy of Grimshaw GM, Thompson JM, Hamer JD: A statistical analysis of the growth of small abdominal aortic aneurysms. *Eur J Vasc Surg* 8:741–746, 1994.)

aneurysms between 4 and 4.5 cm on the initial scan, a once-yearly scanning appears safe. These recommendations seem reasonable. See also Abstract 145-96-3–11.

Unoperated Aortic Aneurysm: A Survey of 170 Patients
Perko MJ, Nørgaard M, Herzog TM, Olsen PS, Schroeder TV, Pettersson G
(Natl Univ Hosp, Copenhagen)
Ann Thorac Surg 59:1204–1209, 1995   145-96-7–4

Objective.—To determine whether improved surveillance and medical care have improved the outlook for unoperated patients who have aortic aneurysms (AAs), the outcome was examined in 1,053 patients with AA who were admitted in the years 1984–1993, 170 of whom (15%) were not treated surgically. Most often, the patient was considered to be technically inoperable.

Results.—There were no significant differences in survival between patients with dissecting and nondissecting AAs. The overall mortality in the unoperated group was 78%. Fifty-nine percent of deaths were caused by rupture, which occurred on average about 3½ years after they were seen. Dissecting AAs were twice as likely as nondissecting aneurysms to rupture within 5 years. The risk of rupture was comparable for type A and type B dissections, but aneurysms measuring 6 cm or more in diameter were fivefold more likely to rupture. Renal failure was a risk factor for both rupture and death, and arterial hypertension was a mortality risk factor.

Implications.—An aggressive approach is warranted for patients who have an AA measuring 6 cm or more in size or a type A dissection. Further data are needed to confirm that patients with type B dissections have better results if they undergo surgery. Early elective surgery may be indicated for older patients and those who have small aneurysms.

▶ This is a curious paper, which, although proving nothing, is at least interesting. During a 10-year period, 170 of 1,053 patients who were seen with AAs were deemed to be inoperable for a variety of subjective reasons, usually the surgeon's preference. During follow-up, which averaged approximately 3 years, 132 of these 137 patients died, with 59% of the deaths being caused by an AA rupture at a mean of about 3 years after diagnosis.

In this unusual series, dissecting AA ruptured twice as often as nondissecting aneurysms, and a diameter greater than 6 cm was associated with a fivefold increase in the risk of rupture. Although interesting, these results are statistically meaningless because of the nonstandarized requirements for study entry.

Nonruptured Abdominal Aortic Aneurysm: Six-Year Follow-Up Results From the Multicenter Prospective Canadian Aneurysm Study
Johnston KW, and the Canadian Society for Vascular Surgery Aneurysm

Study Group (Univ of Toronto; The Toronto Hosp)
J Vasc Surg 20:163–170, 1994   145-96-7–5

Background.—Previous reports of data from the Canadian Society for Vascular Surgery Aneurysm Registry have described the early results and complications of patients undergoing repair of nonruptured abdominal aortic aneurysms. The late survival of these patients was determined, and the causes of death and prognostic factors associated with survival were identified.

Methods.—The prospective analysis defined the 5-year survival of 680 patients who underwent repair of a nonruptured abdominal aortic aneurysm (AAA) and compared it with that of an age- and sex-matched population. The causes of late death were analyzed, including the influence of heart-related death on late survival. Kaplan-Meier analysis and Cox regression analysis were used to determine the prognostic variables associated with late survival. Up-to-date patient follow-up information was provided by the registry.

Results.—During follow-up, survival decreased from 90.7% at 1 year to 87.1% at 2 years, 81% at 3 years, 74% at 4 years, 67.7% at 5 years, and 60.2% at 6 years. By contrast, 6-year survival in a matched normal population was 79.2% (Fig 7–4). Forty-four percent of the deaths in the AAA group were heart related compared with 34.1% of those in the normal population; figures for cerebrovascular causes were 8.3% and 5.8%, respectively. The 5-year heart-related mortality was calculated as

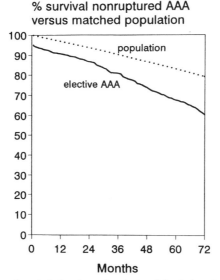

% survival nonruptured AAA
versus matched population

Months

Fig 7–4.—Comparison of survival of patients after elective abdominal aortic aneurysm (*AAA*) repair vs. age- and sex-matched population. (Courtesy of Johnston KW, and the Canadian Society for Vascular Surgery Aneurysm Study Group: Nonruptured abdominal aortic aneurysm: Six-year follow-up results from the Multicenter Prospective Canadian Aneurysm Study. *J Vasc Surg* 20:163–170, 1994.)

being 14.3% for the AAA group vs. 6.4% for the matched population; therefore, the risk of heart-related death for the AAA group increased by nearly 2% per year. Few patients died of the vascular complications of AAA repair or of recurrent aneurysmal disease. Advanced age, evidence of previous myocardial infarction on the preoperative ECG, and increased serum levels of creatinine were all significant predictors of a poorer late survival.

Conclusions.—The late survival of patients undergoing repair of non-ruptured AAA was defined, including an analysis of the causes of late death. The risk of heart-related death for these patients was somewhat higher than that of the general population. Cardiac operative risk might be reduced by identifying high-risk patients before AAA repair. However, any strategy in which all patients are screened and treated would be unlikely to prevent late heart-related deaths in a cost-effective manner.

▶ Another small slice of salami rolls off the meat cutter of the Canadian Society Aneurysm Study Group, which is currently reporting survival after AAA repair in comparison to an age- and sex-matched population without aneurysm. Postoperative survival was 60.2% at 6 years, significantly less than an age-and-sex matched normal population 6-year survival rate of 79.2%, a finding that has been repeatedly shown by others (1, 2). The survival numbers in the earlier studies are almost identical to those previously reported. We are in debt to the Canadian Society for confirming what we already knew.

References

1. 1995 YEAR BOOK OF VASCULAR SURGERY, p 169.
2. 1995 YEAR BOOK OF VASCULAR SURGERY, p 177.

Morphology of Small Aneurysms: Definition and Impact on Risk of Rupture
Faggioli GL, Stella A, Gargiulo M, Tarantini S, D'Addato M, Ricotta JJ (Univ of Bologna, Italy; State Univ of New York, Buffalo)
Am J Surg 168:131–135, 1994   145-96-7–6

Background.—The indications for surgical repair of aneurysms measuring less than 5 cm in diameter are open to debate. Available diagnostic imaging techniques can provide a detailed picture of the aneurysmal morphology before surgery, but the parietal characteristics of small aneurysms associated with a higher risk of rupture are unknown. The results of a prospective morphologic study of small abdominal aortic aneurysms were reported.

Methods.—The analysis included 135 consecutive patients with abdominal aortic aneurysms that measured less than 5 cm. Twelve patients required emergency surgery because of aneurysmal rupture; the other 123 underwent ultrasonography, angiography, and intraoperative evaluation during elective aneurysm repair. Computed tomography was performed in

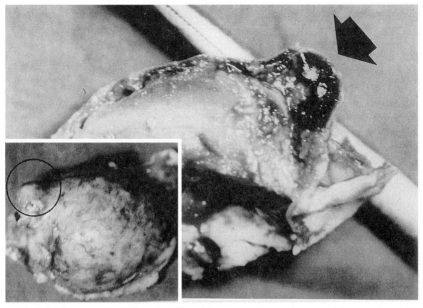

Fig 7–5.—Intraoperative finding of a blister. The arrow points to the area of discontinuity of the arterial wall. (*Inset*) The outpouching, as seen from the outside, is encircled (*circle*). (Courtesy of Faggioli GL, Stella A, Gargiulo M, et al: Morphology of small aneurysms: Definition and impact on risk of rupture. *Am J Surg* 168:131–135, 1994. Reprinted with permission from *American Journal of Surgery*.)

78% of patients. The morphologic assessment included the thickness of the endoluminal thrombus and arterial wall; the presence of saccular outpouchings, or blisters (Fig 7–5); and any areas of impending rupture, which were defined as arterial wall discontinuities in which only a thrombus was preventing a rupture.

Results.—Intraoperative evaluation revealed blisters in 12 aneurysms, 3 of which were detected by preoperative digital subtraction angiography. Blisters were also detected before operation in 3 of 11 patients undergoing CT scanning. Computed tomography permitted the measurement of endoluminal thrombus and wall thickness, whereas ultrasonography did not. Impending rupture was detected in 71% of patients with blisters vs. 29% of those without. This incidence was little affected by the presence of more or less than 2 cm of endoluminal thrombus, 57% vs. 40%, or aneurysmal walls thicker or thinner than 0.3 cm, 14% vs. 20%. On logistic regression analysis, the presence of a blister was the only morphologic characteristic that independently predicted impending rupture.

Conclusion.—Blisters in patients with small aortic aneurysms are a significant predictor of impending rupture. Increased efforts are needed to detect these blisters before operation.

▶ This article indicates—or suggests—that the risk of rupture in small aneurysms of less than 5 cm is something in the order of 14%. This is not in accordance with the majority of reports and must be unusually high. The figures are based on what the authors term "impending" rupture, without any evidence that this would actually occur. I do not think this article proves that blisters are associated with rupture.—P.R.F. Bell, M.D.

▶ I agree.—J.M. Porter, M.D.

Combined Disease

Optimal Timing of Abdominal Aortic Aneurysm Repair After Coronary Artery Revascularization
Blackbourne LH, Tribble CG, Langenburg SE, Mauney MC, Buchanan SA, Sinclair KN, Kron IL (Univ of Virginia Health Sciences Ctr, Charlottesville)
Ann Surg 219:693–698, 1994   145-96-7–7

Background.—Coronary artery disease commonly co-exists with abdominal aortic aneurysm (AAA), and its significance is heightened by the need to cross-clamp the aorta before repairing the aneurysm. Fatal rupture of an asymptomatic AAA has been described in patients undergoing coronary bypass graft surgery. Presently, most patients have an asymptomatic aneurysm repaired within 6 months after myocardial revascularization.

Objective.—The operative results were reviewed in 23 patients who were scheduled to have an asymptomatic AAA repaired within 6 months after coronary bypass surgery.

Results.—None of the 14 patients who had aneurysm repair at the time of coronary revascularization or within 2 weeks afterward died. By contrast, 3 of 9 patients who were scheduled for aneurysm repair longer than 2 weeks after coronary bypass surgery died of aneurysmal rupture. These deaths occurred 16–29 days after myocardial revascularization.

Conclusion.—Patients who have an AAA and require coronary bypass surgery should have the aneurysm repaired electively at the same session or within 2 weeks afterward.

▶ These authors raise the haunting question as to when an aortic aneurysm should be repaired after coronary bypass in a patient with AAA who has a preoperative bypass performed. They find that repair up to 14 days after coronary artery bypass grafting appears to be safe, whereas in their experience, a delay in repair of more than 14 days resulted in one third of patients experiencing aortic rupture with death.

Their conclusion that elective AAA repair should be undertaken either simultaneously or within 2 weeks of coronary revascularization appears reasonable. I certainly prefer to wait several weeks. I find no persuasive indication to perform simultaneous procedures. Dr. Richard H. Dean's discussion of this paper, which was presented at the Southern Surgical Association, appears to be right on target, as usual.

Combined Coronary Artery Bypass Grafting and Abdominal Aortic Aneurysm Repair

Vicaretti M, Fletcher JP, Richardson A, Chard R, Klineberg P, Nicholson I (Univ of Sydney, Australia; Westmead Hosp, Australia)
Cardiovasc Surg 2:340–343, 1994   145-96-7–8

Background.—When patients die postoperatively or subsequent to having an abdominal aortic aneurysm repaired, cardiac complications are most often responsible. Myocardial infarction may explain half of all postoperative deaths in these patients. Whether high-risk patients should undergo coronary bypass graft surgery at the time the aneurysm is repaired was investigated.

Methods.—Fifteen patients (average age, 65 years) underwent combined coronary bypass grafting and repair of an abdominal aortic aneurysm. All but 2 of the patients had angina, and all had coronary angiographic evidence of significant disease. Bypass grafting was done first. Placement of a median of 4 grafts was done during a median aortic cross-clamp time of 39 minutes. The aneurysm then was repaired in a median aortic cross-clamp time of 66 minutes. Nine patients received bifurcated grafts, and 6 received straight grafts. The median total operating time was approximately 6½ hours.

Results.—Patients remained in the cardiothoracic ICU for a median of 5 days postoperatively. The median total hospital time was 2 weeks. One patient (6.7%) died of noncardiac causes.

Conclusion.—In carefully selected patients, it is feasible to repair an abdominal aortic aneurysm and perform coronary bypass graft surgery at the same session.

▶ The issue of performing simultaneous coronary bypass and infrarenal abdominal aortic aneurysm surgery is again raised. This anecdotal, retrospective series reported on 15 patients who were undergoing combined procedures with a median total operating time of 6½ hours. One patient died, for a mortality of 6.7%. I am not sure what the authors are trying to prove. Their conclusion, "... combined CABG and AAA repair is advocated in carefully selected patients," is somewhat difficult for me to understand, because several patients in their current series had no coronary symptoms at all. I am not convinced.

Rupture of a Known Abdominal Aneurysm Following Cardiac Stress Testing

Feldman AY, Davies AH, Wilkins DC (Derriford Hosp, Plymouth, England)
J Cardiovasc Surg 35:541, 1994   145-96-7–9

Introduction.—Cardiac risk status is an important correlate of 5-year survival in patients who have surgical repair of an abdominal aortic aneurysm (AAA). Few complications have been reported after exercise or inotropic stress testing before elective repair of an AAA.

Case Report.—Woman, 72, was referred for cardiac assessment after ultra-sonography demonstrated an infrarenal aneurysm 6 cm in diameter. She had recovered well from an anterior myocardial infarction 14 years earlier. Long-standing hypertension was controlled by atenolol. A dobutamine stress test was done, during which the blood pressure reached a peak of 183/110 mm Hg and the heart rate increased to 141 beats/min. Significant ST segment depression was noted, but the patient did not report chest pain. Pain did occur in the center of the abdomen immediately after the test and radiated to the back, but it resolved within 5 minutes. Pain recurred 2 hours later. Emergency surgery was done to repair a leaking 7-cm aneurysm that extended into the iliac arteries. An aortobifemoral graft was inserted. The patient recovered uneventfully.

Conclusion.—If a patient with an AAA experiences any abdominal or back pain in conjunction with cardiac stress testing, immediate admission is necessary to detect expansion or rupture of the aneurysm.

▶ This case report described a 72-year-old female with a known 6-cm infrarenal aneurysm who was referred for prophylactic cardiac stress testing with dobutamine before aneurysm surgery. Immediately after the stress test, the patient complained of abdominal pain, and 2 hours later a diagnosis of a ruptured aneurysm was made. Thankfully, the patient survived. I will add this to the list of reasons why we at Oregon Health Sciences University do not favor routine extensive coronary evaluation preoperatively in patients with aneurysm.

Coexistence of Abdominal Aortic Aneurysm in Patients With Carotid Stenosis
Karanjia PN, Madden KP, Lobner S (Marshfield Clinic, Wis)
Stroke 25:627–630, 1994   145-96-7–10

Background.—Although carotid artery atherosclerosis is known to be associated with coronary artery disease, its association with other forms of arterial disease is less clear. The incidence of concomitant abdominal aortic aneurysm was evaluated in patients who had carotid artery stenosis diagnosed.

Methods.—The study sample comprised 89 consecutive patients who were referred for evaluation of symptomatic or asymptomatic carotid artery disease. All underwent abdominal ultrasonography and physical examination to screen for abdominal aortic aneurysm. The patients with transverse infrarenal aortic dilatation greater than 2.5 cm and clear focal dilatation, as judged by the ultrasonographer, were considered to have an abdominal aortic aneurysm. The frequency of this finding in the study population was compared with its incidental frequency in age- and sex-matched patients who had abdominal ultrasonography for reasons unrelated to the vascular system.

Results.—Of the 89 patients with carotid stenosis, 18 had abdominal aortic aneurysms on ultrasonography. By contrast, only 3 of 89 matched

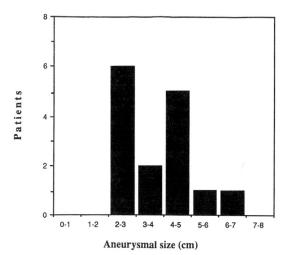

Aneurysmal size (cm)

Fig 7–6.—Bar graph shows size of abdominal aortic aneurysms in patients with carotid stenosis. (Courtesy of Karanjia PN, Madden KP, Lobner S: Coexistence of abdominal aortic aneurym in patients with carotid stenosis. *Stroke* 25:627–630, 1994. Reproduced with permission. *Stroke* Copyright 1994, American Heart Association.)

patients had incidentally detected aneurysms. The findings of abdominal physical examination were abnormal in 12 of 18 patients with abdominal aneurysms. The average size of the ultrasound-detected aneurysms was 3.7 cm (Fig 7–6).

Conclusion.—One fifth of the patients with carotid stenosis may also have abdominal aortic aneurysm. A careful abdominal physical examination of patients with known carotid artery stenosis, along with consideration of routine screening abdominal ultrasonography, was recommended.

▶ The finding of an increased incidence of aneurysms in such patients is hardly a surprise, because we know that all patients with vascular disease have a higher incidence of aneurysms.—P.R.F. Bell, M.D.

Technical Considerations

The Juxtarenal Abdominal Aortic Aneurysm: A More Common Problem Than Previously Realized?

Taylor SM, Mills JL, Fujitani RM (Univ of South Florida, Tampa; Wilford Hall US Air Force Med Ctr, San Antonio, Tex)
Arch Surg 129:734–737, 1994   145-96-7–11

Objective.—A 5-year review of aortic operations was undertaken to determine the frequency with which juxtarenal infrarenal aneurysms were removed and to evaluate the outcome.

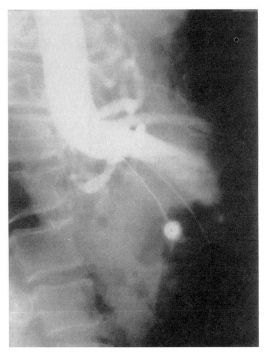

Fig 7-7.—A lateral aortic arteriogram showing the proximal extent of a typical juxtarenal abdominal aortic aneurysm. (Courtesy of Taylor SM, Mills JL, Fujitani RM: The juxtarenal abdominal aortic aneurysm: A more common problem than previously realized. *Arch Surg* 129:734–737, 1994. Copyright 1994/95, American Medical Association.)

Patients.—A total of 174 infrarenal aortic aneurysms were removed during the period reviewed. Twenty-seven (15.5%) involved the juxtarenal aorta (Fig 7–7). In only 2 of these cases was juxtarenal involvement suspected before aortography.

Results.—Twenty of the juxtarenal aneurysms were resected by a transabdominal approach, 7 of them retroperitoneally. There were no deaths at surgery, but the morbidity rate was 19% and included transient renal failure in 7% of patients. Eighty-nine percent of the patients were living after an average follow-up of 18 months.

Conclusion.—Juxtarenal infrarenal aortic aneurysms may be more prevalent than previously thought, and they can be effectively dealt with outside large referral centers.

▶ The authors define a juxtarenal aneurysm as one that extends to—and sometimes involves—the lower margins of the renal arteries. Using this definition, they found that 27 of 174 (15.5%) of their clinical aneurysm series had juxtarenal aneurysms, which were accurately diagnosed by aortography in 25 of the 27 cases. The authors preferred clamping the aorta at the diaphragm, using the cell saver to replace backbleeding. Their 100% survival rate is admirable.

Our preference is for retroperitoneal aortic exposure, with clamping at a site of convenience in the visceral segment, usually just below the superior mesenteric artery if anatomy permits. In recent years, patients who have been referred to us for aneurysm surgery are older than prior referrals and have larger aneurysms and a higher prevalence of juxtarenal aneurysms. I suppose others must be doing the more straightforward variety of surgery.

Transabdominal Versus Retroperitoneal Incision for Abdominal Aortic Surgery: Report of a Prospective Randomized Trial
Sicard GA, Reilly JM, Rubin BG, Thompson RW, Allen BT, Flye MW, Schechtman KB, Young-Beyer P, Weiss C, Anderson CB (Washington Univ, St Louis)
J Vasc Surg 21:174–183, 1995   145-96-7–12

Background.—It is generally agreed that a retroperitoneal incision (RPI) is advantageous in selected patients who have a juxtarenal or suprarenal aortic aneurysm, an inflammatory aneurysm, or horseshoe kidneys. It also may be helpful in obese patients and in those who have previously had surgery on the aorta or multiple abdominal surgeries. Nevertheless, the standard transabdominal incision (TAI) still is used in most cases.

Methods.—The TAI, which was used in 75 patients with an abdominal aortic aneurysm or aortoiliac occlusive disease, was compared with the RPI, which was used in 70 patients. Those in the 2 groups were comparable with respect to age, sex, type of aortic disease, and comorbidity (except for more frequent chronic obstructive lung disease in the TAI group).

Results.—Intraoperative complications were comparably frequent in the 2 groups, but prolonged ileus and small bowel obstruction were both more frequent in the TAI group. Overall, complications were significantly less prevalent in the RPI group, but there was no difference in pulmonary problems. Both postoperative deaths occurred in the TAI group. Patients in the RPI group had shorter stays in the ICU and tended to be discharged from the hospital sooner. Their hospital charges were correspondingly lower. During an average follow-up of nearly 2 years, patients in the RPI group reported more incisional pain, but there were no group differences in the frequency of incisional hernia or bulging.

Conclusion.—The RPI approach to surgery on the abdominal aorta may cause more incisional pain than the standard TAI, but it is associated with fewer postoperative complications, shorter ICU and hospital stays, and lower costs.

▶ Why the subject of the preferential approach to the abdominal aorta engenders such ardor continues to amaze me. I am not really sure what the debate is. Clearly, if there is a physiologic difference between the 2 approaches (and I suspect that there is not), it is a small one. As co-author of one of the recent studies, I take the position that there is *no* role for a preferential approach to any vascular surgical problem. A competent surgeon should have both techniques in his or her repertoire and should selectively use either of them, depending on the individual patient's needs, which are related to many variables, including body habitus, anastomotic details, and technical requirements. No single approach to the aorta will ever be inherently superior.—W. Abbott, M.D.

▶ Here is another thoughtful, middle-of-the-road, understated opinion from Professor Abbott!—J.M. Porter, M.D.

Surgical Workload as a Consequence of Screening for Abdominal Aortic Aneurysm
Scott RAP, Gudgeon AM, Ashton HA, Allen DR, Wilson NM (St Richard's Hosp, Chichester, England)
Br J Surg 81:1440–1442, 1994   145-96-7–13

Background.—Ultrasound screening to detect abdominal aortic aneurysms (AAAs) has become increasingly widespread. A national screening program was recently proposed. Screening augments the surgical workload to a degree that depends on many factors, including the screening method used, the criteria for operating, and the effect of screening on the need for emergency surgery.

Methods.—Changes in the surgical workload were examined over 8 years, when 8,944 individuals 65–80 years of age were ultrasonographically screened.

Results.—An AAA 3 cm or larger in diameter was discovered in 356 of the patients. A total of 288 outpatient visits were made by 171 of these patients, and 43 (4.8%) ultimately underwent surgery. It was estimated that a fully operational screening program for a population of 250,000, in which 2,000 men and women were screened each year, would result in 9 or 10 operations for AAA annually. Screening men only would yield 34 yearly operations.

Conclusion.—The increase in surgical workload as a result of screening for AAAs is not great and, in view of the high cost of emergency surgery, screening may well reduce surgical costs overall. Screening men at ages 65 and 70 years would reduce the workload.

▶ The authors tell us that if you perform population screening for AAAs in patients between the ages of 65 and 80, at a rate of 2,000 examinations per year, and reserve surgery for those with an aneurysm larger than 6 cm, an expansion rate of 1 cm or more per year, or symptoms, you will produce about 9 or 10 operations for AAA per year from this population. Screening 2,000 men only would increase the annual increment in operations to 34 per year. I wonder whether this would pass a cost/benefit analysis using the politically correct quality-adjusted life years calculation described in the comment after Abstract 145-96-7–1. Almost identical numbers were presented by another group, which reported its screening experience at the Society for Vascular Surgery Annual Meeting in New Orleans in June 1995 (1).

Reference

1. *Society for Vascular Surgery Program 1995, p 52.*

Miscellaneous Topics

Ligation and Extraanatomic Arterial Reconstruction for the Treatment of Aneurysms of the Abdominal Aorta

Pevec WC, Holcroft JW, Blaisdell FW (Univ of California, Davis)
J Vasc Surg 20:629–636, 1994   145-96-7–14

Backgrund.—Axillobifemoral bypass with aortic exclusion remains a controversial approach to treating patients with abdominal aortic aneurysms. Reported patient outcomes have varied widely, and the indications for extra-anatomical surgery remain uncertain.

Methods.—Twenty-six patients whose aneurysms averaged 7 cm in diameter underwent ligation and extra-anatomical reconstruction between 1980 and 1992. One fifth of the lesions were suprarenal. Two thirds of the patients were symptomatic, and all had serious comorbidity. Axillobifemoral bypass and iliac artery ligation were done in all cases, and in 62% of cases, the infrarenal aorta also was ligated.

Results.—Postoperative mortality was 7.75%. Fifty-nine percent of the patients survived 1 year after surgery, and 38% after 2 years. Three patients (11.5%) died of a ruptured aneurysm; 2 of them had not had the aorta ligated. The extra-anatomical bypass graft thrombosed in 5 patients, but no extremities were lost as a result. No patient had colonic ischemia develop, even though both hypogastric arteries were excluded in 42% of cases.

Conclusion.—Axillobifemoral bypass is an effective means of managing patients who have a symptomatic, anatomically complex, or large abdominal aortic aneurysm and those with severe comorbidity. Aortic ligation must be part of the procedure. Only direct replacement of the diseased aorta eliminates the risk of subsequent rupture.

▶ The originator of the aneurysm ligation together with the axillobifemoral bypass describes his experience with 26 patients over 12 years. All patients underwent axillobifemoral bypass with iliac artery ligation. Sixty-two percent had concomitant infrarenal aortic ligation. The 1- and 2-year survival rates were 59% and 38%, respectively. Three patients died of aneurysm rupture, 2 of whom had not had the aorta ligated proximally and 1 in whom it had. Certainly, this survival rate is inferior to that reported in modern series of aneurysm resections.

I agree with the authors that axillobifemoral bypass without aortic ligation does not effectively reduce the risk of aneurysm rupture. Although this procedure using proximal aneurysm ligation may reduce the risk of rupture, the difficulty of proximal ligation is almost identical to that of placing an abdominal aortic graft, and I see no reason for preferring ligation in any patient.

Platelet Count and the Outcome of Operation for Ruptured Abdominal Aortic Aneurysm
Bradbury AW, Bachoo P, Milne AA, Duncan JL (Royal Infirmary Edinburgh, Scotland; Raigmore Hosp, Inverness, Scotland)
J Vasc Surg 21:484–491, 1995   145-96-7–15

Background.—There is reason to believe that disseminated intravascular coagulation, with its hemorrhagic and thrombotic consequences, may underlie a number of complications seen in patients who undergo surgery for abdominal aortic aneurysm (AAA), including persistent bleeding, multiorgan failure, thromboembolism, and myocardial infarction.

Methods.—The platelet count (PC) determined at admission and again postoperatively was related to the outcome of emergency surgery for ruptured AAA in 65 consecutive patients. Sixty of the patients actually underwent surgery. Twelve died at surgery and 13 afterward, leaving 35 survivors.

Results.—Mortality decreased from 93% in patients with an admitting PC of less than 150×10^9/L to 17% in those whose counts exceeded 250×10^9/L. Of 29 patients whose PC was less than 100×10^9/L, 20 had multiorgan failure and 13 (45%) died. Six of these patients required reoperation for hemorrhagic complications. Only 16% of 19 patients whose postoperative PC was 100×10^9/L had multiorgan failure, and all survived; none required further surgery. The higher the PC at the end of surgery, the shorter the time required for receiving ventilation and intensive care and the briefer the overall hospital stay. Deep venous thrombosis developed in 10 of 15 patients who had thrombocytosis postoperatively, as evidenced by a PC greater than 400×10^9/L. Eight patients had pulmonary embolism. No thromboembolism was seen in patients who did not have thrombocytosis develop.

Conclusion.—The PC is a simple means of predicting the outcome in patients who require emergency surgery for a ruptured AAA.

▶ Within the limits of a reasonable emergency room and competent vascular surgeons, I regard the outcome of a ruptured AAA to be significantly dependent upon the condition of the patient when he or she is seen. If the patient is stable with a contained rupture, then survival is likely. If the patient has a wide open intra-abdominal rupture with shock and/or preoperative cardiac arrest, especially if it is combined with old age, then survival is almost impossible. Therefore, I conclude that most studies that report the outcome of ruptured aneurysms are substantially reporting the condition of the patient upon arrival at the health care facility. Although they are interesting, I suspect the contents of this article will have little effect on clinical decision-making.

8   Aortoiliac Disease

Axillofemoral

Axillofemoral Bypass: Compromised Bypass for Compromised Patients
Harrington ME, Harrington EB, Haimov M, Schanzer H, Jacobson JH II
(Mount Sinai Med Ctr, New York)
J Vasc Surg 20:195–201, 1994   145-96-8–1

Background.—In the past, axillofemoral (AXF) bypass grafts have generally been used when reconstructive surgery on the abdominal aorta is contraindicated. The improved results noted in some recent series have suggested that indications might be extended.

Method.—The results of 153 AXF bypass graft procedures performed in the years 1974–1992 were examined. There were 80 axillobifemoral and 73 axillounifemoral bypasses.

Results.—The primary patency rate at 3 years was 49.4%, and the secondary rate was 65.7%. The factors compromising primary patency included superficial femoral artery occlusion, the use of externally supported polytetrafluoroethylene, distal endarterectomy, and distal anastomosis to the deep femoral artery. Whether bifemoral or unifemoral outflow was available was not a factor, and concomitant distal surgery did not affect bypass patency. The operative mortality rate in patients who underwent surgery for claudication and limb salvage was 8.3% overall and 5.9% after 1984. The limb salvage rate was 74.8% both 3 and 5 years postoperatively. Both mortality and limb loss were more frequent when AXF bypass was done for acute ischemia.

Conclusion.—Axillofemoral bypass is a useful alternative for patients requiring surgery on the aorta when aortofemoral bypass is not feasible. It should still be limited, however, to poor-risk patients who have disabling claudication or a threatened limb.

▶ In the past 5 years, we have obtained excellent results from AXF bypass, equalling concurrent results with aortobifemoral bypass. We are achieving 70% to 80% primary patency at 5 years in both patient groups. However, our modern AXF bypasses are performed by a few surgeons using a standardized protocol. The authors of this article have reviewed an 18-year experience with 153 AXF bypasses, one half of which were unifemoral, performed by a large number of surgeons with no standard protocol. Despite this, their

3-year primary patency rate was an acceptable 50%, whereas the secondary patency rate was 66%. Although these authors strangely conclude that their study shows bad results for AXF bypass, I interpret their results quite differently. In the compromised setting over the many years in which their results were obtained, they were actually quite good. We continue to perform fewer and fewer aortofemoral bypasses and more and more AXF bypasses. See the commentary after Abstract 145-96-8-2.

Axillofemoral Grafting With Externally Supported Polytetrafluoroethylene
Taylor LM Jr, Moneta GL, Mcconnell D, Yeager RA, Edwards JM, Porter JM
(Oregon Health Sciences Univ, Portland)
Arch Surg 129:588–595, 1994   145-96-8–2

Objective.—A total of 184 axillofemoral (AXF) bypass operations were performed during a 10-year period, starting in 1984 and involving 164 consecutive patients with ischemic peripheral vascular disease. The patients were prospectively followed for an average of 23 months. The patients were 14–90 years of age, with an average age of 67 years. Ischemia was the indication for 83% of procedures, and aortic sepsis for 16%.

Methods.—All operations used external supported polytetrafluoroethylene (PTFE) prostheses.

Results.—The operative mortality rate was 5%. There were 17 major complications, including 4 nonfatal myocardial infarctions and 1 stroke. The life table primary patency rate at 5 years was 71% (Fig 8–1), and the limb salvage rate was 92% (Fig 8–2). The 5-year survival rate was 52%. Patency was not influenced by the indication for surgery, the state of the superficial femoral artery, or surgery at more than 1 level.

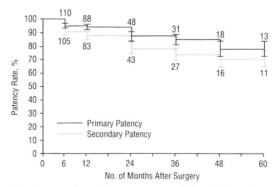

Fig 8–1.—Life-table primary and secondary patency rates of the axillofemoral procedures (*n* = 184). *Vertical bars* indicate standard error of the cumulative patency figure. (Courtesy of Taylor LM Jr, Moneta CL, McConnell D, et al: *Arch Surg* 129:588–595, 1994. Copyright 1994/95, American Medical Association.) Axillofemoral grafting with externally supported polytetrafluoroethylene.

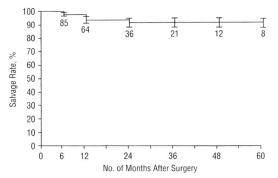

Fig 8–2.—Life-table salvage rates for 149 limbs at risk for loss treated by 127 axillofemoral grafts. *Vertical bars* indicate standard error. (Courtesy of Taylor LM Jr, Moneta GL, McConnell D, et al: Axillofemoral grafting with externally supported polytetrafluoroethylene. *Arch Surg* 129:588–595, 1994. Copyright 1994/95, American Medical Association.)

Conclusion.—Axillofemoral grafting with PTFE prostheses yields results comparable to those achieved by balloon angioplasty, aortofemoral bypass, and infrainguinal bypass.

▶ Dr. Porter has generously asked my opinion of this work from his group, and the temptation is too great to decline. In this paper, the Oregon Health Sciences University group continues to report on their series of patients with AXF grafts with quite good results. A primary patency rate of 71% at 5 years is truly commendable. However, I doubt that AXF grafting, which is a good operation in some patients and is associated with satisfactory results in the hands of those who perform it well, is equivalent to conventional anatomical repair in equivalent patients, as the authors state. Hence, I do not agree that the indications for its use should be liberalized. The authors correctly point out that there is no good contemporary study of aortofemoral reconstruction; however, I will bet a dollar that when one appears, it will remain superior in the current era.—W. Abbott, M.D.

▶ A concurrent series of axillobifemoral and aortobifemoral grafts presented by our Oregon group at the June 1995 Society for Vascular Surgery meeting indicated statistically identical primary patency at 5 years (1). I believe I just won a dollar from Dr. Abbott.—J.M. Porter, M.D.

Reference

1. Passman M: *Society for Vascular Surgery Program,* 1995, p 18.

Acute Disruption of Polytetrafluoroethylene Grafts Adjacent to Axillary Anastomoses: A Complication of Axillofemoral Grafting
Taylor LM Jr, Park TC, Edwards JM, Yeager RA, McConnell DC, Moneta GA, Porter JM (Oregon Health Sciences Univ, Portland)
J Vasc Surg 20:520–528, 1994   145-96-8–3

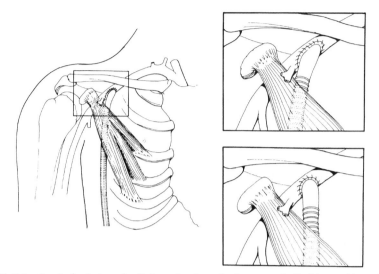

Fig 8–3.—Standard technique of axillofemoral graft proximal anastomosis. Graft is passed beneath the plane of the pectoralis minor and anastomosed to the first portion of the axillary artery, medial to pectoralis minor and to thoracromial artery. *Upper inset:* standard end-to-side anastomosis. *Lower inset:* anastomosis as recommended by graft manufacturer—there is minimal bevel, which equalizes pulling force around suture line. (Courtesy of Taylor LM Jr, Park TC, Edwards JM, et al: Acute disruption of polytetrafluoroethylene grafts adjacent to axillary anastomoses: A complication of axillofemoral grafting. *J Vasc Surg* 20:520–528, 1994.)

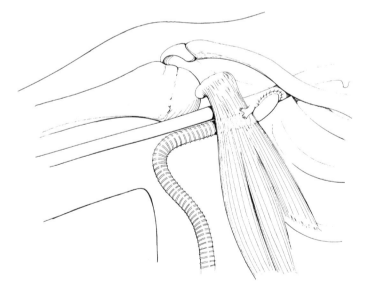

Fig 8–4.—Modified technique of axillofemoral graft proximal anastomosis. Graft is anastomosed in end-to-side fashion to the first portion of axillary artery and is routed parallel and adjacent to the artery beneath the pectoralis minor for 8–10 cm before being directed in gentle and redundant curve in the axilla to lie against the chest wall in the subcutaneous position. (Courtesy of Taylor LM Jr, Park TC, Edwards JM, et al: Acute disruption of polytetrafluoroethylene grafts adjacent to axillary anastomoses: A complication of axillofemoral grafting. *J Vasc Surg* 20:520–528, 1994.)

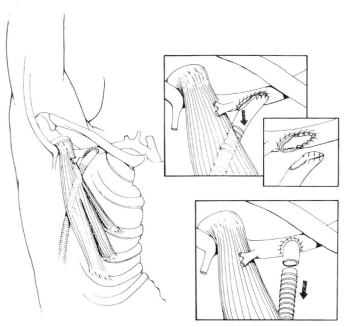

Fig 8–5.—Operative findings in cases of graft disruption. Force producing disruption occurs with arm abduction/shoulder elevation as illustrated. *Upper inset:* combined disruption with "heel" of graft tear and sutures pulling out of "toe" of graft. *Lower inset:* complete circumferential graft disruption adjacent to anastomosis. (Courtesy of Taylor LM Jr, Park TC, Edwards JM, et al: Acute disruption of polytetrafluoroethylene grafts adjacent to axillary anastomoses: A complication of axillofemoral grafting. *J Vasc Surg* 20:520–528, 1994.)

Objective.—Sporadic reports of acute disruption at or adjacent to the axillary anastomosis of an axillofemoral (AXF) graft prompted a review of 202 such grafts placed in the years 1983–1993.

Methods.—Bypass was performed by a standardized technique (Fig 8–3) using 8-mm grafts of externally supported polytetrafluoroethylene. Axillary anastomoses were performed on the first part of the artery with the arm abducted and the graft redundant. Beginning in 1992, the anastomoses were made end-to-side to the anterior surface of the first part of the axillary artery and were entirely medial to the pectoralis minor muscle and thoracoacromial artery. Rather than being directed inferiorly, the graft was routed parallel to the axillary artery for 8–10 cm into the axilla and then, in a gentle curve, inferiorly to the chest wall (Fig 8–4). The goal was to focus tension on the curved part of the graft rather than at the anastomosis.

Results.—Ten patients (5% of those who underwent surgery) had axillary disruption at an average of 3 weeks postoperatively. The longest interval was 46 days. Seven of these patients had surgery for ischemia and 3 for an infected aortic prosthesis. None of the disruptions resulted from infection. Four disruptions occurred when the arm was abducted or the shoulder elevated (Fig 8–5). One patient had a brachial plexus deficit. Four of the 10 disrupted grafts were acutely occluded. In 4 evaluable cases, the sutures had pulled out of the artery, and in 4 others, the graft was torn or sutures had pulled out of it.

Management and Outcome.—In 1 case, the artery was ligated. The remaining 9 patients had the graft revised to restore circulation. One patient had a prolonged hospital course and died 9 months later. No patient has had further disruption. The patient with a brachial plexus deficit failed to improve.

Conclusion.—There continues to be a risk of disruption of the proximal anastomosis of an AXF graft.

▶ This article reveals that complications can occur, even in the best of hands. The authors describe, in great detail, the technical aspects of the creation of their AXF bypass grafts and include a detailed description of the forces at work on the graft–axillary artery anastomosis. It is interesting that there were equal occurrences of arterial and prosthetic or suture line failures in this series, leading the authors and the commentators in the discussion section to speculate on the etiology of this conundrum.—E.S. Weinstein, M.D.

▶ Thankfully, this complication seems to have vanished after adoption of the modified operative approach described in this paper.—J.M. Porter, M.D.

Miscellaneous Topics

The Fate of the Aortofemoral Graft
Raptis S, Faris I, Miller J, Quigley F (Univ of Adelaide, Australia)
Eur J Vasc Endovasc Surg 9:97–102, 1995   145-96-8–4

Objective.—The need for reoperation and the reasons why it was necessary were studied in 301 patients who, in the years 1978–1991, underwent aortofemoral bypass surgery for symptomatic aortoiliac stenosis or occlusion. Fifty patients received aortounifemoral (AUF) grafts, and 251 received aortobifemoral (ABF) grafts.

Observations.—More than half the patients had other surgery. Procedures were performed in 16% of the ABF patients and in 50% of AUF patients before the index operation. Subsequently, 33% of the ABF and 60% of AUF patients had 1 or more additional vascular operations. For up to 10 years after surgery, graft infection or a false aneurysm developed in approximately 1% of patients per year (table). The actuarial 5-year survival rates were 73% for the ABF graft group and 38% in the AUF graft group. The primary 5-year patency rates were 85% for ABF and 81% for AUF patients. Amputation was necessary in 6% of the ABF patients and 20% of those given AUF grafts.

Conclusion.—When aortofemoral bypass surgery is contemplated in a patient with claudication, the significant likelihood that further vascular

Infection and False Aneursym—Classification	
Femoral false aneurysm (no bacteria cultured)	12
Infection in femoral anastomosis, aortic anastomosis intact	7
Infection involving both femoral and aortic anastomosis	4
Aorto enteric fistula	7

(Courtesy of Raptis S, Paris I, Miller J, et al: The fate of the aortofemoral graft. *Eur J Endovasc Surg* 9:97–102, 1995.)

surgery will be necessary should be taken into account. This is especially important for patients who may require surgery to relieve myocardial or cerebral ischemia.

▶ This pedestrian study reports a large number of aortofemoral grafts followed to define the natural history. Most of these patients required subsequent vascular surgery. Graft infections and false aneurysms occurred in approximately 1% of patients per year, at least up to 10 years. A very acceptable 5-year primary patency rate of 85% was noted in the aorto-bifemoral grafts. The patency rate of 85% is identical to our recently experienced patency rate in ABF grafting; it also is no different statistically from our 5-year patency rate for axillobifemoral grafting. We currently place considerably more axillobifemoral grafts than we do ABF grafts, because they seem to behave about the same and because the axillobifemoral grafts can be done in 1 hour with little surgical morbidity. See the commentary after Abstract 145-96-8–2.

Acute Aortic Occlusion: A 40-Year Experience
Dossa CD, Shepard AD, Reddy DJ, Jones CM, Elliott JP, Smith RF, Ernst CB
(Henry Ford Hosp, Detroit)
Arch Surg 129:603–608, 1994   145-96-8–5

Background.—Because of its rarity, the cause, mode of clinical presentation, significance of the ischemic duration, recurrence, and long-term survival of acute aortic occlusion have not been well defined. A 40-year review of patients with aortic occlusion of the abdominal aorta addressed these questions.

Methods.—A retrospective review of the study hospital's records and vascular registry was conducted for the period from June 1953 through May 1993. Only adult patients with aortographic and/or operative confirmation of aortic occlusion plus signs and symptoms of acute ischemia were included.

Results.—Forty-six patients (27 women) were identified, with embolism to the infrarenal aorta being the most common cause of acute aortic occlusion, affecting 30 patients (65%). In the remaining 16 patients, aortic thrombosis was the cause of the occlusion. Twenty-one of the 30 embolic events (70%) occurred in women. The heart was the source of all but 1.

The median duration of ischemia was 7 hours in patients with emboli. The most common procedure performed was aortic embolectomy, and the hospital mortality rate was 37%. Forty-three percent of patients experienced recurrent arterial emboli.

In the thrombotic acute aortic occlusion group, there were 10 men and 6 women. Severe aortoiliac occlusive disease was the cause in 12 patients, hypercoagulable states in 2, abdominal aortic aneurysm in 1, and aortic dissection in 1. The median duration of ischemia was 17 hours in the thrombotic group. One received anticoagulant therapy, 3 had transfemoral balloon catheter thrombectomy, 4 underwent axillobifemoral grafting, and 8 patients underwent aortic reconstruction. In this group, the hospital mortality rate was 31%.

Patients with embolic acute aortic occlusion were more likely to be female and had a significantly greater incidence of heart disease than those with thrombotic occlusion. Any neurologic deficit, other than mild sensory changes, was associated with significant mortality rates, no matter the cause of the occlusion (table). No major impact on hospital mortality among patients with embolic occlusion was seen after the introduction of the Fogarty balloon thromboembolectomy catheter in 1964.

Conclusion.—Long-term survival in both groups of patients with acute aortic occlusion was good. The early mortality probably reflects the advanced cardiac disease in these patients.

▶ The value of this paper is diminished by its retrospective nature and its acquisition of data over an unbelievable 40 years. Two conclusions are inescapable: First, acute aortic occlusion is an extraordinarily morbid condition, with a mortality rate of 35% and a morbidity rate of 75%. Second, it is, thankfully, a rare condition. Although the problem is not mentioned by these authors, in our experience, a distressing number of these patients experience permanent lower extremity neurologic dysfunction after the event.

Effect of Initial Lower Extremity Neurologic Deficit on Mortality Rate

	No. of Patients	No. of Deaths	Mortality Rate, %
Sensory deficit			
None	4	0	0
Moderate*	19	7	37
Severe†	13	5	38
Unknown	10	4	40
Motor deficit			
None	7	0	0
Paresis	17	8	47
Paralysis	18	6	33
Unknown	4	2	50

* Moderate is defined as diminished sensation to light touch.
† Severe is defined as anesthetic.
(Courtesy of Dossa CD, Shepard AD, Reddy DJ, et al: Acute aortic occlusion: A 40-year experience. *Arch Surg* 129:603–608, 1994. Courtesy of 1994/95, American Medical Association.)

Heparin-Related Thrombocytopenia and Adrenal Hemorrhagic Necrosis Following Aortic Surgery
Leschi J-P, Goëau-Brissonnière O, Coggia M, Chiche L (Hôpital Ambroise Paré, Boulogne, France)
Ann Vasc Surg 8:506–508, 1994   145-96-8-6

Background.—Adrenal hemorrhagic necrosis is a rare complication of heparin-related thrombocytopenia that may be difficult to diagnose unless suspected. A favorable outcome depends on detecting the disorder at an early stage.

Case Report.—Man, 63, had severe occlusive disease of the aorta and iliac arteries, and received an aortofemoral bypass graft. Heparin was given intraoperatively in a dose of 25,000 IU and postoperatively in a dose of 150,000 IU in 24 hours. A repeat dose was given 4 days later, after which IV heparin was replaced by daily injections of 40 mg of enoxaparin. The platelets decreased to 85,000/mm^3 8 days postoperatively as evidence of disseminated intravascular coagulation appeared. When platelet aggregation was noted in the presence of both standard and low molecular weight heparin, enoxaparin was withdrawn and ethyl biscoumacetate was substituted. The platelets decreased to 30,000/mm^3 before starting to recover. The patient became comatose and went into cardiocirculatory arrest, which resolved spontaneously but was followed by intractable shock. Abdominal ultrasonography showed a hematoma in the right psoas muscle. The patient died 13 days postoperatively after repeat cardiocirculatory arrest. Bilateral adrenal hemorrhagic necrosis was noted, involving the entire medulla and part of the cortex of each adrenal gland. There were no other abnormalities; the vascular graft was intact.

Conclusion.—Adrenal hemorrhagic necrosis is found most often in connection with hypocoagulable states. Hemodynamic instability and gastrointestinal disorder are characteristic of the condition. Computed tomographic scanning of the adrenal glands is the best means of making the diagnosis.

▶ This extremely interesting case report describes the outcome of a 63-year-old man after aortofemoral grafting. Heparin-associated antibody with a diminished platelet count developed. The patient eventually experienced circulatory collapse and death. Autopsy showed bilateral hemorrhagic necrosis of the adrenal glands, clearly the cause of the patient's circulatory collapse. This association of HAT and adrenal hemorrhagic necrosis with death from circulatory collapse has been previously reported (1). In the future, if we encounter a patient pursuing this course, a test dose of steroids will be given.

Reference

1. Scully RE, Mark EJ, McNeely NF, et al: Case records of the Massachusetts General Hospital. *N Engl J Med* 321:1595–1603, 1989.

Late Complications After Aortic Surgery

Browning N, Barry R, Nel C, Basson S, Linde P (Univ of the Orange Free State, Bloemfontein, South Africa)
Ann Vasc Surg 8:232–237, 1994   145-96-8-7

Background.—Reported rates of false aneurysm formation, anastomotic stenosis, and ureteric obstruction are reported to be low in patients having aortic surgery. Possibly, the long-term identification of such complications should be aided by IV digital subtraction angiography with completion excretory urography (CEU).

Objective.—Complications were studied in 44 patients who, 1–12 years earlier, had undergone surgery on the aorta.

Results.—False aneurysms were detected at 10 distal anastomoses but no aortic anastomoses. They occurred in 16% of patients and 11% of all anastomoses. Both endarterectomy and use of the femoral artery for distal anastomosis disposed to the formation of anastomotic aneurysms, which were found at 18% of aortic anastomoses. No distal anastomoses were stenosed. Two patients, both of whom had emergency surgery on a ruptured aortic aneurysm, had 3 asymptomatic ureteric obstructions.

Conclusion.—Intravenous digital subtraction angiography with CEU is an effective means of detecting clinically silent complications after surgery on the aorta.

▶ Slightly more anastomotic aneurysms were found than would have been predicted, along with an 5% incidence of ureteric obstructions. There was a disconcerting incidence of 18% aortic anastomotic stenoses. The use of IV digital subtraction angiography, at times remote from aortic surgery, to identify complications is noteworthy. I wonder whether most of us would have similar complications if we routinely performed the imaging studies required for their documentation.

The Retroperitoneal Incision: An Evaluation of Postoperative Flank 'Bulge'

Gardner GP, Josephs LG, Rosca M, Rich J, Woodson J, Menzoian JO (Boston Univ)
Arch Surg 129:753–756, 1994   145-96-8-8

Background.—In patients undergoing repair of abdominal aortic aneurysm, the retroperitoneal incisions may be associated with an unsightly laxity, or "bulge," of the ipsilateral abdominal wall musculature. This bulge may result from injury to the ipsilateral intercostal nerve (IN). The possible associations between IN injury, the extent of the retroperitoneal incisions, and postoperative flank bulge were studied.

Methods.—Bilateral dissections of the eleventh IN were performed in 7 cadavers. In addition, the extent of the retroperitoneal incision and the incidence of postoperative flank bulge were analyzed retrospectively in 63

Moving?

I'd like to receive my *Year Book of Vascular Surgery* without interruption.
Please note the following change of address, effective:

Name: _____

New Address: _____

_____

City: _____ State: _____ Zip: _____

Old Address: _____

_____

City: _____ State: _____ Zip: _____

Reservation Card

Yes, I would like my own copy of *Year Book of Vascular Surgery* . Please begin my subscription with the current edition according to the terms described below.* I understand that I will have 30 days to examine each annual edition. If satisfied, I will pay just $75.95 plus sales tax, postage and handling (price subject to change without notice).

Name: _____

Address: _____

City: _____ State: _____ Zip: _____

Method of Payment
○ Visa   ○ Mastercard   ○ AmEx   ○ Bill me   ○ Check (in US dollars, payable to Mosby, Inc.)

Card number: _____ Exp date: _____

Signature: _____

LS-0908

---

*Your *Year Book* Service Guarantee:

When you subscribe to the *Year Book*, we'll send you an advance notice of future volumes about two months before they publish. This automatic notice system is designed to take up as little of your time as possible. If you do not want the *Year Book*, the advance notice makes it quick and easy for you to let us know your decision, and you will always have at least 20 days to decide. If we don't hear from you, we'll send you the new volume as soon as it's available. And, of course, the *Year Book* is yours to examine free of charge for 30 days (postage, handling and applicable sales tax are added to each shipment.).

BUSINESS REPLY MAIL
FIRST CLASS MAIL   PERMIT No. 762   CHICAGO, IL

NO POSTAGE
NECESSARY
IF MAILED
IN THE
UNITED STATES

POSTAGE WILL BE PAID BY ADDRESSEE

Chris Hughes
Mosby-Year Book, Inc.
200 N. LaSalle Street
Suite 2600
Chicago, IL 60601-9981

BUSINESS REPLY MAIL
FIRST CLASS MAIL   PERMIT No. 762   CHICAGO, IL

NO POSTAGE
NECESSARY
IF MAILED
IN THE
UNITED STATES

POSTAGE WILL BE PAID BY ADDRESSEE

Chris Hughes
Mosby-Year Book, Inc.
200 N. LaSalle Street
Suite 2600
Chicago, IL 60601-9981

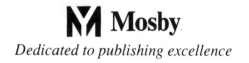

M Mosby

Dedicated to publishing excellence

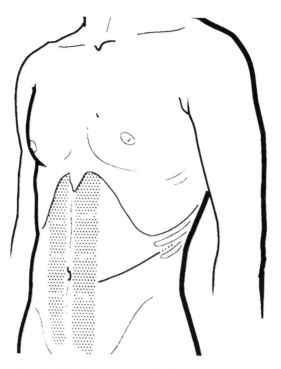

Fig 8–6.—Retroperitoneal incision for postoperative flank bulge. *Solid line* shows the extent of the incision (up to 11th intercostal space) used after modification to reduce the rate of postoperative bulge. *Dotted line* shows extension into this intercostal space. (Courtesy of Gardner GP, Josephs LG, Rosca M, et al: The retroperitoneal incision: An evaluation of potoperative flank "bulge." *Arch Surg* 129:753–756, 1994. Copyright 1994/95, Americal Medical Association.)

consecutive patients undergoing this approach to repair of an abdominal aortic aneurysm. Neurophysiologic evaluation was done in 5 patients—3 with and 2 without a flank bulge. The findings were analyzed to determine whether avoiding extension of the retroperitoneal incision into the intercostal space could reduce the incidence of injury to the eleventh IN.

Results.—Of the 14 cadaver dissections, bifurcations of the main trunk of the eleventh IN were noted within the intercostal space in 4 cases, at the tip of the eleventh rib in 7 cases, and at least 2 cm distal to the tip of the rib in 3 cases. In the 3 patients with a flank bulge, neurophysiologic evaluation showed iterative discharges, polyphasia, fibrillation potentials, and altered recruitment patterns consistent with IN injury. These findings were present neither in the opposite abdominal wall musculature nor in the patients without a flank bulge. In this patient series, the incidence of postoperative flank bulge was 11%. The incision extended into the eleventh intercostal space in 31 patients, 19% of whom had postoperative bulge. In contrast, a bulge developed in only 0.03% of patients in which the incision did not extend into the intercostal space (Fig 8–6).

Conclusion.—Flank bulge after abdominal aortic aneurysm repair is associated with IN injury and subsequent paralysis of the abdominal wall musculature. By avoiding extension of the retroperitoneal incision into the eleventh intercostal space, the surgeon can reduce IN injury and, thus, the incidence of postoperative bulge.

▶ I believe the information is clear. Flank bulges are undesirable and should be avoided. You avoid this by not damaging the posterior portion of the intercostal nerve. Intercostal nerve injury anterior to the end of the 11th and 12th ribs appears to have little effect. We typically end our extraperitoneal incision approximately 1 or 2 cm inferior and posterior to the tip of the 12th rib. To routinely go into the 11th interspace is perfectly acceptable, but one should not go into the posterior aspects of the interspace unless it is absolutely required for surgical exposure.

9 Visceral Renal Artery Disease

Mesenteric Bypass

Isolated Bypass to the Superior Mesenteric Artery for Intestinal Ischemia

Gentile AT, Moneta GL, Taylor LM Jr, Park TC, McConnell DB, Porter JM (Oregon Health Sciences Univ, Portland; Portland Veterans Affairs Hosp, Ore)

Arch Surg 129:926–932, 1994   145-96-9–1

Background.—Several reports have advocated the inclusion of the superior mesenteric artery (SMA) and the celiac artery in revascularization procedures for patients with intestinal ischemia. However, there are no data from controlled or randomized studies to confirm that this approach gives better results than the SMA bypass alone. Experience with isolated bypass to the SMA for patients with intestinal ischemia was reviewed.

Methods.—The analysis included 26 patients who underwent 29 isolated bypasses to the SMA for intestinal ischemia from 1982 through 1993. The operative indications, operative technique, perioperative mortality, and long-term outcomes were examined. All patients had duplex scanning or arteriography to evaluate the patency of the SMA grafts within the previous 6 months. The life-table method was used to compute patient survival and graft patency rates.

Results.—The 16 female and 10 male patients had a mean age of 59 years. Twenty-three bypasses were performed for symptomatic chronic mesenteric ischemia, 5 for acute intestinal ischemia, and 1 for symptomatic SMA occlusion. Three patients died in the perioperative period, for a mortality rate of 10%. All 3 had acute intestinal ischemia and a history of previous mesenteric artery surgery. The primary graft patency rate was 89% and patient survival was 82% at 4 years (Fig 9–1). All patients for whom follow-up data were available had good maintenance of symptomatic improvement.

Conclusion.—An isolated bypass to the SMA yields excellent graft patency rates in patients with intestinal ischemia. Perioperative mortality and long-term patient survival were acceptable in this retrospective series. The

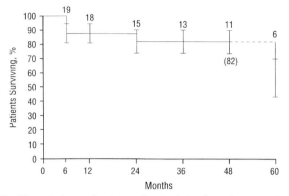

Fig 9–1.—Life-table survival rates of patients undergoing isolated superior mesenteric artery bypass for mesenteric ischemia. The *numbers above the curve* indicate the number of patients at risk; the *number below the curve* indicates the 4-year survival rate. The *dotted line* indicates when the standard error exceeds 10%. (Courtesy of Gentile AT, Moneta GL, Taylor LM Jr, et al: Isolated bypass to the superior mesenteric artery for intestinal ischemia. *Arch Surg* 129:926–932, 1994. Copyright 1994/95, American Medical Association.)

use of the SMA bypass alone appears to produce results as good as those of bypass to multiple visceral vessels.

▶ This report challenges the traditional recommendation of complete (at least 2 of 3) vessel revascularization in the treatment of chronic mesenteric ischemia. The authors present an experience with 29 bypasses in 26 patients with mesenteric ischemia, in whom only the SMA was revascularized. Graft patency was 89% at 4 years, with patient survival of 82% during the same interval.

At first glance, one would conclude that isolated bypass to the SMA is sufficient revascularization in the treatment of these patients. However, careful analysis of this patient population reveals that 7 of the 26 patients had a stenosis of 50% or less in the celiac axis, with 4 patients having a normal celiac artery. Seven additional patients were having a second intervention after either a failed bypass or transluminal angioplasty. Of note is that 3 of the patients who previously had an isolated SMA bypass had acute intestinal ischemia when the bypass failed. In the experience reported by Dr. Ronald J. Stoney in the discussion of this paper, patients who underwent multiple visceral revascularization for the treatment of chronic mesenteric ischemia and who eventually had graft failure fared better than those who had a single artery revascularization; the latter will frequently present with acute intestinal ischemia when the graft fails. This concern has been the basis for the traditional approach.

The authors have documented the durability of bypass grafts to the SMA. Their technique of retrograde bypass is certainly simpler than using the supraceliac aorta as inflow. The mortality was primarily related to the management of acute intestinal ischemia, with all patients undergoing elective surgery for chronic intestinal ischemia surviving the procedure. Overall, these results document the long-term success of bypass to the SMA for intestinal ischemia, which, in selected patients, may be performed as a single-vessel revascularization. In patients with significant occlusive disease of the celiac artery, I still prefer multiple-vessel revascularization of at least 2 of 3 mesenteric arteries.—W. Quiñones-Baldrich, M.D.

Revascularisation of Atherosclerotic Mesenteric Arteries: Experience in 90 Consecutive Patients
Christensen MG, Lorentzen JE, Schroeder TV (Univ Hosp, Copenhagen)
Eur J Vasc Surg 8:297–302, 1994   145-96-9–2

Introduction.—Vascular surgeons are well aware of visceral artery surgery, but most have little personal experience with it. Twenty-five years' experience with patients treated for atherosclerotic lesions of the visceral arteries was reviewed.

Patients.—The experience included 90 patients treated at 1 vascular surgery department. There were 54 men and 36 women, with a median age of 56 years. These patients underwent 109 mesenteric reconstructions. Of the 90 primary procedures, 25 were performed for acute mesenteric ischemia of nonembolic origin, 53 for chronic ischemia, and 12 for prophylactic reconstruction in association with aortic surgery. Revascularization of the superior mesenteric artery (SMA) was performed in 87 patients and of the celiac axis or common hepatic artery in 6; both territories were revascularized in only 3 patients. Fifteen patients had thromboendarterectomy, 30 had transposition of the SMA directly into the infrarenal aorta, and 48 had bypass.

Outcomes.—The 30-day mortality rate was 44% in acutely operated patients, compared with 0% in electively operated patients and 8% in prophylactically operated patients. The overall perioperative mortality rate was 13%. Of 12 deaths, 9 were caused by progressive mesenteric infarction. The cumulative survival rates were 81% at 5 years, 60% at 10 years, and 35% at 20 years. These long-term results suggested a mortality rate 3 times greater than in an age- and sex-matched population. Survival was better for patients who had surgery for chronic ischemia. Thirty patients had recurrent symptoms during follow-up. Recurrences were more likely in patients who had undergone emergency surgery and SMA transposition.

Conclusion.—Mesenteric revascularization can yield good long-term results for patients with atherosclerosis of visceral arteries. Early surgery should be performed, if possible, because the mortality rate is high for patients undergoing acute operation.

▶ The authors' conclusion that SMA bypass alone is adequate in a larger majority of patients is the same as our opinion at Oregon Health Sciences University. The excellent clinical series reported herein will be a model for us all.

Usefulness of Fasting and Postprandial Duplex Ultrasound Examinations for Predicting High-Grade Superior Mesenteric Artery Stenosis

Gentile AT, Moneta GL, Lee RW, Masser PA, Taylor LM Jr, Porter JM (Oregon Health Sciences Univ, Portland; Veterans Affairs Hosp, Portland, Ore)
Am J Surg 169:476–479, 1995   145-96-9–3

Background.—High-grade stenosis—i.e., greater than 70%—of the superior mesenteric artery (SMA) can be accurately depicted by fasting duplex ultrasonography. To find out whether postprandial SMA duplex ultrasonography may provide further information, thereby improving the ability to detect high-grade stenosis, the results of fasting and postprandial duplex scans were compared.

Methods.—Eighty patients undergoing aortography because of vascular disease and 25 healthy controls participated. Aortographic results showed that 61 of the patients had 0% to 30% SMA stenosis (group 1), 10 had 30% to 70% stenosis (group 2), and 9 had 70% to 99% stenosis (group 3). On fasting SMA duplex scanning, a peak systolic velocity (PSV) of 275 cm/sec or greater was defined as indicating high-grade SMA stenosis.

Results.—No significant difference was found in the mean fasting SMA PSV between the controls and the patients with SMA stenosis of less than 70%. All groups showed a significant increase in the postprandial PSV, although this value was not significantly different between groups 1 and 2 and the control group. Patients in group 3 had a significantly greater mean fasting PSV and a significantly lower postprandial increase in PSV (table). For the prediction of high-grade SMA stenosis, the sensitivity was 89% for the fasting duplex scan, 67% for the postprandial scan, and 67% for the combination. Specificities were 89% for the fasting scan, 94% for the postprandial scan, and 100% for the combination; positive predictive values were 80%, 60%, and 100%; negative predictive values were 99%, 96%, and 96%; and accuracies were 96%, 91%, and 96% respectively.

Conclusion.—On duplex scanning, patients with high-grade stenosis of the SMA show a blunted postprandial increase in PSV. However, feeding velocities cannot distinguish among patients with less severe degrees of

Peak Systolic Velocity (PSV) Profiles of Superior Mesenteric Artery (SMA) Stenosis of Patients With Atherosclerosis

	Group 1 (n = 61)	Group 2 (n = 10)	Group 3 (n = 9)
Fasting PSV*	161 ± 56	186 ± 65	355 ± 137
Postprandial PSV*	246 ± 65	280 ± 94	402 ± 125
Mean postprandial increase in PSV	53%	50%	13%

Note: Group 1 includes patients with 0% to < 30% SMA stenosis; group 2, patients with 30% to < 70% SMA stenosis; group 3, patients with 70% to 99% SMA stenosis.
* Values expressed as mean ± standard deviation, cm/sec.
(Courtesy of Gentile AT, Moneta GL, Lee RW, et al: Usefulness of fasting and postprandial duplex ultrasound examinations for predicting high-grade superior mesenteric artery stenosis. *Am J Surg* 169:476–479, 1995. Reprinted with permission from *American Journal of Surgery.*)

SMA stenosis. Stenosis of greater than 70% can be detected by fasting or postprandial PSV; combining both yields some increase in specificity and positive predictive value compared with the fasting study alone. If the fasting scan shows a PSV of 275 cm/sec or more, the postprandial scan need not be done.

▶ This study of duplex criteria for significant SMA stenosis concludes that a fasting PSV of 275 cm/sec or greater most accurately identifies a hemo-dynamically significant (> 70%) stenosis. Postprandial blunting of the antici-pated increase in PSV is noted in patients with severe stenosis, but using this in combination with the fasting criteria only marginally improves overall accuracy. It appears that feeding studies are not necessary for the accurate duplex evaluation of SMA stenosis.

Miscellaneous

Pediatric Renovascular Hypertension: A Thirty-Year Experience of Operative Treatment

Stanley JC, Zelenock GB, Messina LM, Wakefield TW (Univ of Michigan, Ann Arbor)
J Vasc Surg 21:212–227, 1995   145-96-9-4

Objective.—Changing patterns of operative management for renovas-cular hypertension in pediatric patients were reviewed over 30 years. Three eras were highlighted, covering the years 1963–1972, 1973–1980, and 1981–1993.

Patients.—Thirty-three boys and 24 girls, 10 months to 17 years of age, had surgery for renovascular hypertension during the period reviewed. Atypical medial-perimedial dysplasia, often associated with secondary in-timal fibroplasia, was present in 88% of patients, and inflammatory mural fibrosis was seen in 12%. Fifteen patients had narrowing of the abdominal aorta.

Results.—A total of 74 primary operative procedures were done. The most common were aortorenal bypass with autogenous vein grafting and renal artery resection beyond the stenosis, with reimplantation of the remaining vessel into the aorta. Aortorenal bypass with vein grafting accounted for 56.5% of all primary operations done in era I but only 3% of those done in era III. There were no reimplantation operations in era I, but more than half the operations in era III were reimplantations (Fig 9–2). Fourteen patients had 20 secondary operations, 7 of which were neph-rectomies. In all, hypertension was cured operatively in 79% of patients and improved in another 19%. There were no operative deaths.

Conclusion.—Pediatric patients with renovascular hypertension have clearly benefited from the various operative procedures used in the past 3 decades.

▶ This retrospective 30-year institutional experience with pediatric patients undergoing surgery for renovascular hypertension is interesting and impor-

ERA III: 1981 - 1993

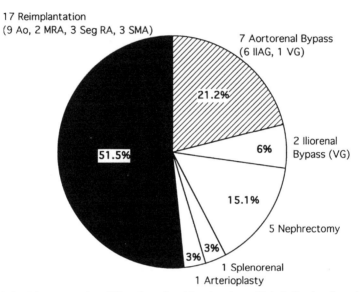

17 Reimplantation
(9 Ao, 2 MRA, 3 Seg RA, 3 SMA)

7 Aortorenal Bypass
(6 IIAG, 1 VG)

21.2%

51.5%

6%

2 Iliorenal
Bypass (VG)

15.1%

5 Nephrectomy

3%

3%

1 Splenorenal

1 Arterioplasty

Fig 9–2.—Primary operations (33) performed on 24 patients in era III, including 1 patient who also underwent primary contralateral renal vascularization in era I. Note predominance of reimplantation procedures and frequent use of internal iliac artery grafts for aortorenal bypasses. *Abbreviations:* Ao, aorta; *MRA*, main renal artery; *Seg RA*, segmental renal artery; *SMA*, superior mesenteric artery; *IIAG*, internal iliac artery graft; *VG*, vein graft. (Courtesy of Stanley JC, Zelenock GB, Messina LM, et al: Pediatric renovascular hypertension: A thirty-year experience of operative treatment. *J Vasc Surg* 21:212–227, 1995.)

tant. Of note is the paucity of ex vivo reconstructions (only 1). In recent years, there has been a trend toward more reimplantations of the transected renal artery and fewer vein grafts. The operative findings of significant improvement in 98% of patients and no operative deaths are exemplary. This experience sets the standards for management of this difficult patient group.

MR Measurements of Mesenteric Venous Flow: Prospective Evaluation in Healthy Volunteers and Patients With Suspected Chronic Mesenteric Ischemia
Burkart DJ, Johnson CD, Reading CC, Ehman RL (Mayo Clinic and Found, Rochester, Minn)
Radiology 194:801–806, 1995   145-96-9-5

Objective.—Blood flow in the portal vein and superior mesenteric vein was quantified by the cine phase-contrast MR technique before and after a standard meal in 10 healthy individuals and 10 patients clinically suspected of having chronic mesenteric ischemia.

Results.—In normal individuals, the postprandial study demonstrated a 245% augmentation of flow in the superior mesenteric vein and a 70% greater flow in the portal vein. The postprandial increase in the superior mesenteric vein flow was significantly less in the 4 patients with confirmed mesenteric ischemia, averaging 64% (Fig 9–3). The 6 patients without mesenteric ischemia had flow augmentation of 206%, not significantly different from that in controls.

Conclusion.—Magnetic resonance estimates of postprandial blood flow augmentation in the superior mesenteric vein may prove to be a useful noninvasive screening measure for detecting chronic mesenteric ischemia.

▶ This is the first study of which I am aware that attempts to evaluate portal venous flow quantitatively after a standardized meal. The authors use the MR quantitative flow measurement previously reported (see Abstracts 145-96-3–3 and 145-96-3–4). Predictably, the investigators noted significant postprandial augmentation of superior mesenteric vein and portal vein flow, with decreased augmentation in the few patients studied who had mesenteric arterial ischemia. The authors conclude that the measurement of postprandial flow augmentation in the superior mesenteric vein with MR flow measurements may be a valuable test for chronic mesenteric ischemia. They had only 10 patients with mesenteric ischemia, so their results must be interpreted in light of this very small patient group.

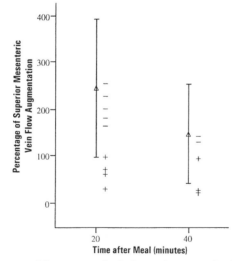

Fig 9–3.—The percentage of flow augmentation in the superior mesenteric vein at 20 and 40 minutes after a standardized meal in volunteers and patients. At 20 minutes, the percentage of change in patients without mesenteric ischemia was not significantly different from that of the volunteers ($P = 0.31$). The percentage of flow augmentation at 20 minutes after a meal in patients with mesenteric ischemia was significantly less than in patients without ischemia ($P = 0.02$) and in volunteers ($P = 0.02$). *Triangles* indicate fasting flow in volunteers ± 2 SD; *plus signs,* fasting flow in patients with mesenteric ischemia; *minus signs,* fasting flow in patients without mesenteric ischemia. (Courtesy of Burkart DJ, Johnson CD, Reading CC, et al; MR measurements of mesenteric venous flow: Prospective evaluation in healthy volunteers and patients with suspected chronic mesenteric ischemia. *Radiology* 194:801–806, 1995.)

10 Leg Ischemia

Leg Bypass

Infrainguinal Reconstruction With Arm Vein, Lesser Saphenous Vein, and Remnants of Greater Saphenous Vein: A Report of 257 Cases

Londrey GL, Bosher LP, Brown PW, Stoneburner FD Jr, Pancoast JW, Davis RK (Virginia Surgical Associates, Richmond)

J Vasc Surg 20:451–457, 1994   145-96-10–1

Background.—Patients who need infrainguinal arterial reconstruction but lack adequate ipsilateral greater saphenous vein (GSV) pose a challenge for the vascular surgeon. Although each of the available options has its limitations, the use of all-autogenous grafts, mainly arm vein grafts, has long been preferred at 1 center. A 17-year experience with this approach was reviewed.

Methods.—The experience included 257 infrainguinal arterial reconstructions with ectopic vein grafts in 240 extremities of 222 patients. All patients had lower extremity ischemia and lacked a suitable ipsilateral GSV. In 83% of cases, the GSV could not be used because of previous bypass surgery, either in the peripheral vasculature or coronary arteries. The reconstructions were performed with the use of arm vein, lesser saphenous vein, and remnants of ipsilateral GSV. Eighty-eight percent of the reconstructions were performed because of rest pain or tissue loss. Seventy percent were secondary reconstructions, and 90% of the distal anastomoses were infrapopliteal. Single-length vein grafts were used in two thirds of the cases, and composite vein grafts were used in one third.

Results.—In the overall series, the secondary graft patency rates were 70% at 1 year, 52% at 3 years, and 43% at 5 years (Fig 10–1). The 1-year patency rate was 78% for single-length grafts vs. 56% for composite vein grafts. This advantage persisted at all follow-up intervals: 60% vs. 39% at 3 years and 52% vs. 29% at 5 years. The 5-year extremity salvage rate was 69%. The 5-year survival rate by the life-table method was 60%, and the 30-day mortality rate was 2%.

Conclusion.—When infrainguinal reconstruction must be performed in patients without suitable ipsilateral GSV, the ectopic vein graft approach is an acceptable alternative. Patency is significantly better for single-length than for ectopic vein grafts. Although better results might have been

PATENCY - ALL GRAFTS

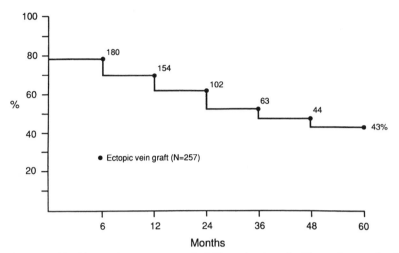

Fig 10–1.—Life-table secondary patency rates for 257 ectopic vein grafts. *The number at each point* represents the number of grafts at risk for that interval. (Courtesy of Londrey GL, Bosher LP, Brown PW, et al: Infrainguinal reconstruction with arm vein, lesser saphenous vein, and remnants of greater saphenous vein: A report of 257 cases. *J Vasc Surg* 20:451–457, 1994.)

achieved by routine use of contralateral GSV, this conduit was not available at the time of ectopic graft placement in most patients.

▶ These authors have had a very large experience using alternate veins for leg bypass. Their overall patency rate is good, but I really wish they had not used the term "secondary patency," as I believe what they mean is primary assisted patency, a term added since the 1986 reporting standards. These authors note, just as we have, that an increased number of alternate veins require revision—in their experience, 20%. In our recent experience, 28% of alternate veins used for tibial bypasses required revision based on postoperative graft surveillance (1). Currently, we find that alternate veins are required in slightly more than 20% of our entire leg bypass operative series, and approximately one quarter of these require revision within 12 months to maintain primary assisted patency. When one performs leg bypass, one accepts the responsibility for ongoing graft surveillance and graft revisions as needed.

Reference

1. Gentile A: Society for Vascular Surgery Program, 1995, p 18.

A Comparison of Endovascular Assisted and Conventional in Situ Bypass Grafts

Cikrit DF, Fiore NF, Dalsing MC, Lalka SG, Sawchuk AP, Ladd AP, Dodson S

(Indiana Univ, Indianapolis; Richard L Roudebush VA Hosp, Indianapolis, Ind)
Ann Vasc Surg 9:37–43, 1995   145-96-10-2

Background.—In situ saphenous vein bypass grafting is a useful technique, but the associated wound complication rates can be quite high. An initial experience with endovascular-assisted in situ (EAI) saphenous vein bypass grafting—developed in an attempt to decrease the length of the surgical wound and, thus, to lessen the chances of flap necrosis—was reported.

Methods.—Thirty-three in situ saphenous vein bypass grafts were performed using a conventional open technique (CI) and 31 in situ bypass grafts using endovascular occlusion of side branches (Fig 10–2). The grafts were performed from the femoral to the popliteal artery in 37 cases and from the femoral artery to a trifurcation artery in 27 cases. The indications were tissue loss in 43 cases, rest pain in 14, and claudication in 7.

Results.—The length of postoperative hospitalization was 8 days in the CI group vs. 4 days in the EAI group. After surgery, missed arteriovenous fistulas were detected in only 1 CI limb compared with 17 EAI limbs. At follow-up, the rate of occlusion or revision surgery was 12% in the CI group and 19% in the EAI group. On life-table analysis, the 18-month cumulative patency rates were 79% with CI and 83% with EAI. The operative time was no shorter with the EAI technique; however, the length of surgical incisions and the duration of postoperative hospitalization were significantly shorter. Wound complications were less frequent with EAI, but missed arteriovenous fistulas were more common.

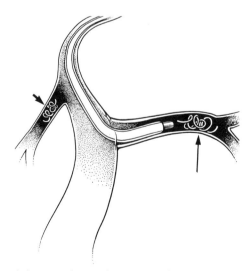

Fig 10–2.—Coil embolization technique showing an occlusion coil in a tributary superior to a saphenous vein branch that has just been cannulated. Another coil (*arrow*) was hydrodynamically delivered to the vessel through the Cynosar (*small arrow*) protruding from the end of the electronically steerable nitinol catheter. (Courtesy of Cikrit DF, Fiore NF, Dalsing MC, et al: A comparison of endovascular assisted and conventional in situ bypass grafts. *Ann Vasc Surg* 9:37–43, March 1995.)

Conclusion.—Initial experience suggests that the EAI and CI techniques for in situ saphenous vein bypass grafting are comparable in terms of patency. The ultimate determinant of the value of the endovascular-assisted technique will be long-term patency.

▶ I continue to be amazed by what we do in the name of progress. To use endovascular methods to assist in in situ bypass construction is to carry absurdity to a new level. These authors have compared endovascular-assisted to conventional in situ bypass grafting and, after searching diligently, have been able to identify only the minimal benefit of marginally decreasing the length of the surgical incision. They conclude that endovascular-assisted and conventional in situ bypass grafts are comparable. I cannot tell you how happy I am to learn this.

Surgical Treatment of Threatened Reversed Infrainguinal Vein Grafts
Nehler MR, Moneta GL, Yeager RA, Edwards JM, Taylor LM Jr, Porter JM (Oregon Health Sciences Univ, Portland; Portland Veterans Affairs Hosp, Ore)
J Vasc Surg 20:558–565, 1994   145-96-10-3

Background.—Most past experience in revising threatened infrainguinal vein grafts has involved in situ conduits. These grafts may be threatened by either intrinsic disease or a stenosed inflow or outflow vessel.

Methods.—The results of revision surgery were examined in 96 patients who had a threatened but patent infrainguinal reversed vein graft in the years 1987–1993. The patients had 69 femoropopliteal and 31 femorotibial grafts, and they underwent a total of 117 operative vein graft revisions or inflow procedures. A large majority of original grafts consisted of a single segment of greater saphenous vein. In all cases, either the graft itself or an adjacent vessel was stenosed by at least 50% (Table 1). Thirteen of the 100 grafts were revised twice, and 2 were revised 3 times. Approximately half the revisions were interposition vein graft placements, whereas one fourth involved extending the vein graft to a new distal anastomotic site.

Results.—The median interval from initial surgery to primary revision was 15 months, and the average time to secondary revision was 21 months. One patient died of postoperative myocardial infarction. The

---

TABLE 1.—Preoperative Angiographic Location of Significant (Greater than 50%) Stenoses in 117 Operative Revisions of Stenotic Reversed Vein Grafts

Inflow (%)	Proximal Graft (%)	Mid Graft (%)	Distal Graft (%)	Outflow (%)	Combination (%)
9%*	42	10	8	20†	11

* Includes 5 grafts with 100% inflow occlusion.
† Includes 13 grafts with 100% outflow occlusion.
(Courtesy of Nehler MR, Moneta GL, Yeager RA, et al: Surgical treatment of threatened reversed infrainguinal vein grafts. *J Vasc Surg* 20:558–565, 1994.)

cumulative assisted primary patency rate of initial grafts revised for stenosis was 99% at 1 year and 92% at 5 years (Table 2). The respective limb salvage rates were 98% and 97% (Table 3).

Conclusion.—Reversed vein grafts in the infrainguinal region that are threatened for any reason may be surgically revised with the expectation of excellent patency and limb salvage rates, with minimal procedural morbidity.

▶ This manuscript summarizes the authors' experience with the management of 100 infrainguinal reversed vein grafts that were identified as failing grafts under an intensive follow-up surveillance protocol using duplex scan. The criteria used for identification of the failing graft included midgraft velocities less than 45 cm/sec, and/or the presence of a peak systolic velocity greater than 200 cm/sec in any portion of the graft or adjacent inflow or outflow artery. All grafts consisted of reversed saphenous vein bypasses, with a few grafts being of segments of vein with venovenostomies. Importantly, no difference in the mechanism of graft failure was identified between these groups.

Most, if not all, grafts were placed in an anatomical plane, which may account for the extremely high use of segmental interposition grafts and/or graft extensions. Herein lies one of the main advantages of subcutaneous placement of saphenous vein grafts, be they in situ or reversed. When the graft is in the subcutaneous location, revision is greatly simplified, and many of the intrinsic lesions that may be identified during surveillance can be treated with patch angioplasty, as opposed to interposition grafting. In this particular series, interposition grafting or graft extensions accounted for 91 of the 117 graft revisions. Most importantly, the authors document the effectiveness of management for intervention in the presence of a failing graft identified in a surveillance protocol. They were able to accomplish an assisted primary patency rate in these conduits of 91% at 5 years.

As the authors point out, this particular series of revised vein grafts has an increased number of patients whose primary indication for reconstruction was claudication (approximately one third), as compared with their previ-

TABLE 2.—Cumulative Assisted Primary Patency for 100 Stenotic Infrainguinal Reversed Vein Grafts

Interval (mo)	At Risk	Occluded	Withdrawn	Interval Patency	Cumulative Patency	Standard Error
0–1	100	0	0	1.000	1.000	0.0000
2–6	100	1	7	0.990	0.990	0.0099
7–12	92	0	4	1.000	0.990	0.0103
13–24	88	1	19	0.987	0.977	0.0158
25–36	68	1	15	0.983	0.960	0.0233
37–48	52	1	8	0.979	0.940	0.0319
49–60	43	1	11	0.973	0.915	0.0407
61–72	31	0	7	1.000	0.915	0.0479
72–84	24	1	10	0.947	0.867	0.0645

(Courtesy of Nehler MR, Moneta GL, Yeager RA, et al: Surgical treatment of threatened reversed infrainguinal vein grafts. *J Vasc Surg* 20:558–565, 1994.)

TABLE 3.—Limb Salvage in 100 Limbs With Surgically Revised Stenotic Reversed
Infrainguinal Vein Grafts

Interval (mo)	At Risk	Amputated	Withdrawn	Interval Salvage	Cumulative Salvage	Standard Error
0–1	100	0	0	1.000	1.000	0.0000
2–6	100	1	7	0.990	0.990	0.0099
7–12	92	1	3	0.989	0.979	0.0148
13–24	88	1	19	0.987	0.966	0.0190
25–36	68	0	16	1.000	0.966	0.0216
37–48	52	0	9	1.000	0.966	0.0247
49–60	43	0	12	1.000	0.966	0.0272
61–72	31	0	7	1.000	0.966	0.0320
73–84	24	0	11	1.000	0.966	0.0364
85+	13	0	13	1.000	0.966	0.0494

(Courtesy of Nehler MR, Moneta GL, Yeager RA, et al: Surgical treatment of threatened reversed infrainguinal vein grafts. *J Vasc Surg* 20:558–565, 1994.)

ously published series in which most conduits were placed for limb salvage. This difference may account for the improved results noted in this series of revised vein grafts. Based on this experience, the authors have provided documentation of the effectiveness of graft surveillance by demonstrating excellent results with relatively minor revisions of these conduits when they are identified in their failing stage before graft thrombosis. The authors suggest that surgical revision may offer advantages over percutaneous endovascular techniques; based on their results, a strong case favoring surgical revision of these failing conduits can be made.—W. Quiñones-Baldrich, M.D.

Return to Well-Being and Function After Infrainguinal Revascularization
Gibbons GW, Burgess AM, Guadagnoli E, Pomposelli FB Jr, Freeman DV, Campbell DR, Miller A, Marcaccio EJ Jr, Nordberg P, LoGerfo FW (New England Deaconess Hosp, Boston; Harvard Med School, Boston; Surgical Specialists Inc, Pawtucket, RI)
J Vasc Surg 21:35–45, 1995   145-96-10–4

Introduction.—Outcome after infrainguinal revascularization has primarily focused on perioperative morbidity, mortality, primary and secondary patency rates, and limb salvage rates, but seldom from the perspective of patient well-being. To address this oversight, functional outcome, symptom relief, well-being, and the overall general health perceptions of patients undergoing infrainguinal revascularization were evaluated.

Patients.—Between 1991 and 1992, 318 patients underwent infrainguinal revascularization for severe peripheral arterial occlusive disease. Of those, 156 of 276 patients (63%) completed questionnaires on symptoms, functional status, and well-being before and 6 months after surgery. The mean age of the patients was 66 years; 67% were men. The majority (84%) had diabetes mellitus, and 83% had various heart-related conditions.

Surgical Procedures.—Distal graft sites were popliteal in 29%, tibial/ peroneal in 40%, and pedal/plantar in 31%. The operative morbidity rate was 21%. At 6 months, the cumulative primary graft patency rate was 93%, the cumulative secondary graft patency rate was 95%, and the limb salvage rate was 97%.

Outcome.—The evaluation of general health status at baseline showed that patients had a very low perception of their overall health, and this measure did not improve at 6 months' follow-up. All other measures of health status—including instrumental activities of daily living, vitality, and mental well-being—improved after surgery. The symptoms of calf cramping and toe or foot pain when walking and at rest improved, and sores or ulcers healed, but leg swelling became worse. The only independent predictor of improved function and well-being was the patients' perception of their function and well-being at baseline. Patients with better functioning or symptom status at baseline reported improved function and well-being at 6 months. Only 47.4% of patients reported feeling "back to normal" at 6 months, and many (74%) still required walking devices.

Conclusion.—Health status at baseline is an important predictor of improved function, mental well-being, and resolution of symptoms after infrainguinal revascularization. Expected return to "normal" may take longer than 6 months. It appears that earlier intervention toward improving patient function and well-being before surgery may additionally maximize patient benefit from infrainguinal revascularization procedures.

▶ We are continually informed that, in the near future, the Washington health care bureaucrats are going to require detailed functional status assessment of postoperative patients to determine whether the expenses related to the procedure will be reimbursed. I am not convinced that this makes much sense. Nonetheless, this threat is stimulating the performance of a number of studies. Basing postoperative functional assessment on patient questionnaires strikes me as a guarantee of dubious results. Keep in mind that if a sick, old arteriopath with a bad heart, bad lungs, and arthritis suddenly has severe leg ischemia and we fix the leg and then do a questionnaire assessment, the patient will undoubtedly note that he still has a bad heart, bad lungs, and arthritis and, not surprisingly, will consider himself little improved.

Should one use these data to conclude that salvage of ischemic legs is without benefit to the patient? I think not. An attempt to make science out of a self-assessment questionnaire besotted with an infinite number of uncontrolled variables strikes me as a futile attempt to make chicken soup out of chicken excrement.

Functional Outcomes in Limb Salvage Vascular Surgery
Duggan MM, Woodson J, Scott TE, Ortega AN, Menzoian JO (Boston Univ)
Am J Surg 168:188–191, 1994   145-96-10–5

Background.—The current health care crisis makes it increasingly important to objectively define what constitutes successful outcomes of medical treatments. Surgeons have come under criticism for relying on concepts of technical success rather than emphasizing functional outcomes.

Methods.—The functional results of extremity salvage surgery were examined in 38 patients aged 65 years and older seen with extremity-threatening ischemia. The general health and functioning of the patients were examined by using the RAND-36-Item Health Assessment Survey, Version 1.

Results.—Extremity salvage was achieved in 80% of cases, but only 58% of patients survived for 3 years, and only 25% retained the operated extremity and were able to walk. Patients who required amputation had RAND scores that did not differ significantly from those of patients whose surgery was successful.

Conclusion.—Greater efforts are needed to precisely define functional outcome goals for patients who require vascular surgery for extremity salvage.

▶ We know, I think, that patients with critical ischemia tend to die, and this paper confirms it. That only 25% were able to walk is a surprise and does not relate to the findings from other publications, which show a much better outcome from limb salvage. Direct comparisons with amputees, involving costs and quality of life, are, of course, important for future studies.—P.R.F. Bell, M.D.

▶ The objective information regarding ambulatory status in this small series is extremely interesting and potentially important. I agree with Dr. Bell that most series have shown better results than this, but I wonder how much better they are. I appreciate that Dr. Menzoian and his group did not rely exclusively on patient questionnaires for outcome assessment.—J.M. Porter, M.D.

The Additional Value of Intraoperative Angiography in Infragenicular Reconstruction

Sayers RD, Naylor AR, London NJM, Watkin EM, Macpherson DS, Barrie WW (Leicester Gen Hosp, England)
Eur J Vasc Endovasc Surg 9:211–217, 1995   145-96-10–6

Background.—Infragenicular reconstruction is capable of revascularizing a severely ischemic lower extremity in which occlusive disease extends below the knee, and it can avoid primary amputation. It is essential to identify a patent below-knee vessel for use in the distal anastomosis, but conventional preoperative angiography has not proved suitable for this purpose.

Methods.—The usefulness of preoperative intra-arterial digital subtraction angiography (IADSA) for determining the feasibility of infragenicular reconstruction was studied in a prospective series of 45 patients with 50 ischemic lower extremities who were potential candidates for the procedure. Intraoperative angiography was done to definitively assess the circulation. The findings were interpreted independently and blindly by a single observer.

Results.—Intra-arterial digital subtraction angiography was 87% accurate in distinguishing between normal, stenosed, and occluded tibial arteries. The adequacy of runoff into the pedal arch was determined with 86% accuracy. The IADSA procedure had a positive predictive value of 100% in determining whether infragenicular reconstruction was feasible, but its negative predictive value in identifying patients in whom reconstruction was not possible was only 73%. When only patients considered to be operable on the basis of IADSA were included, the study identified the correct artery to use for anastomosis in 97% of cases and the correct arterial segment in 92%.

Conclusion.—Only intraoperative angiography can reliably rule out infragenicular reconstruction but, in other patients, an operative approach may be planned by using IADSA. If a good-quality distal vessel is present, a bypass may be done without the need for intraoperative angiography.

▶ I have talked with Dr. P.R.F. Bell about his philosophy of intraoperative arteriography to define the surgical bypass artery, and it is clear that we disagree significantly. At Oregon Health Sciences University, we have world-class arteriographers who can precisely define bypassable infrapopliteal arteries in 99% of all of our patients. We have absolutely no need for intraoperative arteriography to define the bypass target. Dr. Bell tells me he prefers to do it intraoperatively to save time and money. Perhaps so, but, in my opinion, this does not permit optimal surgical planning. This paper tells us that preoperative IADSA is able to predict operative targets in almost all patients. There is nothing new about this. I continue to believe that if you have to rely on an intraoperative arteriogram to define your surgical bypass target, you need better angiographers.

The Popliteal Artery as Inflow for Distal Bypass Grafting

Brown PS Jr, McCarthy WJ, Yao JST, Pearce WH (Northwestern Mem Hosp, Chicago)
Arch Surg 129:596–602, 1994   145-96-10–7

Objective.—The outcome of a saphenous vein bypass from the popliteal artery to a distal vessel was examined in 51 patients with occlusive disease who underwent 52 bypass procedures. The average age at the time of surgery was 62 years. More than two thirds of the patients had gangrene or nonhealing ulceration.

Methods.—The proximal anastomosis was made to the popliteal artery above the knee in 50% of operations and below the knee in the remaining cases. The distal anastomoses were made to tibial arteries in 79% of cases and to pedal arteries in 21%. The average follow-up was 2.7 years.

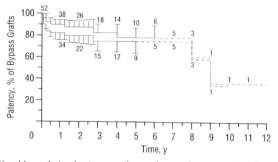

Fig 10–3.—Life-table analysis of primary and secondary graft patency plotted at 3-month intervals. *Bottom line* indicates primary patency; *top line* indicates secondary patency. Numbers at top represent the number of bypass grafts at risk; *bars*, standard error of mean; and *dotted lines*, standard error of mean greater than 10%. (Courtesy of Brown PS Jr, McCarthy WJ, Yao JST, et al: The popliteal artery as inflow for distal bypass grafting. *Arch Surg* 129:596–602, 1994.)

Results.—The perioperative mortality rate was 2%. The primary patency rate decreased from 90% at 1 month after operation to 82% at 1 year and to 50% at 10 years (Fig 10–3). Only 2 of 14 primary graft failures could be ascribed to progressive proximal disease. Five of the grafts failed within the first postoperative month. Six patients gained patency secondarily, yielding a 5-year secondary patency rate of 79%. The extremity salvage rate was 90% at 1 year and 87% at 5 years. Seven major amputations were required. The outcome of bypass surgery could not be related to the level of either anastomosis, the type of vein graft used, or the presence of other illness.

Conclusions.—The popliteal-distal artery bypass provides excellent clinical results in patients with severe ischemic disease in a lower extremity. It is advantageous to use a popliteal artery inflow source when venous segments are scarce, because grafts rarely fail from progressive proximal disease.

▶ The most distal artery with unobstructed inflow should be the preferential site of arterial inflow for a bypass graft. Much fewer than 50% of our lower extremity bypass grafts originate from the common femoral artery. Our artery of preference is the profunda or the superficial femoral, but we are delighted to use the popliteal in appropriate patients and, even, a tibial artery on occasion. The authors' conclusion that an unimpeded popliteal artery is a good origin for a leg bypass graft, although hardly revolutionary, is correct. (See also Abstract 145-96-13–1).

Infrainguinal Bypass in Patients With End-Stage Renal Disease
Baele HR, Piotrowski JJ, Yuhas J, Anderson C, Alexander JJ (Case Western Reserve Univ, Cleveland, Ohio)
Surgery 117:319–324, 1995 145-96-10–8

Introduction.—The demand for arterial reconstruction by patients receiving dialysis is likely to increase. The safety and effectiveness of infrainguinal bypass in patients with end-stage renal disease and limb-threatening ischemia were assessed.

Methods.—The retrospective study included 44 patients receiving maintenance hemodialysis who underwent a total of 57 infrainguinal bypass procedures during 7 years. Seventy-two percent of the procedures were tibial or pedal bypasses and 28% were femoropopliteal bypasses. Autogenous conduit was used in 82% of the cases, prosthetic material in 12%, and composite graft materials in 6%. Seventy-nine percent of the operations were performed for ischemic ulceration or gangrene and 21% were performed for rest pain. Angiography revealed single-vessel runoff in 56% of the cases.

The mean patient age was 63 years. Seventy-five percent were diabetic, 93% had hypertension, 52% had coronary artery disease, and 39% were smokers. Twenty percent of the patients had a history of myocardial infarction, and 18% had undergone contralateral amputation. Thirty-nine percent of the limbs were infected.

Results.—Thirty-day surgical morbidity was 39%; wound breakdown occurred in 19% of the cases, graft thrombosis in 9%, and major amputation in 4%. Nine percent of the patients died in the perioperative period. The cumulative primary graft patency rate was 71% at 1 year and 63% at 2 years. Secondary patency rates were 80% and 66%, and limb salvage rates were 70% and 52%, respectively. Preoperative infection was the best predictor of limb loss. The 2-year patient survival rate was 52%.

Conclusion.—For properly selected patients with end-stage renal disease, infrainguinal bypass can yield acceptable limb salvage rates. Life expectancy continues to be poor for these patients. Arterial reconstruction should not be performed if severe limb infection is present preoperatively.

▶ We seem to have poked a hornet's nest with our early report on the outcome of arterial bypass for limb salvage in patients with end-stage renal disease (1). We not only found poor results in these patients, we found that patients who had a large ischemic ulcer on the foot failed to heal with a disturbing frequency, even with a patent bypass. Although it is reasonable to attempt repair in selected patients with end-stage renal disease and leg ischemia, it is important to keep in mind that this is the most significantly disadvantaged group of patients requiring leg bypass that we are called on to treat.

Reference

1. Edwards JM, Taylor LM Jr, Porter JM: Limb salvage in end-stage renal disease (ESRD). *Arch Surg* 123:1164–1168, 1988.

Microscope-Aided Pedal Bypass Is an Effective and Low-Risk Operation to Salvage the Ischemic Foot
Gloviczki P, Bower TC, Toomey BJ, Mendonca C, Naessens JM, Schabauer AM, Stanson AW, Rooke TW (Mayo Clinic and Found, Rochester, Minn)
Am J Surg 168:76–84, 1994   145-96-10–9

Background.—Infrainguinal revascularization is an alternative to amputation for lower extremity vascular disease that can be performed with low risk and the expectation that 75% to 80% of the extremities can be salvaged. This procedure has been extended to the inframalleolar arteries. It has been reported that pedal bypass surgery has resulted in salvage of the ischemic foot in 75% of patients. To determine the current risks and durability of this procedure, as well as the factors that affect long-term outcome, 100 pedal bypass surgeries were observed prospectively in patients with chronic critical extremity ischemia.

Methods.—Between September 15, 1987 and July 15, 1993, a total of 96 patients underwent 100 surgeries using autogenous vein grafts. Ninety-one of the extremities had ischemic ulcers or gangrene, and 9 produced rest pain only. Sixty-four of the 96 patients were diabetic, 61 had hypertension, 50 had a history of smoking, 36 had coronary artery disease, and 21 had renal failure; 7 of these 21 were receiving chronic dialysis.

Results.—No patient died within 30 days of surgery, and 2 had hemodynamically insignificant myocardial infarctions. Early wound complications developed in 12 patients. There were 10 early graft failures, and 6 of these were salvaged with a second surgery; 96 of the 100 grafts were patent at patient discharge. There were 17 major amputations. After operation, 16 of 33 failing or failed grafts were successfully revised, but 7 of the 16 failed again within 15 months. At 3 years, primary and secondary patency rates were 60% and 69%. The factors associated with better secondary patency were diabetes and an intraoperative graft flow rate of at least 50

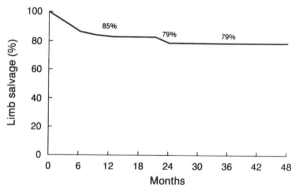

Fig 10–4.—Cumulative foot salvage rates for 100 extremities with pedal bypasses. (Courtesy of Gloviczki P, Bower TC, Toomey BJ, et al: Microscope-aided pedal bypass is an effective and low-risk operation to salvage the ischemic foot. *Am J Surg* 168:76–84, 1994. Copyright 1994/95, American Medical Association.)

mL/min. At 3 years, the cumulative survival rate was 83% and the cumulative foot salvage rate was 79% (Fig 10–4).

Discussion.—Without pedal bypass surgery, most of these patients would have undergone major amputation. Pedal bypass surgery is effective and durable and is safe for high-risk patients. This procedure should be considered for all patients with critical extremity ischemia.

▶ This very competent pedal bypass series has 3-year primary and secondary patency rates of 60% and 69%, respectively. I find no convincing advantage to using an operating microscope, which, indeed is something the authors do not emphasize in this article, despite its curious title.

Dorsalis Pedis Arterial Bypass: Durable Limb Salvage for Foot Ischemia in Patients With Diabetes Mellitus
Pomposelli FB Jr, Marcaccio EJ, Gibbons GW, Campbell DR, Freeman DV, Burgess AM, Miller A, LoGerfo FW (New England Deaconess Hosp, Boston; Harvard Med School, Boston)
J Vasc Surg 21:375–384, 1995   145-96-10–10

Background.—Pedal artery bypass is a technically feasible approach to limb salvage in patients with peripheral artery disease, but indications for the procedure and the durability of the results remain uncertain.

Methods.—A total of 384 vein bypass grafts were made to the dorsalis pedis artery for limb salvage in 367 consecutive patients treated in an 8-year period. All but 5% of the patients had diabetes mellitus, and more than half had infection complicating ischemia. The dorsalis pedis artery was patent in 93% of the extremities preoperatively. Veins were used in all cases. Inflow was from the superficial femoral or popliteal artery in more than half of the patients (table).

Results.—When the dorsalis pedis artery was patent preoperatively, 98.6% of 362 bypasses were successful. Of 28 operations done when no arteries were demonstrated but pedal Doppler signals were audible, 16 succeeded. Eleven of 12 patients whose angiographic status was unknown had a successful outcome. The perioperative mortality rate was 1.8%, and myocardial infarction developed in 21 patients (5.4%). Nineteen of 29 failed grafts were successfully revised, but 8 of the remaining 10 patients required major amputation. Of 39 subsequent graft failures, 17 were successfully revised. Seventeen patients required major amputation later in their course. The actuarial primary and secondary patency rates at 5 years were 68% and 82%, respectively, and the limb salvage rate was 87%. Patency rates were comparable for in situ and translocated saphenous vein grafts. The actuarial patient survival at 5 years was 57%.

Conclusion.—Vein graft bypass of the dorsalis pedis artery is an effective and durable approach to limb salvage. The results are similar to those achieved when distal vein grafts are placed in more proximal arteries.

Operative Details for Dorsalis Pedis Bypass in 384 Extremities

	No.	%
Inflow source		
Common femoral	129	34
SFA/Pop	231	60
Tibial artery	5	1
Previously placed graft	19	5
Total	384	100
Conduit		
ISSV	148	39
RSV	110	29
NRSV	68	18
Arm	27	7
Composite	31	8
Total	384	100

Abbreviations: SFA, superficial femoral artery; *Pop,* popliteal; *ISSV,* in situ saphenous vein; *RSV,* reversed saphenous vein, *NRSV,* nonreversed saphenous vein.
(Courtesy of Pomposelli FB Jr, Marcaccio EJ, Gibbons GW, et al: Dorsalis pedis arterial bypass: Durable limb salvage for foot ischemia in patients with diabetes mellitus. *J Vasc Surg* 21:375–384, 1995.)

▶ The surgical group at New England Deaconess Hospital provides vascular support for an enormous number of patients with diabetes. We have learned a considerable amount about diabetic bypass from their experience. In this article, the group reports performing a remarkable 384 vein graft procedures to the dorsalis pedis over 8 years. The perioperative death rate of only 1.8% in this group is remarkable. The primary and secondary patency and limb salvage rates at 5 years were 68%, 82%, and 87%, respectively—outstanding results indeed. Dr. LoGerfo and his group at New England Deaconess Hospital have set the standard for pedal bypass in diabetics.

Distal Wound Complications Following Pedal Bypass: Analysis of Risk Factors
Robison JG, Ross JP, Brothers TE, Elliott BM (Univ of South Carolina, Charleston)
Ann Vasc Surg 9:53–59, 1995   145-96-10–11

Background.—Complications of pedal incisions occasionally compromise the results of aggressive revascularization performed for limb salvage.

Series.—Fourteen of 142 patients who underwent pedal bypass with autogenous vein for limb salvage (9.8%) had significant disruption of the distal wound. Tissue necrosis was present in approximately half the patients, and three fourths of the patients had diabetes. All but 8 of the patients either had diabetes or had used tobacco.

Management and Outcome.—Eight of the 14 disrupted wounds were salvaged, with maintenance of a patent graft after follow-up that extended from 5 months to 5 years. Three patients in whom a patent graft was exposed required amputation, as did 1 with an occluded graft. One graft

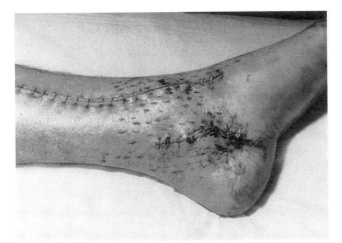

Fig 10–5.—Posterior tibial incision after "pie-crusting." (Courtesy of Robison JG, Ross JP, Brothers TE, et al: Distal wound complications following pedal bypass: Analysis of risk factors: *Ann Vasc Surg* 9:53–59, 1995.)

was revised to the peroneal artery and salvaged, and another was covered by a local bipedicled flap. Diabetes, age older than 70 years, and rest pain all disposed to wound complications. In patients at risk, the use of such ancillary methods as "pie-crusting" (Fig 10–5) did not produce distal wound problems.

Recommendations.—Pedal wound complications may be minimized by careful distal tunneling of the graft and by closing the wound to reduce tension. In addition, swelling may be controlled by avoiding dependency and by using gentle elastic compression.

▶ These authors accurately note that wound complications accompanying pedal bypass occur with disturbing frequency and may seriously threaten the graft. They report a 9.8% incidence of significant distal wound disruption, which led to amputation in 3 patients, graft occlusion in an additional patient, and revision of the graft to a different artery in another patient. The authors present a very interesting method of pie crusting the adjacent skin to relieve tension on the skin closure. I shall consider using this. I notice that in the preceding paper (Abstract 145-96-10–10) from New England Deaconess Hospital a wound complication rate of 5.7% was reported.

Infrapopliteal Polytetrafluoroethylene and Composite Bypass: Factors Influencing Patency
Fichelle J-M, Marzelle J, Colacchio G, Gigou F, Cormier F, Cormier JM (Clinique Bizet, Paris; Hôpital Saint-Joseph, Paris; Clinique de la Défence, Nanterre, France; et al)
Ann Vasc Surg 9:187–196, 1995   145-96-10–12

Patients.—The outcome of infrapopliteal polytetrafluoroethylene (PTFE) bypass surgery was examined in 145 patients who underwent surgery from 1979 to 1988 for chronic but limb-threatening ischemia. They represented slightly more than one fourth of all infrapopliteal bypass operations done during the period evaluated. The average patient age was 71.8 years. More than two thirds of the patients had gangrenous changes at the time of surgery.

Methods.—A composite PTFE-saphenous vein graft was used in 53 patients. The distal anastomosis of prosthetic bypasses was done using vein patch angioplasty in 65 instances and directly in 31.

Results.—The hospital mortality rate was 3.3% in this series. The actuarial survival rate was 68% at 3 years and 57% at 5 years. Primary patency rates were 41% and 35%, respectively; secondary patency rates are given in the table. Limb salvage rates were 68% at 3 years and 65% at 5 years. The primary patency rates 3 years after repair could not be related to the type or site of distal anastomosis, whether the bypass was placed laterally or medially, or whether previous surgery had been done.

Conclusion.—Patency rates after infrapopliteal PTFE bypass surgery are not impressive. Limb salvage rates are, however, encouraging and warrant routine distal revascularization, even if autogenous vein grafting is not possible.

▶ These authors accurately note that patency with PTFE bypass below the popliteal artery is extremely poor. I continue to note that we are able to achieve an all-autologous vein bypass conduit in 94% of all patients, despite the observation that more than 50% of our patients had preceding vascular surgery before reaching our institution. The vigorous use of lesser saphenous, cephalic, basilic, and even, on occasion, superficial femoral veins, dramatically reduces the need for prosthetic leg bypasses. If more than 10% of your leg bypasses are being performed with prosthetic grafts, you are not looking hard enough for veins.

Life-Table Analysis of Overall Secondary Patency After Infrapopliteal Polytetrafluoroethylene Bypass

Interval (mo.)	Bypasses at Risk	Occluded	Excluded Duration of Follow-Up	Died	Lost to Follow-Up	Interval Patency	Cumulative Patency (%)	Standard Deviation (%)
0–1	149	32	0	2	8	0.79	100	
1–6	115	25	0	6	11	0.78	79	3
7–12	73	13	2	2	0	0.82	61	4
13–24	56	10	5	7	0	0.82	51	5
25–36	34	3	9	1	1	0.91	41	5
37–48	20	2	4	4	0	0.90	38	7
49–60	10	1	2	0	0	0.90	34	9
61–72	7	0	3	2	0	1.00	31	10
73–84	2	0	1	0	0	1.00	31	18
85–96	1	0	1	0	0	1.00	31	26

(Courtesy of Fichelle J-M, Marzelle J, Colacchio G, et al: Infrapopliteal polytetrafluoroethylene and composite bypass: Factors influencing patency. *Ann Vasc Surg* 9:187–196, 1995.)

Low-Molecular Weight Heparin Versus Aspirin and Dipyridamole After Femoropopliteal Bypass Grafting

Edmondson RA, Cohen AT, Das SK, Wagner MB, Kakkar VV (Thrombosis Research Inst, London)

Lancet 344:914–918, 1994   145-96-10-13

Background.—Theoretically, low–molecular-weight heparin should maintain the patency of vascular grafts more effectively than aspirin and dipyridamole, because of both its potent antithrombotic action and its antiproliferative effect on vascular smooth-muscle cells.

Methods.—Two hundred patients with femoropopliteal bypass grafts of autologous vein, polytetrafluoroethylene, or Dacron were randomly assigned to receive either injections of 2,500 IU of low-molecular-weight heparin or 300 mg of aspirin combined with 100 mg of dipyridamole every 8 hours for 3 months. The patients were stratified by the indication for surgery. Ninety-four patients assigned to receive heparin and 106 given aspirin and dipyridamole were followed for 1 year.

Results.—Eighty-seven percent of grafts in patients receiving heparin and 72% of grafts in patients given aspirin and dipyridamole remained patent at 6 months. The respective patency rates at 1 year were 78% and 64% (Fig 10–6). The added benefit from heparin was limited to patients requiring salvage surgery. No patient in either group had major bleeding.

Conclusion.—Low-molecular-weight heparin is preferable to aspirin and dipyridamole for maintaining the patency of all types of femoropopliteal bypass grafts in patients with critical limb ischemia.

▶ In this very interesting study, 200 patients undergoing femoropopliteal bypass grafting were randomly assigned to receive low-molecular-weight

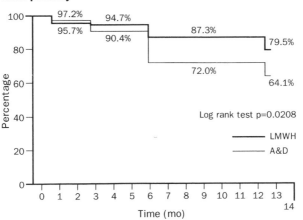

Graft patency

Fig 10–6.—Kaplan-Meier plot of the effect of treatment group on graft patency. *Abbreviations: A&D,* aspirin and dipyridamole; *MWH,* low-molecular-weight heparin. (Courtesy of Edmondson RA, Cohen AT, Das SK, et al: Low-molecular-weight heparin versus aspirin and dipyridamole after femoropopliteal bypass grafting. *Lancet* 344:914–918, 1994. Copyright by The Lancet Ltd.)

heparin or aspirin and dipyridamole for 3 months postoperatively. Twelve-month patencies were 78% in the heparin group and 64% in the aspirin/dipyridamole group, with a highly significant *P* value in those patients undergoing surgery for limb salvage. Difficulties with this study include the wide variety of graft materials used, apparently without stratification in the randomization matrix, as well as the generally low 12-month patency rate. These problems cause me to place far less importance on this study than I would had the patients all received vein grafts and the 1-year patency rate been 90% or so, which it should have been.

Treatment and Outcome of Severe Lower-Limb Ischaemia
Sayers RD, Thompson MM, Hartshorne T, Budd JS, Bell PRF (Leicester Royal Infirmary, England)
Br J Surg 81:521–523, 1994   145-96-10–14

Objective.—There are few data on the overall limb salvage and mortality outcomes of patients with severe lower-limb ischemia. The treatment and results of 232 severely ischemic legs in 209 patients were described.

Findings.—The patients were managed by an aggressive policy of revascularization. Revascularization was attempted in 89% of the legs, with a primary amputation rate of 8%. There was a 79% 30-day limb salvage rate and a 20% patient mortality rate. The limb salvage rates were 74% at 12 months and 71% at 24 months (Fig 10–7). The patient survival rates were 75% and 73%, respectively. None of the preoperative risk factors evaluated by life-table analysis affected limb salvage and mortality.

Conclusion.—For patients with severe leg ischemia, an aggressive policy of revascularization yields excellent results. The results of treatment are unaffected by age, sex, pain at rest, tissue necrosis, diabetes, or preoperative ankle systolic pressure.

▶ This short article provides an interesting update on the current state of affairs in the United Kingdom. Dr. Bell's group at Leicester is one of the best informed and most aggressive vascular groups in the United Kingdom. In the

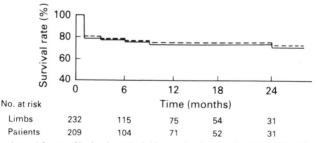

No. at risk	Time (months)			
	0	6	12	18	24
Limbs	232	115	75	54	31
Patients	209	104	71	52	31

Fig 10–7.—Actuarial rates of limb salvage (*solid line*) and patient survival (*dashed line*) for all patients. The standard error of the mean is less than 10% at all time points. (Courtesy of Sayers RD, Thompson MM, Hartshorne T, et al: Treatment and outcome of severe lower-limb ischaemia. *Br J Surg* 81:521–523, 1994. Reprinted by permission of Blackwell Science Ltd.)

group of patients with difficult limb salvage, they attempted revascularization in 89% of patients seen with a 30-day limb salvage rate of 79% and a patient mortality rate of 20%. At 12 and 24 months, the limb salvage rates were 74% and 71%, respectively. I find the patient survival rate of these authors to be right on the mark, but I find their limb salvage rate to be a bit less than we have come to expect in the United States. It is important to note that, to date, aggressive referral from general practitioners to vascular centers has been the exception, not the rule, in the United Kingdom. Within the limitations of the referral matrix there, I believe these results are truly outstanding.

Trends in Vascular Surgery Since the Introduction of Percutaneous Transluminal Angioplasty
Pell JP, Whyman MR, Fowkes FGR, Gillespie I, Ruckley CV (Univ of Edinburgh, Scotland; Royal Infirmary, Edinburgh, Scotland)
Br J Surg 81:832–835, 1994   145-96-10–15

Introduction.—The past decade has seen an increase in the use of lower-limb percutaneous transluminal angioplasty (PTA), on its own or in combination with surgical arterial reconstruction. At the same time, because PTA is both an alternative and adjunct to surgery, its implications for surgical workload and health care resources have proven difficult to predict. The impact of PTA on rates of vascular surgery—including arterial reconstruction and major amputation for critical lower-limb ischemia—was assessed.

Methods.—The study was conducted at a specialist vascular surgery unit that receives almost all outpatient referrals for peripheral arterial disease from 2 United Kingdom health boards. These referrals were added to emergency admissions to determine the total numbers of referrals for peripheral arterial disease. The rates of vascular operations and PTAs per referral for the years 1986 to 1992 were calculated (table).

Findings.—The procedure rate per referral increased by 2.6-fold. Although the proportion of total procedures performed for critical ischemia decreased, the overall rate of procedures for critical ischemia doubled. The rate of PTA for peripheral arterial disease increased by ninefold overall, including a fivefold increase in the rate of angioplasty for critical ischemia. For all patients with peripheral arterial disease, the rate of aortic reconstruction increased by 40% and the rate of femoral reconstruction increased by 100%. However, there was no change in the rate of reconstructive procedures performed for critical ischemia. The major amputation rate increased by 47% from 1986 to 1990, remaining stable thereafter.

Conclusion.—Although the use of PTA increased in recent years, the number of vascular operations performed has not decreased. This situation likely results from several causes: the use of PTA as an adjunct to surgery, failed angioplasty leading to subsequent surgery, and the use of PTA in patients with milder symptoms who are not surgical candidates. The use of

Annual Numbers of Angiograms and Peripheral Arterial Procedures Performed Per Total Referrals for Peripheral Arterial Disease From 1986 to 1992

Year	No. of referrals*	Angiography		Aortic reconstruction		Vascular procedures				PTA		Total	
						Femoral reconstruction		Major amputation					
		No.	Rate†	No.	Rate‡	No.	Rate†	No.	Rate†	No.	Rate†	No.	Rate†
1986	589	295	0.50	60	0.10	63	0.11	86	0.15	28	0.05	237	0.40
1987	593	308	0.52	56	0.09	70	0.12	98	0.17	47	0.08	271	0.46
1988	665	322	0.48	68	0.10	71	0.11	99	0.15	40	0.06	278	0.42
1989	582	392	0.67	64	0.11	77	0.13	108	0.19	86	0.15	335	0.58
1990	513	475	0.93	66	0.13	80	0.16	112	0.22	125	0.24	383	0.75
1991	544	489	0.90	73	0.13	87	0.16	112	0.21	165	0.30	437	0.80
1992	540	533	0.99	77	0.14	120	0.22	117	0.22	241	0.45	555	1.03

* Elective plus emergency referrals for peripheral arterial disease.
† $P < 0.001$
‡ $P < 0.05$ (χ^2 test for linear trend in proportions).
Abbreviation: PTA, percutaneous transluminal angioplasty.
(Courtesy of Pell JP, Whyman MR, Fowkes FGR, et al: Trends in vascular surgery since the introduction of percutaneous transluminal angioplasty. Br J Surg 81:832–835, 1994. Reprinted by permission of Blackwell Science Ltd.)

PTA for critical lower-limb ischemia has not reduced the frequency of amputation or arterial reconstruction.

▶ I am hardly surprised to note that a dramatic increase in the use of angioplasty at a single institution was not associated with a reduction in the number of vascular operations performed. Studies such as this have no way of accounting for the increasing recognition of vascular disease in the medical community as years pass. In our institution, most leg angioplasties are performed in patients for whom we would recommend no vascular intervention at all. The performance of angioplasty in this patient group will have no effect at all on the number of operations that we perform, unless it increases it somewhat as a result of the emergency treatment of complications caused by angioplasty.

Outpatient Clinic Review After Arterial Reconstruction: Is it Necessary?
Dunn JM, Bell A, Elliott TB, Kernick VFM, Lavy JA, Campbell WB (Royal Devon and Exeter Hosp, Exeter, England)
Ann R Coll Surg Engl 76:304–306, 1994   145-96-10–16

Background.—Traditionally, vascular surgeons follow patients after arterial reconstruction at outpatient clinics, frequently for a protracted period. The stated goals are to reassure the patient, reinforce desired lifestyle changes, and detect graft failure.

Objective.—For several years, a policy of limited clinical follow-up, providing "open access" when graft failure was suspected, was followed. Recently, duplex scanning has been used to monitor vein graft function. The efficacy of this self-referral policy was examined in a series of 173 patients having reconstructive arterial surgery for occlusive disease in the lower extremity from 1987 to 1989. Forty-eight proximal grafts and 131 infrainguinal grafts were constructed.

Results.—Thirty-five percent of patients died after a median follow-up of 50 months, and 25% required amputation. Of the patients whose limbs were salvaged, 86% described ongoing symptomatic improvement. Their graft patency rate was 80%. Twenty-seven patients referred themselves

Number of Follow-Up Visits Per Patient	
Number of visits	Number of patients
0	2
1	29
2	19
3	7
4	4
5	2
6	1

(Courtesy of Dunn JM, Bell A, Elliott TB, et al: Outpatient clinic review after arterial reconstruction: Is it necessary? *Ann R Coll Surg Engl* 76:304–306, 1994.)

because they suspected graft occlusion, and 14 of them required surgery. Seventy percent of patients found a single postoperative visit to be helpful (table). A majority believed that further visits would not have been helpful.

Conclusion.—Knowledgeable patients can be relied on to visit the clinic if signs of graft occlusion develop. Little is gained from insisting on regular long-term follow-up at the vascular surgery clinic. This policy is easier for elderly patients, and it gives the surgeons more time to deal with new referrals.

▶ This is a classic example of trying to put a high gloss on dung. If we operate on patients, we have the absolute obligation to follow them post-operatively, because by doing so at frequent intervals and intervening for appropriate indications, we may prevent 30% to 50% of postoperative graft thromboses. The message contained in this article represents a giant step backward and is condemned. If, for the authors' own reasons, they do not wish to follow their patients postoperatively, they should not attempt to impose this behavior on the rest of us.

Popliteal Aneurysm

A Multicenter Study of Popliteal Aneurysms
Varga ZA, Locke-Edmunds JC, Baird RN, and the Joint Vascular Research Group (Bristol Royal Infirmary, England)
J Vasc Surg 20:171–177, 1994   145-96-10–17

Background.—The advent of thrombolysis encourages a policy of monitoring small, asymptomatic aneurysms by ultrasound examination, reserving bypass for lesions that enlarge or begin producing symptoms. Thrombolytic treatment is available should acute limb ischemia develop.

Methods.—A prospective survey was conducted to learn how popliteal aneurysms (PAs) presently are managed. Information was obtained from 19 vascular surgeons who, in a 4-year period starting in 1989, managed 200 PAs in 137 patients.

Clinical Aspects.—A majority of the aneurysms had ischemia in the lower extremity. Both claudication and acute limb-threatening ischemia were frequent findings. Digital atheroembolism developed in 11 extremities. Forty-three PAs caused no symptoms, and 32 others produced symptoms limited to the popliteal fossa.

Management and Outcome.—Sixty-two patients required emergency measures. Bypass was performed in 56 of them, including 10 who experienced early bypass occlusion. Thrombolysis was used alone or in conjunction with bypass in 23 instances and was successful in 16. Elective bypass was performed for 80 PAs, with 1 early occlusion. Of 58 patients who were initially observed, 18 subsequently had bypass during a median follow-up of 22 months. The indication was either expansion of a small asymptomatic aneurysm or the development of distal ischemia.

Conclusions.—When a PA causes acute limb-threatening ischemia, distal runoff can be restored by intra-arterial thrombolysis before undertaking bypass. The present experience does not justify a policy of expectant management for patients with asymptomatic Pas.

▶ I have trouble understanding the anguish the British apparently have regarding elective treatment of Pas. When we encounter a PA we recommend surgery, excise the aneurysm, and replace it with an interposition vein graft, recognizing little difficulty with this approach. Patency has been excellent and the complications few. When a patient is seen with a thrombosed PA with no definable outflow tract, we have found intra-arterial thrombolysis to be a reasonable choice; we have used it with success in some, but by no means all, patients (1). In short, PA is a dangerous condition amenable to straightforward surgical therapy. What is the problem?

Reference

1. Taylor LM Jr, Porter JM, Baur GM, et al: Intraarterial streptokinase infusion for acute popliteal and tibial artery occlusion. *Am J Surg* 147:583–588, 1984.

Asymptomatic Popliteal Aneurysm: Elective Operation *Versus* Conservative Follow-Up
Dawson I, Sie R, van Baalen JM, van Bockel JH (Univ Hosp Leiden, The Netherlands)
Br J Surg 81:1504–1507, 1994   145-96-10–18

Background.—A significant risk of limb loss is associated with popliteal aneurysm (PA), so prophylactic operative treatment is generally recommended for asymptomatic lesions. Some, however, believe that patients should undergo surgery only if limb-threatening complications develop.

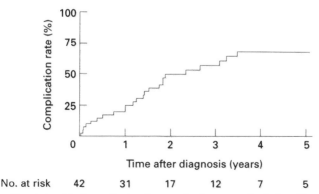

| No. at risk | 42 | 31 | 17 | 12 | 7 | 5 |

Fig 10–8.—Cumulative risk of complications from popliteal aneurysm developing. All patients (*n* = 42). (Courtesy of Dawson I, Sie R, van Baalen JM, et al: Asymptomatic popliteal aneurysm: Elective operation *versus* conservative follow-up. *Br J Surg* 81:1504–1507, 1994. Reprinted by permission of Blackwell Science Ltd.)

Objective.—Complications were monitored in 42 patients with asymptomatic PAs who were followed without having surgery for an average of 6.2 years. The aneurysms initially had an average diameter of 3.1 cm. Eighteen of 42 extremities had abnormal ankle pulses.

Results.—Twenty-five patients had complications after a mean interval of 18 months. Three patients had limb loss, and 2 required fasciotomy. The cumulative risk of complications increased from 24% at 1 year to 68% after 5 years of follow-up (Fig 10–8). The risk of complications was greatest for patients whose ankle pulses were absent and those who had previously had surgery for an abdominal aortic aneurysm. Survival was not compromised.

Conclusion.—Elective surgery may be indicated for patients having an asymptomatic PA because of the significant risk of complications developing. Patients with a history of aortic aneurysm and those who lack an ankle pulse are at the highest risk.

▶ I simply cannot believe that 42 patients with PAs were followed without surgery. In 25 patients, complications developed at a mean of 18 months, resulting in 3 amputations, 1 patient with peroneal nerve palsy, and 8 with claudication, 2 of whom needed fasciotomies. Amazingly, these authors conclude that asymptomatic aneurysms of the popliteal artery are potentially dangerous and may justify elective surgery! What next? Surgery for appendicitis? I wonder whether CNN has picked up on this story.

Does Infrapopliteal Arterial Runoff Predict Success for Popliteal Artery Aneurysmorrhaphy?
Hagino RT, Fujitani RM, Dawson DL, Cull DL, Buehrer JL, Taylor SM, Mills JL
(Uniformed Services Univ of Health Sciences, Lackland Air Force Base, Tex)
Am J Surg 168:652–658, 1994   145-96-10–19

Objective.—A 6-year experience in operating on popliteal artery aneurysms (PAs) was reviewed to learn how the quality of the infrapopliteal outflow vessels influences long-term outcome.

Methods.—Twenty-eight patients underwent 45 popliteal aneurysmorrhaphies during the period reviewed. Thirty-two extremities were operated on electively, but 13 required emergency surgery for acute limb-threatening ischemia. In all cases, the PA was excluded and a reversed autologous saphenous vein graft was placed. Runoff was evaluated by arteriography, and graft patency was monitored by serial duplex scanning.

Results.—Only 20 of the operated extremities (44%) had a patent trifurcation with 3 continuous vessels to the ankle. Two continuous tibial vessels were present in 13 limbs and a single patent runoff vessel was present in 10. In 2 instances, there was no vessel running continuously to the foot. During an average follow-up of 19 months, the 5-year primary graft patency rate (life-table analysis) was 95%, and the 5-year assisted primary patency rate was 97%. One vein graft was secondarily revised on an elective basis. One graft thrombosed, necessitating secondary bypass. All extremities were salvaged. The final outcome did not correlate with the state of the runoff vessels.

Conclusion.—Suboptimal runoff vessels do not preclude an excellent clinical outcome after removal of a PA. Autologous saphenous vein grafts are preferred to prosthetic grafts.

▶ This superb paper presents the results one can expect with careful surgery on PAs. Only 44% of the patients had a patent trifurcation, and 4% had no vessels at all continuous to the foot. Despite this, the 5-year primary patency rate of reversed vein grafting in this setting was 95%. One patient died perioperatively of myocardial infarction, for an overall mortality rate of 3.6%. With results like this, it seems inappropriate to electively follow PAs. Of course, there is some real concern as to just what constitutes an aneurysm. I favor the definition indicating a popliteal artery that is larger than the incoming and outgoing arteries, with a diameter of at least 1.5 cm.

Amputation

Results of Lower Extremity Amputations in Patients With End-Stage Renal Disease
Dossa CD, Shepard AD, Amos AM, Kupin WL, Reddy DJ, Elliott JP, Wilczewski JM, Ernst CB (Henry Ford Hosp, Detroit)
J Vasc Surg 20:14–19, 1994   145-96-10–20

Objective.—The influence of end-stage renal disease (ESRD) on the clinical course of patients requiring lower-limb amputation was examined in 459 patients having amputation over 4½ years. Eighty-four patients with ESRD underwent 137 amputations, whereas 375 without ESRD had a total of 442 amputations.

Results.—The hospital mortality rate was 24% in patients with ESRD and 7% in the others, which is a significant difference (table). Patients with ESRD who had minor amputations had a mortality rate 3 times higher than those without ESRD who required major amputations. More than 40% of patients with ESRD who had bilateral above-knee amputations

Mortality and Survival Rates Among Patients Undergoing Dialysis, Transplantation, and Patients Without End-Stage Renal Disease (ESRD)

Group	No. of Patients	Mortality Rate	Survival* 1-Year	2-Years
Transplant	11	0%	82% ± 4%	61% ± 16%
Dialysis	74	27%	38% ± 6%	20% ± 6%
Total ESRD	85	24%	44% ± 6%	27% ± 6%
Total nonESRD	375	7%	79% ± 3%	68% ± 3%

* Kaplan-Meier survival estimates with standard error.
(Courtesy of Dossa CD, Shepard AD, Amos AM et al: Results of lower extremity amputations in patients with end-stage renal disease. *J Vasc Surg* 20:14–19, 1994.)

died. During an average follow-up of 17 months, patients with ESRD were 7 times more likely to have bilateral amputations. No renal transplant recipient died after amputation.

Conclusion.—Because of the very negative impact of ESRD on survival after lower-limb amputation, every attempt should be made—through patient education and aggressive foot care—to preclude the need for amputation in this high-risk group.

▶ The authors of this retrospective review examined the hospital records of 84 patients with ESRD undergoing 137 limb amputations and compared the results with those in 375 patients without ESRD who underwent lower-extremity limb amputation. The hospital mortality rate was 24% in the patients with ESRD vs. 7% in the non-ESRD group. The patients with ESRD were 7 times more likely to require bilateral amputation than patients without ESRD. The authors' conclusion that ESRD has a profoundly negative impact on morbidity, mortality, and survival after lower extremity amputation is obviously completely correct. As stated previously, these patients are, in my opinion, the single most difficult group of patients whom vascular surgeons are called on to treat. I sometimes wonder where we are going with our transplant programs. See also the commentary on Abstract 145-96-10–8.

Rehabilitation Outcome 5 Years After 100 Lower-Limb Amputations
McWhinnie DL, Gordon AC, Collin J, Gray DWR, Morrison JD (University of Oxford, England; John Radcliffe Hosp, Oxford, England; Disablement Services Centre, Oxford, England)
Br J Surg 81:1596–1599, 1994   145-96-10–21

Background.—It is generally agreed that, to achieve primary healing while assuring the ability of the patient to walk with an artificial limb, it is desirable to maximize the ratio of below-knee to above-knee amputations in patients with end-stage peripheral vascular disease.

Methods.—The long-term results of this policy were examined in 96 patients who underwent 100 consecutive lower limb amputations and were evaluated annually for 5 years. There were 67 below-knee, 14 Gritti-Stokes, and 19 through-thigh amputations. The ratio of primary below-knee to all above-knee amputations was 2:1.

Results.—Nine percent of below-knee amputations were revised to a higher level. Only 26% of the patients were able to walk out of doors 2 years after amputation. Forty percent of the patients had died by this time. At 5 years, two thirds of the patients had died and only 9% were still able to walk outdoors with an artificial limb. Another 8% of patients still used their artificial limbs at home (table). Stump healing was problematic in 25% of below-knee amputations compared with 45% of 193 previous cases, where the below-knee to above-knee ratio was 1:2. In the earlier series, one third of the patients were able to walk at 2 years.

Walking Rates in Patients Who Survived Below-Knee and Above-Knee Amputation, Including Those Not Fitted With Prostheses

Time After Amputation	Below-Knee		Above-Knee		$P*$
	Survivors	Walkers	Survivors	Walkers	
3 months	49	33 (67)	30	9 (30)	< 0·01
1 year	46	32 (70)	27	14 (52)	n.s.
2 years	37	24 (65)	21	9 (43)	n.s.
3 years	31	20 (65)	15	6 (40)	n.s.
4 years	24	15 (62)	13	6 (46)	n.s.
5 years	21	12 (57)	11	5 (45)	n.s.

Values in parentheses are percentages.
* Yates' χ^2 test; *n.s.*, not significant.
(Courtesy of McWhinnie DL, Gordon AC, Colin J, et al: Rehabilitation outcome 5 years after 100 lower-limb amputations. *Br J Surg* 81:1596–1599, 1994. Reprinted by permission of Blackwell Science Ltd.)

Conclusion.—It appears that increasing the proportion of below-knee amputations does not augment the chances of rehabilitating patients with occlusive arterial disease. The true sign of success is the proportion of patients who regain mobility, either walking with an artificial limb or using a self-propelled wheelchair.

▶ For those of you who do not know, Dr. Jack Collin of Oxford University is a delightfully irreverent vascular surgeon. In this study, the Oxford group examines the 5-year performance of 100 consecutive lower extremity ischemic amputations. The below-knee/above-knee ratio was an admirable 2:1. Unfortunately, 2 years after amputation, only 26% of the patients were walking outdoors and 40% were dead. By 5 years, 67% had died and only 9% continued to walk outdoors with an artificial limb.

This group concludes that increasing the proportion of below-knee to above-knee amputations does not improve rehabilitation. The authors accurately observe that "received wisdom" on the desirability of a high below-knee/above-knee ratio may be completely incorrect. In general, Americans have been lulled into a false sense of security by selective reports from enthusiastic amputation centers that have indicated a very high rate of postoperative ambulatory rehabilitation. In the real world, this does not occur. With all-too-infrequent exceptions, a leg amputation for ischemia dooms the patient to a nonambulatory future. Information such as this underlies our vigorous attempt to achieve limb salvage, even if it requires more and more difficult procedures.

Below-Knee Amputation Using a Medially Based Flap

Jain AS, Stewart CPU, Turner MS (Univ of Dundee, Scotland)
Br J Surg 81:516, 1994   145-96-10–22

Introduction.—In elderly patients with severe peripheral vascular disease, salvaging the knee is very important for successful rehabilitation. At many centers, the rate of above-knee amputation remains discouragingly high. A technique of below-knee amputation using a medially based flap was described.

Technique.—A skin flap is mapped out based on the Thermoscan findings and pattern of cutaneous blood flow. The bone is sectioned as far proximally as is feasible, usually 7–12 cm distal to the tibial tuberosity. The base of the flap is usually 30–70 degrees medial to that of a standard long posterior flap. The flap is 12–15 cm in length and includes about half the circumference of the leg. An anterolateral skin incision passes horizontally around the leg just below the planned level of bone sectioning (Fig 10–9). After dividing the soft tissues and bone, considerable muscle is trimmed to comfortably close the stump without tension. The soleus muscle is sacrificed. Suction drainage is instituted, and the stump is encased in plaster for 2–4 weeks. Prosthetic fitting as soon as the skin has healed is facilitated.

▶ This article describes a below-knee amputation using a curious medially based flap, based on the assumption that there is greater skin flow medially than laterally in the average ischemic calf. I suppose if you want to do a medially based below-knee amputation flap, this is a good way to do it. I

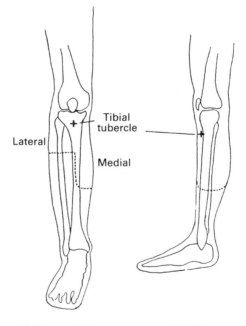

Anteroposterior　　　　Medial

Fig 10–9.—Diagram of the skin incision. (Courtesy of Jain AS, Stewart CPU, Turner MS, et al: Below-knee amputation using a medially based flap. *Br J Surg* 81:516, 1994. Reprinted by permission of Blackwell Science Ltd.)

really do not know whether the blood supply is inherently superior in the medial area, but these doctors believe that has been established beyond doubt.

Nonoperative Treatment

Chelation Therapy for Intermittent Claudication: A Double-Blind, Randomized, Controlled Trial
van Rij AM, Solomon C, Packer SGK, Hopkins WG (Univ of Otago, Dunedin, New Zealand)
Circulation 90:1194–1199, 1994   145-96-10–23

Background.—Chelation therapy, combining repeated infusions of ethylenediaminetetraacetic acid (EDTA) and vitamin supplements, has been suggested as a useful approach to a wide range of disorders, including intermittent claudication. A number of reports have cited excellent results in a significant number of patients, but well-controlled studies are lacking.

Trial Design.—A double-blind, randomized trial enrolled 32 patients with claudication, 15 of whom were randomized to receive 20 infusions of 3 g of disodium EDTA, given twice weekly over 10 weeks. The remaining 17 patients received saline infusions, and patients in both groups received a multivitamin preparation. The chief end point was the distance the patient could walk at 4 km/hr on a treadmill at 10% gradient.

Results.—Walking distances had improved significantly in both groups at the end of the infusion program (table). After 3 months, resting ankle/brachial indices showed some improvement in both the better and worse

Main Outcome Measures at Various Stages of the Trial Comparing the Chelation and Control Groups

Parameter	Group	Screening	End of Treatment	3 Months After Treatment
ABI (exercise), better leg	Chelation	0.55 ± 0.24	0.58 ± 0.30	0.58 ± 0.28
	Control	0.61 ± 0.32	0.61 ± 0.32	0.67 ± 0.34
ABI (exercise), worse leg	Chelation	0.31 ± 0.16	0.32 ± 0.18	0.34 ± 0.18
	Control	0.32 ± 0.14	0.34 ± 0.17	0.32 ± 0.17
ABI (resting), better leg	Chelation	0.74 ± 0.16	0.76 ± 0.2	0.78 ± 0.12
	Control	0.75 ± 0.19	0.86 ± 0.36	0.73 ± 0.21*
ABI (resting), worse leg	Chelation	0.59 ± 0.13	0.70 ± 0.36	0.62 ± 0.15
	Control	0.61 ± 0.11	0.60 ± 0.15	0.58 ± 0.15*
Measured WD, m	Chelation	185 ± 117	208 ± 135	233 ± 138
	Control	196 ± 121	223 ± 149	230 ± 195
Measured WD to onset of pain, m	Chelation	92 ± 64	101 ± 50	104 ± 62
	Control	98 ± 67	121 ± 89†	123 ± 108†
Subjective WD, m	Chelation	170 ± 213	413 ± 775	448 ± 556
	Control	182 ± 115	327 ± 461†	381 ± 473†

* Significant changes between groups ($P < 0.05$).
† Significant overall effect for both groups combined ($P < 0.05$).
Abbreviations: ABI, ankle/brachial index; *WD,* walking distance
(Courtesy of van Rij AM, Solomon C, Packer SGK, et al: Chelation therapy for intermittent claudication: A double-blind, randomized, controlled trial. *Circulation* 90:1194–1199, 1994. Reprinted with permission. *Circulation* Copyright 1994, American Heart Association.)

legs of patients given chelation therapy. There were no significant changes in lifestyle at the end of the treatment period, but at 3 months the actively treated patients were more active and exercised more.

Conclusion.—The encouraging results obtained with chelation therapy in previous series of patients with intermittent claudication were not substantiated.

▶ It is always refreshing to see quack therapies laid to rest. Chelation therapy appears to be on the run in America, but it is not yet dead. We continue to see the occasional patient who is receiving chelation therapy for atherosclerosis. An early randomized trial indicated no benefit whatsoever (1). This study is another carefully controlled prospective, randomized trial showing absolutely no benefit of chelation therapy compared with placebo. There should be no need for any more articles on chelation therapy.

Reference

1. 1993 YEAR BOOK OF VASCULAR SURGERY, p 40.

Epidural Spinal Cord Stimulation in the Treatment of Severe Peripheral Arterial Occlusive Disease
Horsch S, Claeys L (Academic Teaching Hosp, Cologne-Porz, Germany)
Ann Vasc Surg 8:468–474, 1994   145-96-10–24

Background.—Epidural spinal cord stimulation (ESCS) was intended to relieve intractable pain in patients with multiple sclerosis. Early observations suggested markedly improved blood flow in the lower extremities.

Methods.—The clinical effects of ESCS were examined in 177 patients with occlusive peripheral artery disease who had ischemic pain but were not amenable to vascular reconstruction. Chronic ischemic rest pain was present in 114 patients, whereas 63 had, in addition, ulcers or dry gangrene. Arteriosclerotic disease was the prevailing pathology, but 36 patients had diabetic vascular disease as well.

Results.—During an average observation of 3 years, 110 of the 177 patients had greater than 75% pain relief and retained their limbs. Eleven other patients achieved limb salvage and had 50% to 70% relief of pain. Fifty-six patients eventually underwent major amputation. The cumulative limb salvage rate at 4 years was 66%. The ESCS did not alter the systolic ankle/brachial blood pressure index, but oxygenation on the dorsum of the foot—measured transcutaneously—improved in the patients who did well clinically. An increase of more than 50% in transcutaneous oximetry in the first 3 months predicted a good outcome.

Complications.—Dislocated and broken leads were a frequent problem, and 7 patients had device-related infections. In 2 patients, a CSF fistula developed.

▶ There is no evidence that ESCS improves pain in chronic ischemia or reduces amputation. Nonreconstructibility is not defined in this paper. A total of 177 patients were seen in 6 years. We need to know what percentage this represents of the total number seen with critical ischemia at this center. Significantly, most successes occurred in patients in Fontaine stage III. This is a notoriously difficult group to define in terms of critical ischemia. The purported limb salvage rate of 66% at 4 years in these so-called inoperable patients is extraordinary and, I suspect, inaccurate.

We need to know who said the patients were inoperable and we need to compare such patients, receiving either no treatment or medical treatment, in a properly randomized study. Without such randomization, no conclusions can be drawn. The authors state this in their last paragraph, and one wonders why, with such large numbers of patients at their disposal, the authors did not perform a trial. These devices are extremely expensive, and we have to know whether they are effective before they are used indiscriminately.—P.R.F. Bell, M.D.

▶ I could not have said it better.—J.M. Porter, M.D.

Intensive Vascular Training in Stage IIb of Peripheral Arterial Occlusive Disease: The Additive Effects of Intravenous Prostaglandin E, or Intravenous Pentoxifylline During Training
Scheffler P, de la Hamette D, Gross J, Mueller H, Schieffer H (Univ Hosp of Saarland, Homburg/Saar, Germany; Rehabilitation Clinic, Blieskastel, Germany)
Circulation 90:818–822, 1994   145-96-10–25

Background.—In patients with intermittent claudication, a program of regular walking promotes vascular proliferation and collateral vessel formation and, thereby, enhances exercise tolerance. Prostaglandin E_1 (PGE_1) improves peripheral perfusion in this setting and can increase walking distance.

Methods.—Forty-four patients with stage IIb peripheral arterial occlusive disease were randomly assigned either to intensive vascular training alone or to training combined with IV pentoxifylline or PGE_1 treatment. Pentoxifylline was given in a dose of 200 mg twice daily, and PGE_1 was given in a dose of 40 µg twice daily. Both drugs were administered over 2 hours. All patients underwent a demanding exercise program over 4 weeks, using supine pedal ergometry, treadmill exercise, and ball games.

Results.—Walking distance was significantly increased in all groups. In patients undergoing exercise training only, symptom-free walking distance increased by 119%. Pentoxifylline had no additive effect, but PGE_1 combined with exercise resulted in a 604% increase in walking distance. Walking ability decreased in all groups over the ensuing year, but it remained 149% better than baseline in PGE_1-treated patients. Nine of 14 patients in this group remained in stage IIa 1 year after treatment.

Conclusion.—Patients with stage II arterial occlusive disease benefit from intensive vascular training combined with PGE$_1$ injections.

▶ The exercise training consisted of 30 minutes of general exercise, including ball games and pedal ergometry, and 30 minutes of treadmill exercise daily. In addition, a 30-minute rate-controlled walking exercise was done twice daily, with the duration of therapy being 4 weeks. Both exercise and exercise plus pentoxifylline produced improvement of 100% to 120%. In contrast, exercise combined with PGE$_1$ infusion achieved a remarkable 604% improvement in walking distance.

During the 1 year after treatment, maintained improvement in the exercise-only group and in the exercise-plus-pentoxifylline group was 30%, whereas in the PGE$_1$ group, maintained improvement was 149%. I continue to note with interest multiple reports of prolonged clinical improvement after PGE$_1$ infusion long after complete drug metabolism must have occurred. Although it has repeatedly been noted, no satisfactory mechanism of benefit has ever been presented.

Miscellaneous

Acetylcholine Sweat Test: An Effective Way to Select Patients for Lumbar Sympathectomy
Altomare DF, Regina G, Lovreglio R, Memeo V (Univ of Bari, Italy)
Lancet 344:976–978, 1994   145-96-10–26

Background.—Some patients with critical ischemic changes in an extremity benefit from lumbar sympathectomy, but others do not. Pre-existing injury of the sympathetic nerve fibers may be responsible.

Methods.—The acetylcholine sweatspot test was used to evaluate sympathetic nerve function before and after lumbar sympathectomy in 31 patients who had critical ischemia in a lower extremity. All the patients had rest pain, 10 had claudication, and 15 had superficial ischemic lesions of the foot. Sympathectomy was done operatively in 27 patients, and it was done chemically, using phenol, in 4. The sweatspot test was done just before sympathectomy and 2–3 months after by injecting 0.1 mL of 10% acetylcholine solution into the dorsum of the foot.

Results.—Individual changes in sweatspot scores are shown in Figure 10–10. All but 1 of 9 patients whose sympathetic function was normal or nearly normal preoperatively improved clinically. In the exceptional patient, denervation was not achieved. Of 22 patients whose scores indicated marked or complete sympathetic denervation, only 1 improved after lumbar sympathectomy. In the 9 patients who also had oximetry, the preoperative sweatspot score correlated with the change in tissue oxygen pressure.

Conclusion.—The acetylcholine sweatspot test is a reliable means of predicting the outcome of lumbar sympathectomy in patients with critical limb ischemia.

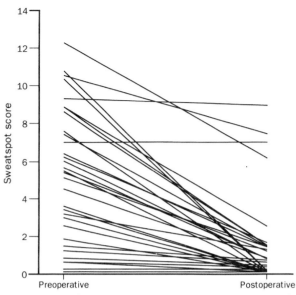

Fig 10–10.—Preoperative and postoperative sweatspot scores in 31 patients undergoing lumbar sympathectomy. (Courtesy of Altomare DF, Regina G, Lovreglio R, et al: Acetylcholine sweat test: An effective way to select patients for lumbar sympathectomy. *Lancet* 344:976–978, 1994. Copyright 1994, The Lancet, Ltd.)

▶ This article is interesting, albeit irrelevant. We long ago decided that lumbar sympathectomy was of no benefit in the treatment of critical limb ischemia, and we have found no reason to modify our position. These authors claim that this modification of the old starch/iodine test allows one to predict which patients are likely to benefit, based on preselection of patients who have a normal or presumed normal, functional, intact autonomic nervous supply. Perhaps, but we are not likely to begin performing this archaic operation.

Reduction of Free Radical Generation Minimises Lower Limb Swelling Following Femoropopliteal Bypass Surgery
Soong CV, Young IS, Lightbody JH, Hood JM, Rowlands BJ, Trimble ER, Barros D'Sa AAB (Royal Victoria Hosp Belfast, Northern Ireland; Queen's Univ of Belfast, Northern Ireland)
Eur J Vasc Surg 8:435–440, 1994   145-96-10–27

Purpose.—In patients who have undergone femoropopliteal bypass grafting, oxygen-derived free radicals may play a role in the development of lower limb edema. The occurrence of free radical–induced lipid peroxidation after femoropopliteal bypass, and the effects of allopurinol in decreasing free radical injury and lower leg edema, were studied.
Methods.—Twenty-nine patients undergoing femoropopliteal bypass surgery were studied. They were randomly selected to receive the xanthine

oxidase inhibitor allopurinol, 200 mg, orally at 24 and 2 hours preoperatively and at 24 hours postoperatively, or placebo. Femoral vein blood samples were taken to measure malondialdehyde (MDA)—an end product of lipid peroxidation—before the arterial clamp was applied, just before and after its release, and every 20 minutes after clamp release for 1 hour.

Results.—Lower limb volume increased by 8.9% in the placebo group vs. 4.6% in the allopurinol group (Fig 10–11). The lower limb increased by at least 10% of its original volume in 6 of 14 patients in the placebo group compared with 1 of 15 in the allopurinol group. For the placebo group, the concentration of MDA increased from 1,168 pmol/mL before clamp release to 1,480 pmol/mL 60 minutes after reperfusion. The corresponding values in the allopurinol group were 864 and 1,060 pmol/mL. The MDA changes were associated with reciprocal changes in vitamin A, vitamin E, and β-carotene concentrations.

Conclusion.—Free radical–induced peroxidation appears to be an important contributor to the lower limb edema that occurs after femoropopliteal bypass grafting. Treatment with allopurinol helps to minimize this complication of femoropopliteal bypass.

► I thought that we at Oregon Health Sciences University definitively showed 23 years ago that leg edema after femoropopliteal bypass resulted from lymphatic disruption (1). Clearly, however, this is not the only reason. Patients with profound ischemia who receive adequate revascularization and who sustain a postoperative "hot foot" invariably show significant edema, even if they remain faithfully in the supine position or even the leg elevated position. In these patients, other factors must be at work.

Allopurinol was randomly given to certain patients undergoing leg bypass because of its presumed benefit in decreasing oxygen-derived free radicals.

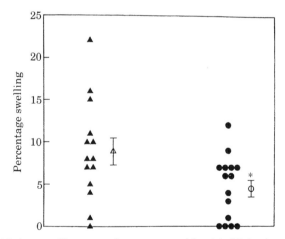

Fig 10–11.—Maximum swelling, expressed as a percentage of the original limb volume, in the 2 groups of patients. *Filled triangles* represent placebo group (*n* = 14); *filled circles* represent allopurinol group (*n* = 15). *Open symbols* represent mean ± SEM. *Asterisk* indicates *P* < 0.05 by Mann-Whitney U-test. (Courtesy of Soong CV, Young IS, Lightbody JH, et al: Reduction of free radical generation minimises lower limb swelling femoropopliteal bypass surgery. *Eur J Vasc Surg* 8:435–440, 1994.)

The other group received placebo. The increase in limb volume was twice as great in the placebo group as in the allopurinol group; also, a significant increase in MDA, an end product of lipid peroxidation, was noted in the placebo group. These authors conclude, and I suspect correctly, that free-radical–induced peroxidation plays a role in the development of lower extremity ischemia after leg bypass grafting. However, I still think lymphatic disruption is the most important mechanism.

Reference

1. Porter JM, Lindell TD, Lakin PC: Leg oedema following femoropopliteal autogenous vein bypass. *Arch Surg* 105:883–888, 1972.

Combined Coronary and Femoral Revascularization Using an Ascending Aorta to Bifemoral Bypass
Jebara VA, Fabiani JN, Acar C, Chardigny C, Julia P, Carpentier A (Hôpital Broussais, Paris)
Arch Surg 129:275–279, 1994   145-96-10–28

Background.—It is common for coronary atherosclerotic disease and aortoiliac disease to co-exist, and a rare patient may require simultaneous revascularization at both sites.

Series.—Ten men with co-existing coronary artery and aortoiliac occlusive disease were followed prospectively after simultaneous coronary and aortoiliac revascularization.

Methods.—The ascending aorta served as the source of inflow to the femoral arteries. A 10-mm polytef graft was joined to the ascending aorta during cardiopulmonary bypass, and, after the patient was weaned off the pump, the graft was passed through the preperitoneal abdominal space lateral to the right rectus muscle where it was joined to the femoral artery. A crossover femorofemoral bypass was then done.

Results.—The single hospital death was unrelated to surgery. All 9 surviving patients recovered well and were free of symptoms. None had symptoms of coronary artery disease or peripheral vascular disease during a mean follow-up of 18 months. Doppler sonography confirmed that all the aortofemoral grafts remained patent. One patient required a femoropopliteal bypass.

Conclusion.—This operative approach is feasible for selected patients with severe coronary and lower limb ischemia. No intraperitoneal surgery is required, and the hospital stay is shortened.

▶ This curious report from Remulac (France) concludes that, occasionally, patients requiring simultaneous coronary bypass grafting and lower extremity revascularization may benefit from simultaneous operation using the ascending aorta for a coronary artery bypass graft and as inflow for lower extremity revascularization. The lower extremity graft was a 10-mm polytef passed in the preperitoneal pararectus space. This procedure worked well in

9 of 10 patients. Although there is nothing new in this study, it is an interesting combination of existing procedures.

I am not at all convinced that the use of the ascending aorta is superior to use of the subclavian artery, and if I were going to perform a coronary artery bypass graft and a leg revascularization simultaneously, I am certain I would choose an axillary-bifemoral bypass. I have had modest experience in taking care of the complications of ascending aorta to bilateral femoral artery bypass performed elsewhere, and I do not identify this as a particularly satisfactory procedure.

11 Upper Extremity Vascular and Hemoaccess

Subclavian Artery

Subclavian Revascularization: A Quarter Century Experience
Edwards WH Jr, Tapper SS, Edwards WH Sr, Mulherin JL, Martin RS III, Jenkins JM (St Thomas Hosp, Nashville, Tenn; Vanderbilt Univ, Nashville, Tenn)
Ann Surg 219:673–678, 1994   145-96-11–1

Background.—There is general agreement that stenosis of the proximal subclavian artery should be treated extrathoracially when possible, but which particular procedure is best is unknown. The options include a subclavian carotid bypass, a subclavian-to-subclavian or axilloaxillary bypass, and subclavian carotid transposition (SCT).

Methods.—Experience over 26 years at a specialty clinic performing extrathoracic subclavian revascularization was reviewed. The 190 procedures included only 12 bypass operations, most of which were subclavian carotid bypasses. These patients were treated primarily for ischemic symptoms in the upper extremity. Subclavian carotid transposition was performed 178 times on 175 patients; more than half the patients experienced dizziness. About half the patients experienced ischemic symptoms in the arm or hand.

Results.—All but 1 of the patients undergoing SCT had patent anastomoses after an average follow-up of 46 months. Five patients were lost to follow-up. The mortality rate was 2.2% overall and 1.1% in patients having SCT. Nonfatal complications occurred in 17% of patients; the most common were transient Horner's syndrome and temporary hoarseness.

Conclusion.—Not only is SCT safe and effective in the short term, but long-term patency is exceptional. It is, therefore, the preferred treatment for most patients with occlusive disease of the proximal subclavian artery.

▶ A remarkable 190 subclavian revascularizations were performed in a single clinic over 26 years. By far, the most common procedure was SCT, which was used in 175 patients. The most frequent single indication for surgery, according to the authors, was dizziness. Another frequent complaint was syncope. I must say I am amazed by this experience. In a rather busy vascular surgery practice, we routinely perform 4–6 subclavian revascularizations per year, and almost all are done for treatment of severe arm ischemia. I do believe SCT is a good procedure, but for me it is difficult. (See the commentary after Abstract 145-96-11–2.)

Subclavian Artery Revascularization: A Decade of Experience With Extrathoracic Bypass Procedures
Salam TA, Lumsden AB, Smith RB III (Emory Univ, Atlanta, Ga)
J Surg Res 56:387–392, 1994   145-96-11–2

Objective.—Patients with symptoms of subclavian artery disease are most often managed by extrathoracic revascularization. The results of 41 such operations were reviewed in 37 patients having stenosis or occlusion of the proximal subclavian artery.

Patients.—Twenty-five women and 12 men averaging 56 years of age underwent surgery. Nineteen patients had symptoms of upper limb ischemia, 4 had vertebrobasilar insufficiency, and 11 had both. In 3 patients, angina developed after coronary artery bypass with the internal mammary artery, reflecting a coronary-subclavian steal syndrome. In all patients, the proximal subclavian artery was markedly narrowed or totally occluded.

Methods.—The most frequent procedure was carotid-subclavian bypass, which most often used a prosthetic graft (table).

Results.—No patient died or had a stroke perioperatively. The average follow-up was 3 years. Patency rates decreased from 95% 1 year after surgery to 86% at 3 years and 73% at 5 years. At 5 years, 83% of the patients in whom the common carotid artery had served as the donor vessel had patent repairs compared with only 46% of those in whom the contralateral subclavian or axillary artery had been used. Two patients with a patent graft nevertheless had recurrent symptoms. The 1 death was unrelated to revascularization.

Conclusion.—Extrathoracic bypass is an effective and safe means of ensuring long-term patency in patients with symptoms of proximal subclavian artery disease. If possible, the ipsilateral common carotid should be used as the donor vessel.

Types of Bypass Procedures and Conduit for Subclavian Artery Revascularization

Type of Procedure	No.	Bypass Conduit
Carotid-subclavian bypass	28	22 prosthetic, 6 vein
Subclavian-carotid transposition	6	—
Axilloaxillary bypass	4	4 prosthetic
Subclavian-subclavian bypass	3	3 prosthetic
Total	41	29 prosthetic, 6 vein

(Courtesy of Salam TA, Lumsden AB, Smith RB III: Subclavian artery revascularization: A decade of experience with extrathoracic bypass procedure. *J Surg Res* 56:387–392, 1994.)

▶ Dr. Smith's group at Emory University prefers carotid-subclavian bypass for upper extremity revascularization, although subclavian-carotid transposition and axilloaxillary bypass are used on occasion. A majority of their patients undergo surgery for symptoms of upper extremity ischemia and only a few for presumed vertebrobasilar insufficiency. The overall patency rate was 73% at 5 years. I currently believe that transposition is the better operation if technically feasible; however, one has to be careful to pick patients in whom a considerable segment of the proximal subclavian artery is undiseased. When transposition is performed, one had best be careful to avoid kinking the proximal vertebral artery, which we have seen happen on occasion. This is best avoided by performing the transposition anastomosis somewhat low behind the sternum; this is inconvenient for the surgeon, but it is less likely to kink the proximal vertebral artery.

Carotid-Subclavian Bypass: A Twenty-Two–Year Experience
Vitti MJ, Thompson BW, Read RC, Gagne PJ, Barone GW, Barnes RW, Eidt JF (Univ of Arkansas, Little Rock; John L McClellan VA Med Ctr, Little Rock, Ark)
J Vasc Surg 20:411–418, 1994   145-96-11–3

Objective.—The results of carotid-subclavian bypass surgery were reviewed in 124 patients who underwent surgery in 1968–1990.

Patients.—The average patient age at surgery was 58 years. The indication for surgery was vertebrobasilar insufficiency in 19% of patients, limb ischemia in 27%, and transient ischemic attacks in 11%. Both vertebrobasilar insufficiency and limb ischemia called for surgery in 25% of cases, and 18% of patients had both transient ischemic attacks and extremity ischemia. Dacron grafts were used in 65% of the patients, and polytetrafluoroethylene prostheses were used in 35%. One fourth of the patients underwent ipsilateral carotid endarterectomy at the same time.

Results.—One patient died intraoperatively, and 10 patients (8%) had complications. All surviving patients had a patent bypass and were free of symptoms 30 days postoperatively. Among 60 patients followed for 5 months or longer, there were 3 graft occlusions, for a primary patency rate of 95% at both 5 and 10 years. Patient survival was 83% at 5 years but decreased to 59% at 10 years. The symptoms recurred in 10% of the patients followed; 3 of the 6 had an occluded graft. In no patient did drop attacks or transient ischemic attacks recur. Limb ischemia recurred in 5% of patients, always in association with an occluded graft. Dizziness recurred in some of those affected, despite maintenance of a patent graft.

Conclusion.—Carotid-subclavian bypass reliably and safely provides long-lasting symptomatic relief in patients with occlusive disease of the subclavian artery. Those seen with drop attacks or upper extremity ischemia are especially likely to do well.

▶ This complex series of 124 patients undergoing carotid-subclavian bypass had many indications for surgery. Carotid endarterectomy was combined with the bypass in 26% of patients. The excellent patency, lack of complications, and excellent resolution of symptoms are noteworthy.

Effect of Subclavian Syndrome on the Basilar Artery

de Bray JM, Zenglein JP, Laroche JP, Joseph PA, Lhoste Ph, Pillet J, Dubas F, Emile J (Univ Hosp, Angers, France; General Hosp, Colmar, France; Univ Hosp, Nîmes, France)

Acta Neurol Scand 90:174–178, 1994   145-96-11–4

Objective.—The usefulness of transcranial Doppler sonography in estimating the risk of stroke was examined in a prospective series of 55 patients in whom a continuous-wave Doppler study had demonstrated intermittent or permanent subclavian steal syndrome. Twenty-five of the patients had no vertebrobasilar symptoms; 8 had such symptoms; and 22 had hemodynamic evidence of vertebrobasilar ischemia.

Methods.—The velocity of blood flow in the basilar artery was recorded by transcranial Doppler sonography under baseline conditions and again after a humeral cuff had been inflated for 3 minutes and deflated to produce hyperemia.

Results.—Spontaneous incomplete basilar steal was demonstrated at baseline in 7 patients and complete basilar steal in 1, totaling 14.5% of patients. After hyperemia, 18 other patients exhibited incomplete basilar steal. All but 1 of the patients with vertebrobasilar symptoms had findings of basilar steal, as did 5 of the 6 symptomatic patients in whom the opposite vertebral artery was more than 50% stenosed.

Conclusion.—Transcranial Doppler sonography is a reliable way of detecting patients with subclavian steal syndrome and vertebral artery stenosis, who may be at high risk of stroke.

▶ Using transcranial Doppler sonography, these investigators defined retrograde flow in the basilar artery in patients with permanent or intermittent subclavian steal. In general, basilar steal was more frequent in patients with vertebrobasilar symptoms and less frequent in asymptomatic patients. Without doubt, transcranial Doppler sonography can define a group of subclavian steal patients with retrograde flow in the basilar arteries. The authors' assumption that this predicts stroke is unproven.

The Effect of Arm Exercise on Regional Cerebral Blood Flow in the Subclavian Steal Syndrome

Webster MW, Downs L, Yonas H, Makaroun MS, Steed DL (Univ of Pittsburgh, Pennsylvania)

Am J Surg 168:91–93, 1994   145-96-11–5

Background.—It is not uncommon for the vertebral arterial blood flow to be reversed distal to a subclavian obstruction, although this rarely leads to stroke. A small number of these patients, however, have an obstruction elsewhere in the extracranial or intracranial circulation, and, in this circumstance, arm exercise may decrease regional cerebral blood flow to a critical level, resulting in a true vascular "steal."

Methods.—Regional cerebral blood flow was mapped by using a stable xenon technique with CT in 6 symptomatic patients with subclavian steal syndrome. Five of the patients had at least 1 other extracranial vessel that was narrowed or occluded. Four patients had hemodynamically significant disease of the ipsilateral internal carotid artery, and 2 had stenosis of the contralateral vertebral artery. The measurements were repeated as patients lifted a weight and squeezed a ball with the arm ipsilateral to the reversed vertebral flow.

Results.—All patients had normal cerebral blood flow at baseline, but after arm exercise, the flow decreased by 13% or more at 1 or more sites in all patients. In all but 1 of them, the flow in at least 1 region decreased more than 30%. One patient with a tight stenosis of the contralateral vertebral artery had a flow of less than 18 mL/min/100 g of tissue at several sites after exercise. In all the patients but 1, the blood flow decreased in both hemispheres.

Conclusion.—Patients with true vascular steal may well be at risk of having a stroke, and regional cerebral blood flow measurements may help detect those who would be expected to benefit from revascularization. Correcting reversed vertebral flow is not likely to lessen symptoms when the blood flow is normal at baseline and responds normally to arm exercise. Instead, any significant carotid obstruction should first be corrected.

▶ Using a sophisticated xenon blood flow technique, combined CT, and cerebral blood flow mapping, these investigators examined intracranial circulation after arm exercise in patients with subclavian steal. A decrease in flow between 13% and 90% in 1 or more regional vascular intracranial territories was found after arm exercise. These authors hypothesize that showing an actual decrease in regional brain circulation with arm exercise may more accurately predict the patients at higher risk for stroke with subclavian steal. This is similar to the prediction in the previous article (Abstract 145-96-11-4). Unfortunately, clinical correlations of these predictions are not presently available.

Embolism

Thromboembolism From Occult Subclavian Arterial Stenosis During Chemotherapy for Breast Carcinoma
Donaldson MC, Whittemore AD (Harvard Med School, Boston)
Arch Surg 130:224–226, 1995   145-96-11–6

Objective.—Hypercoagulability and thromboembolic complications can occur in patients with cancer who are receiving chemotherapy. Three cases of thromboembolism resulting from occult subclavian arterial stenosis in patients with breast cancer undergoing chemotherapy were reported.

Case 1.—Woman, 25, with a history of modified radical mastectomy and adjuvant chemotherapy for breast cancer, was seen with right arm ischemia of 30 hours' duration. On arteriography, she was found to have stenosis of the midsection of the right subclavian artery with post-stenotic dilatation and brachial artery obstruction. The thrombus was dissolved with intra-arterial urokinase, and the patient had surgery. Her anterior scalene muscle was tightly binding the subclavian artery over the cervical rib, which protruded behind the artery. After the muscle insertion was divided and the cervical rib was excised, the artery was opened into the area of poststenotic dilatation. There was no remaining thrombus or intrinsic fibrous stenosis, and the artery was closed primarily. The patient recovered with 3 months of warfarin sodium and discontinuation of chemotherapy.

Case 2.—Woman, 51, who had previously undergone lumpectomy and radiation therapy and was receiving chemotherapy, was seen with recurrent ischemia of the left fifth finger. A left-sided stenosis of the subclavian artery in the area of the anterior scalene muscle, with complete occlusion of the ulnar artery, was seen on angiography. The ulnar artery and hand were disobliterated with intra-arterial urokinase, and the patient was taken to surgery. The anterior scalene muscle was found to be constricting the subclavian artery. The artery showed intimal hyperplasia and residual thrombus, requiring vein patch closure. The patient recovered with 3 months of warfarin anticoagulation therapy and discontinuation of chemotherapy.

Case 3.—Woman, 52, had an abrupt onset of digital ischemia of the left hand. She had a history of modified radical mastectomy, chemotherapy, and radiation therapy for breast cancer and subsequent chemotherapy for bone metastases. Stenosis of the lateral portion of the left subclavian artery and occlusion of 2 digital arteries were seen on arteriography. The subclavian lesion was improved and blood flow to the fingers was restored with intra-arterial urokinase. The subclavian artery appeared normal after surgical release from the anterior scalene muscle. Palliative chemotherapy was restarted 1 month after recovery, including oral anticoagulant therapy.

Discussion.—Three unusual but remarkably similar cases of thromboembolic complications in patients undergoing breast cancer chemotherapy were reported. In all 3 women, the suspected source of distal thromboembolism was a previously asymptomatic, extrinsically caused subclavian artery stenosis. Transient hypercoagulability and underlying arterial disease may interact in the pathogenesis of arterial thromboembolism.

▶ These 3 cases are interesting. The first patient had a cervical rib, the second patient had stenosis of the subclavian artery, apparently caused by the anterior scalene muscle, and the third patient had subclavian stenosis, also in the region of the anterior scalene muscle. Clearly, the unifying factor in all 3 of these patients was mechanical subclavian stenosis. I really do not know whether the chemotherapy had anything to do with the thromboembolic episodes experienced by these patients, but the association is sufficiently interesting for us all to watch for this in the future.

Upper Extremity Thromboembolism Caused by Occlusion of Axillofemoral Grafts

McLafferty RB, Taylor LM Jr, Moneta GL, Yeager RA, Edwards JM, Porter JM
(Oregon Health Sciences Univ, Portland)
Am J Surg 169:492–495, 1995   145-96-11-7

Background.—For high-risk patients with lower extremity ischemia caused by aortoiliac occlusion, axillofemoral bypass grafting (AxFG) has become an accepted treatment alternative. Because of reports of symptom-

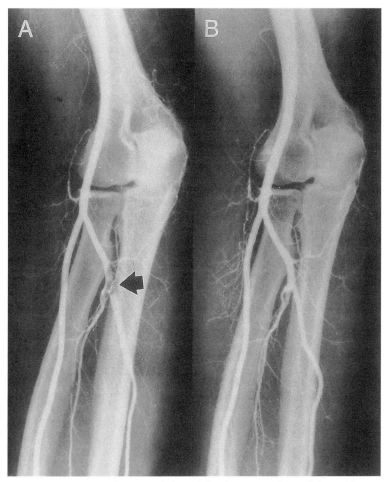

Fig 11–1.—A, arteriogram showing embolism of the ulnar artery after axillofemoral bypass graft occlusion. B, arteriogram showing lysis of the embolus after urokinase infusion. Graft material was externally supported using 8-mm polytetrafluoroethylene. (Courtesy of McLafferty RB, Taylor LM Jr, Moneta GL, et al: Upper extremity thromboembolism caused by occlusion of axillofemoral grafts. *Am J Surg* 169:492–495, 1995. Reprinted with permission from *American Journal of Surgery.*)

atic thromboembolism of the upper extremity caused by occluded AxFG, further study of this complication and its treatment was undertaken.

Methods.—The patients were prospectively followed up by means of a vascular registry of all patients undergoing AxFG from 1984 to 1994. A total of 202 such grafts were performed in 182 patients. A standardized operative technique, including an externally supported 8-mm polytetrafluoroethylene graft, was followed for each procedure.

Results.—Twenty patients had occlusion of a graft during follow-up. In 15 of these cases, revision of the occluded graft was carried out immediately. In 2 patients, upper extremity thromboembolism developed at the same time as graft occlusion; immediate graft revision was done in 1 patient and brachial embolectomy in the other. In the latter patient and 4 others, representing 25% of the patients with an occluded graft, the graft was left in place. All but 1 of these 5 patients experienced upper extremity thromboembolism within 1 month to 7 years (Fig 11–1). The 5 patients had a total of 6 thromboembolic complications of the upper extremity.

Conclusion.—Thromboembolism of the upper extremity may occur in 3% of patients undergoing AxFG and in 25% of those with occluded grafts. It thus appears to be a significant and specific complication. For patients with an occluded graft that does not require immediate revision, the best approach may be to detach the axillary portion of the graft prophylactically and repair the axillary artery. The use of an anastomosis that reduces the angle between the graft and the artery may help to prevent the development of a Y-shaped deformity of the axillary artery (Fig 11–2).

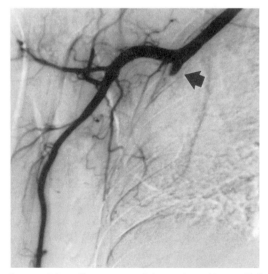

Fig 11–2.—Arteriogram of the axillary anastomosis in a patient with an axillofemoral bypass graft. The *arrow* points to the blind pouch at the proximal end of the occluded axillofemoral graft. Note the Y-shaped deformity of the axillary artery, presumably because of tension. (Courtesy of McLafferty RB, Taylor LM Jr, Moneta GL, et al: Upper extremity thromboembolism caused by occlusion of axillofemoral grafts. *Am J Surg* 169:492–495, 1995. Reprinted with permission from *American Journal of Surgery*.)

▶ We have experienced a disturbingly frequent occurrence of ipsilateral upper extremity embolism from occluded axillofemoral grafts left in place. The embolism was noted 26 days to 7 years after the occlusion. It has been sufficiently worrisome, in our experience, that we are currently contemplating prophylactic detachment of the axillary portion of the occluded graft in patients who do not require immediate graft revision or replacement.

Dialysis Access

Thrombolysis Versus Thrombectomy for Occluded Hemodialysis Grafts
Schuman E, Quinn S, Standage B, Gross G (Good Samaritan Hosp, Portland, Ore)
Am J Surg 167:473–476, 1994   145-96-11–8

Background.—Graft thrombosis is the most common complication resulting from the use of polytetrafluoroethylene grafts for hemodialysis. Surgical thrombectomy is the standard treatment for graft thrombosis. However, recently the use of fibrinolytic agents has shown varying rates of success. To evaluate the safety and efficacy of both methods for declotting a dialysis graft and to investigate whether they permit a patient to promptly and efficiently initiate dialysis, thrombolysis was compared with thrombectomy.

Method.—Thirty-one patients with occluded polytetrafluoroethylene grafts were randomly assigned to have thrombolysis or surgical thrombectomy. After either treatment, the patients proceeded to undergo dialysis. The procedure was considered successful if the patient was able to initiate dialysis that day.

Results.—Fifteen patients underwent thrombolysis and 16 had thrombectomy. The success rate for the thrombolysis group was 67% compared

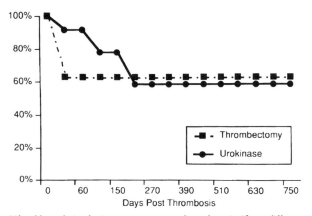

Fig 11–3.—Life-table analysis of primary patency rates showed no significant difference. (Courtesy of Schuman E, Quinn S, Standage B, et al: Thrombolysis versus thrombectomy for occluded hemodialysis grafts. *Am J Surg* 167:473–476, 1994. Reprinted with permission from *American Journal of Surgery*.)

with a 94% success rate for the thrombectomy group. No significant differences in primary and secondary patency rates were seen between the 2 groups (Fig 11–3), but the complication rates were higher and the time to completion was longer in the thrombolysis patients. The charges for surgical treatment were $3,383 for thrombectomy compared with $2,830 for thrombolysis.

Conclusion.—Although both thrombolysis and surgical thrombectomy can be used successfully, thrombectomy remains the optimal choice in the management of occluded dialysis grafts, showing a more rapid and successful initiation of dialysis and a lower rate of complications.

▶ These very experienced access surgeons compared thrombolysis with conventional thrombectomy in a prospective, randomized trial in patients with hemodialysis graft occlusion. In general, their experience favored surgical thrombectomy. Despite the efforts made by many to find a clearly indicated role for thrombolytic therapy in peripheral vascular surgery, the goal, to date, remains elusive.

Thrombosed Dialysis Access Grafts: Percutaneous Mechanical Declotting Without Urokinase
Trerotola SO, Lund GB, Scheel PJ Jr, Savader SJ, Venbrux AC, Osterman FA Jr (Indiana Univ, Indianapolis; Johns Hopkins Med Insts, Baltimore, Md)
Radiology 191:721–726, 1994   145-96-11–9

Background.—Clotted access grafts are a major factor in morbidity and hospitalization among hemodialysis patients. Percutaneous thrombolysis with urokinase yields excellent results, but urokinase is expensive and may be associated with complications. A simple percutaneous technique for declotting dialysis access grafts without urokinase was reported.

Methods and Results.—The experience included 34 clotted grafts treated in 24 patients. The percutaneous mechanical declotting technique used balloon catheters to macerate the clot and push it into the central circulation. Declotting was successful in 94% of patients. In 4 patients with poor venous outflow, the procedure was abandoned after successful declotting; thus, the 24-hour success rate was 82%. The procedure took a mean of 116 minutes to perform. The rate of clinical success—defined as successful dialysis after 1 week—was 59%. The mean primary patency was 126 days. Two cases of brachial artery embolus were successfully managed with urokinase; there were no symptomatic pulmonary emboli.

Conclusion.—Thrombosed dialysis access grafts can be managed by mechanical thrombolysis using currently available catheters and without urokinase. This percutaneous declotting technique is simple, safe, relatively inexpensive, and well tolerated.

▶ In this remarkable study (which could only have been dreamed up by an interventionalist), a clot within a hemodialysis graft was macerated and pushed into the central venous circulation. Occasionally, external massaging was used to facilitate clot maceration. I have never before seen patency results reported in hours, but in this article the radiologists report a 24-hour patency rate of 82%, although a substantial number were lost within the first week. It is gratifying to note that the authors do indicate in their discussion that they recognize that this procedure may result in pulmonary embolization but are relatively certain that this will not be significant in a majority of patients. I continue to be amazed by the procedures conjured up by noncli-nicians.

Proximal Venous Outflow Obstruction in Patients With Upper Extremity Arteriovenous Dialysis Access
Criado E, Marston WA, Jaques PF, Mauro MA, Keagy BA (Univ of North Carolina, Chapel Hill)
Ann Vasc Surg 8:530–535, 1994   145-96-11–10

Objective.—The effects of central venous obstruction on failure of hemodialysis access in the upper extremity were examined in 122 patients who, over 1 year, underwent a total of 158 access procedures.

Findings.—Fourteen patients (11.5%) had marked arm swelling or a thrombotic or malfunctioning graft as the result of central vein obstruction. All these patients had received temporary bilateral subclavian vein dialysis catheters, and all had failed arteriovenous access in the upper extremity.

Management and Outcome.—The 21 procedures included 17 percutaneous transluminal balloon angioplasties, 13 of which were accompanied by stent placement. There were 2 axillary-to-innominate vein bypasses and 2 axillary-to–internal jugular vein bypasses. Symptoms resolved in all patients, but in 4 instances it was not possible to recanalize the vein. Eight angioplasties provided functional hemodialysis access for 2–9 months. Two again became stenosed and were successfully dilated. Two other angioplasties occluded and could not be recanalized, and 1 failed immediately after successful angioplasty. Four patients in whom angioplasty failed underwent venous bypass, and the bypasses remained patent and provided functional access 7 to 13 months afterward (Fig 11–4). Six of 9 stenotic vein lesions were successfully dilated and remained open. In contrast, only 2 of 8 occluded veins were successfully opened without recurrent stenosis.

Conclusion.—In patients with arteriovenous access in the upper extremity, temporary central hemodialysis catheters produce a significant number of symptomatic central vein stenoses and occlusions. Access function often can be prolonged by percutaneous dilatation of venous lesions, with or without stent placement and surgical bypass.

▶ Without question, percutaneous subclavian vein dialysis catheters have a lethal effect on the subclavian vein. High-grade stenoses or venous occlu-

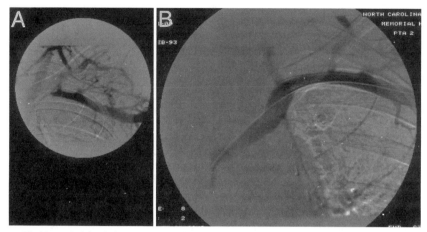

Fig 11-4.—A, left subclavian venogram from a woman, 40, with left upper arm arteriovenous fistula and complete subclavian vein occlusion, who was initially seen with massive left arm swelling. B, after percutaneous transluminal balloon angioplasty and placement of a 10-mm Wallstent, the swelling improved, and the access remains functional at 6 months after dilatation. (Courtesy of Criado E, Marston WA, Jaques PF, et al: Proximal venous outflow obstruction in patients with upper extremity arteriovenous dialysis access. *Ann Vasc Surg* 8:530–535, 1994.)

sions seem to be more the rule than the exception. Subsequent attempts to place hemodialysis access shunts in the same arm are then met with severe complications of venous obstruction. The authors of this article present a variety of imaginative ways to deal with these venous stenoses. Percutaneous transluminal balloon angioplasty does not appear to be particularly successful. Vein bypass appears to be reasonably successful but, of course, is a formidable procedure in this area. These authors make a logical appeal to avoid the use of subclavian vein hemodialysis catheters in patients who may later require permanent hemodialysis access.

Subclavian Vein Repair in Patients With an Ipsilateral Arteriovenous Fistula
Gradman WS, Bressman P, Sernaque JD (Cedars-Sinai Med Ctr, Los Angeles)
Ann Vasc Surg 8:549–556, 1994   145-96-11–11

Background.—The subclavian vein is often catheterized for temporary hemodialysis, but the catheterized vein occasionally becomes stenotic or occluded. Occlusive disease at this site may present a difficult treatment problem when an arteriovenous fistula is present ipsilaterally.

Patients.—Nine patients, 8 with polytetrafluoroethylene grafts and 1 with a Brescia-Cimino fistula, were seen with subclavian vein obstruction and underwent repair. Five of the patients had intractable arm edema as

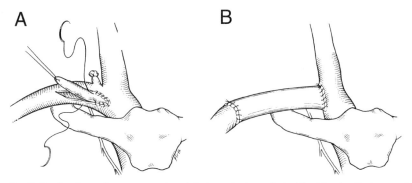

Fig 11–5.—**A,** after endovenectomy, the subclavian vein is patched with either locally harvested external jugular vein or polytetrafluoroethylene (PTFE). **B,** a PTFE interposition graft is used if the segment of diseased vein is too long for a patch. (Courtesy of Gradman WS, Bressman P, Sernaque JD: Subclavian vein repair in patients with an ipsilateral arteriovenous fistula. *Ann Vasc Surg* 8:549–556, 1994.)

their chief symptom. Occlusions occurred anywhere from the midsubclavian vein to the proximal innominate vein. The pathology ranged from a focal occluding web to a long segment of intimal fibroplasia. Five veins were occluded and 4 were stenotic.

Management.—The medial half of the clavicle was resected to gain access to the subclavian vein. As complete an endovenectomy as possible was done to remove intraluminal fibroplasia, bands, or webs, and the defect was patched with external jugular vein when possible (Fig 11–5). A

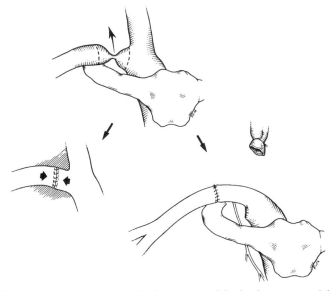

Fig 11–6.—After a stricture is resected, either the veins are mobilized and reanastomosed (**lower left**) or the internal jugular vein is divided and transposed for an end-to-end anastomosis to the subclavian vein (**lower right**). (Courtesy of Gradman WS, Bressman P, Sernaque JD: Subclavian vein repair in patients with an ipsilateral arteriovenous fistula. *Ann Vasc Surg* 8:549–556, 1994.)

patch or interposition graft of polytetrafluoroethylene was sometimes used. A focal hourglass stricture was managed as shown in Fig 11–6. The most common procedure was endovenectomy with placement of a vein patch.

Results.—Contrast venography showed a patent subclavian vein in all 8 surviving patients. One patient died postoperatively of unrelated causes. Two patients died with functioning fistulas 8 and 12 months, respectively, after repair. Two grafts became infected and were removed, and 1 deteriorated graft was abandoned because of repeated thrombosis. Only 3 grafts are still in use.

Conclusion.—Vein repair may retain a role in treating occlusions, especially in patients having a Brescia-Cimino fistula.

▶ Nine patients undergoing significant surgical procedures for correction of subclavian vein occlusive disease ipsilateral to an arteriovenous fistula are reported. The results generally were moderately successful. I have reservations about using medial clavicular resection as recommended in this article. These are very significant operations and in my opinion, should be reserved for most unusual patients. (See also Abstract 145-96-11–10.)

Hemodialysis Access in the Pediatric Patient Population
Lumsden AB, MacDonald MJ, Allen RC, Dodson TF (Emory Univ, Atlanta, Ga)
Am J Surg 168:197–201, 1994   145-96-11–12

Objective.—Twenty-four children aged 3–17 years, all of whom were significantly below expected body weight, were evaluated for placement of permanent hemodialysis access. In 7 cases, hemodialysis was elected after peritoneal dialysis had failed. Seventeen patients received a renal transplant, but 7 have resumed hemodialysis.

Methods.—Hemodialysis was established using an arteriovenous fistula in 15 instances, an expanded polytetrafluoroethylene bridge graft in 37, a bovine arteriovenous bridge graft in 9, and a central venous catheter in 29.

Results.—The fistulas remained functionally patent for an average of 6.2 months. One third of the fistulas failed to mature enough to be used for dialysis. The 21 polytetrafluoroethylene grafts implanted in the upper extremity remained functionally patent for an average of 11 months. Sixteen groin loop grafts were patent for only 4.1 months on the average. Thrombectomy was done in 25 cases, and the mean duration of secondary patency was 10.5 months. On average, each procedure provided dialysis access for a mean of 7.3 months. Eight polytetrafluoroethylene grafts became infected and all but 1 of them were lost. Other complications included superior vena caval occlusion and axillo-subclavian vein occlusion in 2 patients each and 1 case of inferior caval thrombosis.

Conclusion.—All children with renal dysfunction should be viewed as potential candidates for long-term dialysis, and an attempt should be made to gain maximum use from each access site. Distal sites should be used before proximal ones, and autogenous methods should be used before prostheses.

▶ A rather significant experience with hemodialysis access procedures in a pediatric population is presented. The authors accurately note that this is a time-consuming and, at times, frustrating undertaking. The authors' advocacy of distal before proximal and autogenous before prosthetic dogma in pediatric hemodialysis appears entirely reasonable. I am not sure that these authors have anything new to say, but their significant experience and the pathos of their presentation are noteworthy.

Ischemic Monomelic Neuropathy: An Under-Recognized Complication of Hemodialysis Access
Hye RJ, Wolf YG (Univ of California, San Diego)
Ann Vasc Surg 8:578–582, 1994   145-96-11–13

Background.—In patients with advanced atherosclerotic disease or diabetic complications requiring hemodialysis, ischemia most often results from a "steal" syndrome or a "venous sink" phenomenon, whereby the access diverts blood into the low-resistance venous system, and distal arterial perfusion becomes deficient. Patients may have distal ischemic rest pain and mild sensory loss, and they may later experience tissue loss and muscle weakness. Alternately, marked sensorimotor dysfunction may develop, which could be irreversible in the absence of distal tissue necrosis. The latter disorder, termed ischemic monomelic neuropathy (IMN), is the more disabling condition.

Patients.—Over 3 years, 5 patients (Table 1) were seen with 6 episodes of IMN complicating a dialysis graft in the upper extremity. The patients all had insulin-dependent diabetes of long standing and peripheral neuropathy. Three of the 5 had peripheral vascular disease. All the patients had polytetrafluoroethylene grafts originating in the brachial artery, in either the forearm or upper arm. Five episodes of IMN occurred just after graft placement, whereas 1 resulted from graft-related thromboembolism. Often the diagnosis was delayed when the findings were ascribed to

---

TABLE 1.—Clinical Characteristics of Patients With Ischemic Monomelic Neuropathy

Patient	Age (yr)	Sex	Diabetic complications	Insulin dependent (yr)	Vascular disease
1	64	M	N,K	30	Yes
2	62	M	R,N,K	20	Yes
3	51	F	?N,K	8	No
4 (a and b)	64	M	R,N,K	22	Yes
5	56	F	R,N,K	25	No

Abbreviations: R, retinopathy; N, neuropathy; K, nephropathy.
(Courtesy of Hye RJ, Wolf YG: Ischemic monomelic neuropathy: An under-recognized complication of hemodialysis access. *Ann Vasc Surg* 8:578–582, 1994.)

TABLE 2.—Treatment and Outcome of Patients With Ischemic Monomelic Neuropathy

Patient	Time to diagnosis	Diagnostic criteria	Treatment	Outcome
1	6 wk	EMG/NCV	Proximal angioplasty	Unimproved
2	4 wk	EMB/NCV	None	Unimproved
3	7 days	Clinical	Graft ligation	Significant improvement
4a	1 day	EMG/NCV	Graft ligation	Unimproved
4b	2 yr	EMG/NCV	None	Moderate improvement
5	4 days	Clinical	Embolectomy	Unimproved

(Courtesy of Hye RJ, Wolf YG: Ischemic monomelic neuropathy: An under-recognized complication of hemodialysis access. *Ann Vasc Surg* 8:578–582, 1994.)

anesthesia, positioning, or operative trauma. Electrophysiologic studies demonstrated marked multifocal neuropathy distal to the graft. Digital pressures were decreased, but no critical ischemia was evident.

Management and Outcome.—In 3 instances, ischemia was totally corrected, but only 1 of these patients improved (Table 2). One patient failed to improve after proximal balloon angioplasty. One of the 2 untreated patients improved slightly.

Conclusion.—Ischemic monomelic neuropathy is a rare and unpredictable complication of dialysis access in patients with diabetes who are uremic. The best hope is to find better ways of identifying patients at risk.

▶ These authors have introduced me to the concept of sensorimotor dysfunction without tissue necrosis distal to an arterial anastomosis, a condition termed "ischemic monomelic neuropathy" by my good friend Dr. Asa Wilbourne in Cleveland. The authors describe 5 patients experiencing the onset of severe dysfunctional IMN shortly after placement of a dialysis graft. Electromyographic studies showed diabetic neuropathy. Digital pressure indices were reduced, but critical ischemia was not present. The authors conclude that IMN is a rare but disabling complication of access in selected patients with diabetes. I must confess that I was not aware of this complication before reading this paper, but I shall look for it in the future.

Hyperhidrosis

Endoscopic Transthoracic Sympathectomy in the Treatment of Primary Hyperhidrosis: A Review of 290 Sympathectomies
Shachor D, Jedeikin R, Olsfanger D, Bendahan J, Sivak G, Freund U (Univ of Tel Aviv, Israel)
Arch Surg 129:241–244, 1994   145-96-11–14

Background.—Primary palmar hyperhidrosis, a condition of unknown etiology, afflicts 0.6% to 1% of the population. It occurs primarily in adolescents. Medical treatment of this condition seems to succeed in only the mildest cases. The outcomes of endoscopic transthoracic sympathectomy (ETS) in 1 series of patients with palmar hyperhidrosis was reviewed.

Methods.—One hundred fifty consecutive patients underwent 290 ETSs. With the patients under general anesthesia, the surgeon used a trocar and endoscope inserted into the chest cavity to identify, cauterize, and cut the sympathetic chain and the second, third, and fourth ganglia. This procedure was repeated on the other side after reinflation of the lung.

Outcome.—The success rate was 98%. Complications included pneumothorax in 2.4%, hemothorax in 1%, and temporary Horner's syndrome in 0.7%. Treatment was needed for severe postoperative pain 2–4 hours after the procedure. Of 60 patients followed for 1 year, compensatory sweating developed in half, and rebound sweating developed in 8.3%. In 3 patients, hyperhidrosis recurred.

Conclusion.—Endoscopic transthoracic sympathectomy is an effective way to treat palmar primary hyperhidrosis. The procedure is associated with low morbidity and can be done on an ambulatory basis.

▶ Clearly, a large number of patients in Israel have hyperhidrosis.

Endoscopic Thoracic Sympathectomy for Primary Hyperhidrosis of the Upper Limbs
Herbst F, Plas EG, Függer R, Fritsch A (Univ of Vienna)
Ann Surg 220:86–90, 1994   145-96-11–15

Background.—Primary hyperhidrosis, which can affect various areas of the body, is a distressing and often socially disabling condition. A number of surgical and nonsurgical treatment approaches have been used. Endoscopic thoracic sympathectomy (ETS) is the treatment of choice for patients with palmar or axillary hyperhidrosis, but there are few data on the long-term results. The outcomes of a large series of patients with primary hyperhidrosis of the upper limbs treated by ETS were reported, with an emphasis on long-term patient satisfaction.

Methods.—From 1965 to 1992, 323 patients with palmar and axillary hyperhidrosis underwent ETS. Two hundred seventy patients responded to a questionnaire, for a response rate of 84%. The patients underwent a total of 480 sympathectomies, which were performed from below D1 to D4, using a single-site access technique. The mean follow-up was 16 years. The questionnaire addressed the early postoperative results; side effects; complications resulting from the operation; and long-term results, especially in terms of patient satisfaction.

Findings.—Postoperative mortality was nil, and there were no major complications requiring surgical intervention. The operation was considered successful in 98% of patients, and 96% were initially satisfied. Permanent side effects were common, including compensatory sweating in 67% of patients, gustatory sweating in 51%, and Horner's syndrome in 2.5%. Although the recurrence rate was only 1.5%, patient satisfaction decreased over time. As a result, only 67% of patients were satisfied, and 27% were partially satisfied. The most common reasons for dissatisfaction were compensatory and gustatory sweating. The satisfaction rate was significantly lower for patients undergoing ETS for axillary hyperhidrosis without palmar involvement (33% vs. 46%).

Conclusion.—For patients with hyperhidrosis of the upper limbs, ETS yields a high success rate, a high initial satisfaction rate, and reasonably long-term outcomes. However, compensatory hyperhidrosis and gustatory sweating may cause long-term dissatisfaction. These side effects should be discussed with the patients in detail before the operation.

▶ This and the prior paper (Abstract 145-96-11–14) report 570 thoracic sympathectomies for hyperhidrosis. Because we annually see approximately 1 patient with hyperhidrosis, I am amazed at the number of patients in these 2 series. I have several opinions on this subject: First, surgery for hyperhidrosis should never be attempted until exhaustion of nonoperative measures, including topical application of aluminum chloride preparations and consideration of axillary sweat gland excision. Second, the procedure of choice includes removal of the second, third, and fourth thoracic ganglia, without disturbance of the stellate ganglion at all. Third, the procedure is best performed currently with endoscopic technology. Fourth, a supraclavicular stellate ganglionectomy for this problem is not indicated. Finally, because we do not recommend upper extremity sympathectomy for causalgia or Raynaud's phenomenon, we will never achieve experience in endoscopic sympathectomy on our vascular unit. For that reason, when we encounter our 1 patient with hyperhidrosis, we refer the patient to an endoscopic center.

Miscellaneous

Complications and Failures of Subclavian-Vein Catheterization
Mansfield PF, Hohn DC, Fornage BD, Gregurich MA, Ota DM (MD Anderson Cancer Ctr, Houston)
N Engl J Med 331:1735–1738, 1994   145-96-11–16

Introduction.—Subclavian vein catheterization is a common procedure used to enable administration of chemotherapy, total parenteral nutrition, perioperative fluids, or long-term antibiotics. With the exception of the physician's experience, the risk factor for complications and failures of this procedure are poorly understood. The use of ultrasound guidance has been recommended for the placement of central venous catheters. The value of ultrasound guidance in locating the subclavian vein and in reducing the rate of complications and failures was examined.

Methods.—Catheters were inserted in the subclavian vein under controlled, nonemergency conditions, either using ultrasound guidance (411 patients) or using standard insertion techniques (410 patients). Demographic, clinical, and technical factors, as well as the physician's experience and medical history data, were evaluated to determine their association with the rate of complications and failures.

Results.—There were complications in 9.7% of the ultrasound group and 9.8% of the control group, and there were failed attempts in 12.4% of the ultrasound group and 12% of the control group. Univariate analysis identified previous major surgery or radiotherapy in the region, prior catheterization, prior catheterization attempts, the physician's lack of experience, a high body-mass index, and more than 2 needle passes as factors associated with failure. Prior surgery, a body-mass index above 30 or below 20, and prior catheterization were independently associated with failure in multivariate analysis. Univariate analysis of the factors associated with complications identified gender, body-mass index, and the number of needle passes. Only a body-mass index lower than 20 was significantly associated with complications in multivariate analysis. However, failed attempts at catheterization were the strongest predictor of complications.

Discussion.—Ultrasound guidance did not improve location of the subclavian vein or reduce the complication and failure rates of catheterization. Patients with a high (above 30) or low (below 20) body-mass index or a history of previous catheterization or prior surgery or radiotherapy on the catheterization side are at higher risk for failed attempts and complications. Therefore, only experienced physicians should place catheters in these patients.

▶ Despite the frequency of use, subclavian vein catheterization has numerous complications and, not infrequently, is met with failure. It has been suggested that ultrasound guidance may be helpful in the placement of these catheters. These authors conducted a large, prospective, randomized trial of ultrasound-guided subclavian catheterization vs. non–ultrasound-guided subclavian catheterization. They found that ultrasound guidance conveyed no demonstrable benefit. They gratuitously conclude that experienced physicians should perform these procedures.

Long-Term Outcome of Surgery for Thoracic Outlet Syndrome
Lindgren K-A, Oksala I (Kuopio Univ, Finland)
Am J Surg 169:358–360, 1995   145-96-11–17

Background.—Thoracic outlet syndrome remains a controversial concept; some even question its existence. Surgery is frequently viewed as the best primary approach, but reported rates of good results range widely from 24% to 100%.

Methods.—The results of surgery for symptoms of thoracic outlet syndrome were reviewed in 45 patients who were evaluated by an independent clinician 8 years on average after treatment. Forty-two patients had transaxillary resection of the first rib. Six patients had a cervical rib resected, 2 of them bilaterally.

Results.—Forty-three percent of operations were clinically successful. The presence of nocturnal pain and neck pain preoperatively correlated with an unsuccessful outcome, but no other preoperative features pre-

Preoperative Characteristics and Long-Term Outcome of Surgery

	Asymptomatic ($n = 23$)*	Symptomatic ($n = 30$)*	P Value†
Sex (F/M)	14/9	21/9	
Neck pain	15	25	< 0.05
Nocturnal pain	11	21	< 0.001
Headache	11	21	NS
Heavy work	10	21	NS
Sedentary work	9	5	NS
Previous physiotherapy	16	22	NS
Previous surgery	3	4	NS

* Number of ribs resected.
† Fisher's exact test and the chi-square test were used, as appropriate, and unavailable data were excluded.
Abbreviation: NS, nonsignificant difference.
(Courtesy of Lindgren K-A, Oksala I: Long-term outcome of surgery for thoracic outlet syndrome. *Am J Surg* 169:358–360, 1995. Reprinted with permission from *American Journal of Surgery.*)

dicted the outcome (table). The radiographic and neurophysiologic findings at baseline also failed to predict the outcome.

Conclusion.—These results suggest that the feasibility of conservative management be considered before deciding on surgery for symptoms of thoracic outlet syndrome.

▶ Based on considerable clinical experience, I have concluded that there is probably no such thing as neurogenic thoracic outlet syndrome in the absence of bony abnormalities and abnormal nerve conduction testing. I am further convinced that the pain for which certain centers are removing hundreds of first ribs, is likely a variant of fibromyalgia. The all-too-frequent absence of long-term pain relief in patients undergoing surgery compared with a control group having no surgery, has permanently marred the database of the proponents of this procedure.

This article is a typical paper on thoracic outlet syndrome. Forty-five patients were examined at a considerable time after thoracic outlet syndrome surgery, and a miserable 43% of the operations were deemed "successful." I wonder how many people in a randomized, nonoperative control group would also have been successful at 8 years. I suspect the number would likely have been 43%.

Although the problem of chronic neck, shoulder, and arm pain is worldwide and afflicts an estimated 5% of the individuals in the working population, America is the only country to date that has attempted to remedy this condition by surgery. As this surgery is of no proven benefit and is frequently associated with long-term litigation, I strongly suspect our future managed care environment will decree that very little of this surgery will be performed.

Arterial Injuries in the Thoracic Outlet Syndrome
Durham JR, Yao JST, Pearce WH, Nuber GM, McCarthy WJ III (Northwestern Univ, Chicago)
J Vasc Surg 21:57–70, 1995   145-96-11–18

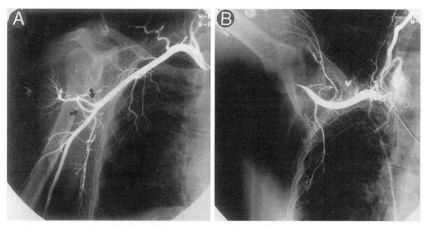

Fig 11–7.—A, right subclavian-axillary angiogram of a weight lifter in neutral position. Note the generous size of the circumflex humeral arteries (*arrows*) and the arterial loop they form around the surgical neck of the humerus. **B,** angiogram of the same patient during hyperabduction–external rotation maneuver. Note the beaklike occlusion of the axillary artery at the level of the humeral head. The circumflex humeral arteries are also occluded. (Courtesy of Durham JR, Yao JST, Pearce WH, et al: Arterial injuries in the thoracic outlet syndrome. *J Vasc Surg* 21:57–70, 1995.)

Objective.—Pathogenetic factors related to athletic activity and work were sought in 34 patients 13 to 67 years of age who had upper extremity symptoms or ischemic complications of thoracic outlet syndrome.

Methods.—Occupational and recreational activities were closely examined, and the patients underwent duplex ultrasound studies and contrast angiography with provocative maneuvers.

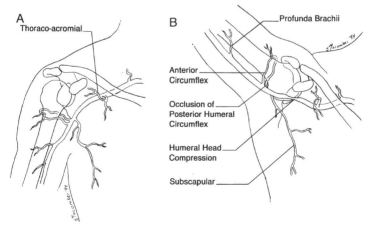

Fig 11–8.—A, diagrammatic representation of the axillary artery, its major branches, and the adjacent bony structures in neutral position. **B,** depiction of compression of the axillary artery and posterior circumflex humeral artery by the humeral head as the arm is abducted and externally rotated. Branch arteries tether the axillary artery in a fixed position, leading to compression by downward displacement of the humeral head. Note the arterial loop formed by anterior and posterior circumflex humeral arteries. (Courtesy of Durham JR, Yao JST, Pearce WH, et al: Arterial injuries in the thoracic outlet syndrome. *J Vasc Surg* 21:57–70, 1995).

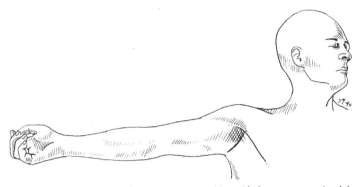

Fig 11–9.—Operative positioning of a patient: supine position with the upper extremity abducted and prepared into operative field. Note the site of a transverse incision just below the axillary hairline. (Courtesy of Durham JR, Yao JST, Pearce WH, et al: Arterial injuries in the thoracic outlet syndrome. *J Vasc Surg* 21:57–70, 1995.)

Results.—Twenty-two patients had subclavian artery injuries in 27 extremities. A cervical rib was responsible in 16 instances, an anomalous first rib in 2, and both a cervical rib and an anomalous first rib in 2. Distal embolization occurred in 14 extremities. In all cases, the subclavian artery was decompressed operatively, and 15 patients also required arterial reconstruction. The other 12 patients, 9 of whom were athletes, had axillary artery injuries resulting from compression by the humeral head during abduction (Figs 11-7 and 11-8). In all cases, the posterior circumflex humeral artery was also compressed. Two of these patients had an aneurysm and 1 had thrombosis. Three patients had operative decompression and 4 underwent direct arterial repair (Fig 11–9). All subclavian and axillary reconstructions were patent when last evaluated, an average of 31 months postoperatively.

Conclusion.—Most patients with thoracic outlet syndrome and subclavian artery compression have bony anomalies. When the axillary artery is involved, compression by the humeral head during hyperabduction is often responsible.

▶ The Northwestern University group has had an unusual experience in dealing with chronic work-related arterial injuries between the subclavian and the brachial artery. A large majority of these 34 patients had obvious bony abnormalities of the thoracic inlet region, including the cervical rib and anomalous first rib. The interesting part of this article is the 12 additional patients who had axillary artery involvement, presumably resulting from compression by the head of the humerus during abduction maneuvers, primarily involving baseball pitching. This unusual site of injury is one that I have never seen. On the other hand, we have very few major league baseball pitchers in Portland. For that matter, we appear to have very few decent professional basketball players.

12 Carotid and Cerebrovascular Disease

Natural History

Improved Survival of Stroke Patients During the 1980's: The Minnesota Stroke Survey

Shahar E, McGovern PG, Sprafka M, Pankow JS, Doliszny KM, Luepker RV, Blackburn H (Univ of Minnesota, Minneapolis)

Stroke 26:1–6, 1995   145-96-12–1

Background.—Stroke deaths decreased in the 1960s and more rapidly in the following decade, the time when the National High Blood Pressure Education Program began and population levels of cardiovascular risk

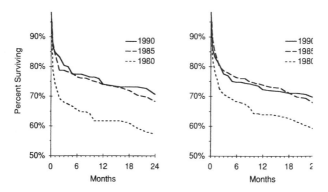

Fig 12–1.—Line graphs show age-adjusted 2-year survival of men hospitalized for acute stroke, by survey year. *Abbreviations: WHO,* World Health Organization; *MSS,* Minnesota Stroke Survey. (Courtesy of Shahar E, McGovern PG, Sprafka M, et al: Improved survival of stroke patients during the 1980's: The Minnesota Stroke Survey. *Stroke* 26:1–6, 1995. Reproduced with permission. *Stroke* Copyright 1995, American Heart Association.)

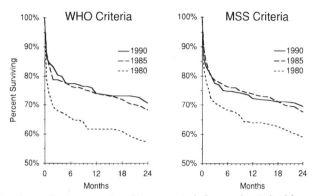

Fig 12–2.—Line graphs show age-adjusted 2-year survival of women hospitalized for acute stroke, by survey year. *Abbreviations: WHO*, World Health Organization; *MSS*, Minnesota Stroke Survey. (Courtesy of Shahar E, McGovern PG, Sprafka M, et al: Improved survival of stroke patients during the 1980's: The Minnesota Stroke Survey. *Stroke* 26:1–6, 1995. Reproduced with permission. *Stroke* Copyright 1995, American Heart Association.)

factors decreased. The reduction in stroke mortality appears to have slowed in the 1980s; stroke remains the third leading cause of death in the United States.

Objective and Methods.—Trends in stroke mortality in the Minneapolis–St. Paul region were examined for the years 1980, 1985, and 1990. Standard criteria for stroke were applied to a 50% random sample of men and women 30–74 years of age. Each period cohort of hospitalized patients with stroke was followed for 2 years or longer. Patients with acute stroke totalled 564, 598, and 691, respectively, in the 3 periods reviewed.

Results.—After controlling for age, the risk of dying within 2 years of stroke was about 40% lower in 1990 than in 1980. The relative risk of dying within 2 years in 1990, compared with 1980, was 0.65 for men and 0.60 for women (Figs 12–1 and 12–2). The overall trend was largely explained by the improved survival of patients with ischemic stroke and those with no apparent cardioembolic source. The proportion of patients who were comatose when admitted to the hospital did not change during the decade reviewed.

Conclusion.—A decreasing incidence of stroke likely contributes to the decline in stroke deaths noted in the 1970s and earlier, but there is no firm evidence for a reduced incidence of stroke in the 1980s. Improved supportive care and rehabilitation may be responsible, as well as a possible change in the natural course of the condition.

▶ Major epidemiologic trends, which have a profound influence on our practice patterns, are frequently not perceived by practitioners in the short term. For example, the incidence of pulmonary tuberculosis was declining markedly before the introduction of INH. Peptic ulcer disease, which was the most prominent surgical condition seen during my residency, precipitously declined before the advent of H-2 blockers. Postoperative gastrointestinal stress bleeding also precipitously declined before the advent of H-2 blockers. In recent years, we have seen a dramatic decline in mortality from coronary artery disease and also from stroke. It is not at all clear that anything we have done has resulted in this decline.

In this paper, the authors examine the cause of the dramatic reduction in stroke mortality that has occurred in America during the past 30 years. The authors conclude that no one really knows why the mortality from stroke has declined so dramatically. Although the declining incidence of stroke has contributed to the decrease in stroke mortality, a much more dramatic reason for such a decline is the remarkably improved survival after stroke that occurs for reasons that are completely unclear. On balance, this is another example of a major unexplained epidemiologic happening.

Trends in Stroke Incidence and Mortality in Hawaiian Japanese Men
Kagan A, Popper J, Reed DM, MacLean CJ, Grove JS (Kuakini Med Ctr, Honolulu, Hawaii; Buck Ctr for Research in Aging, Novato, Calif; Virginia Commonwealth Univ, Richmond; et al)
Stroke 25:1170–1175, 1994   145-96-12–2

Objective.—The mortality rate from stroke in the United States has decreased sharply since the late 1960s. There are no data to determine whether this change represents a decreased incidence of disease or a lower case-fatality rate. An even steeper decrease in stroke mortality has been noted in Japan, where the initial level was higher. Trends in the incidence and mortality of stroke among Hawaiian men of Japanese ancestry were reported.

Methods.—Since 1966, the Honolulu Heart Program has been monitoring the incidence and mortality of coronary heart disease in a target population of 11,136 men of Japanese ancestry living on the island of Oahu. The trends in the incidence and mortality of stroke from 1969 through 1988 were analyzed.

Results.—During this 20-year follow-up, 530 first episodes of stroke occurred in 7,893 men who were 45–68 years of age and free of stroke at their first examination. There were 389 thromboembolic strokes, 124 hemorrhagic strokes, and 17 strokes of unknown type. In the first 3 years of the study, the age-adjusted annual incidence of stroke was 5.1 per 1,000 person-years. By the last 3 years, this figure had decreased to 2.4 per 1,000 person-years (Fig 12–3). The yearly reduction in incidence was 3.5% for thromboembolic stroke, 4.2% for hemorrhagic stroke, and 4.4% for total stroke. The annual decrease in 30-day case-fatality rates was 3.7% for thromboembolic stroke, 8.7% for hemorrhagic stroke, and 7.3% for total stroke.

Conclusion.—The trend toward decreased stroke mortality appears to result from decreasing incidence rates and early case-fatality rates of thromboembolic stroke, hemorrhagic stroke, and stroke of unknown origin. These decreases may stem from changes in risk factors—including reductions in blood pressure and cigarette smoking—and from improved

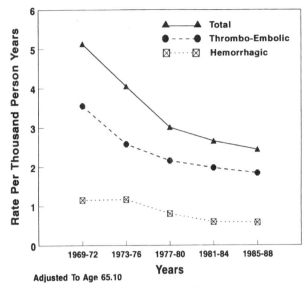

Fig 12–3.—Line graph shows average annual incidence of stroke during successive 4-year follow-up periods. (Courtesy of Kagan A, Popper J, Reed DM et al: Trends in stroke incidence and mortality in Hawaiian Japanese men: *Stroke* 25:1170–1175, 1994. Reproduced with permission. *Stroke* Copyright 1995, American Heart Association.)

diagnosis and treatment. There is no way to tell whether there will be further improvements in stroke mortality.

▶ For the past 30 years, the Honolulu Heart Program has monitored the incidence and mortality of both coronary disease and stroke in a large population of men of Japanese ancestry living on the island of Oahu in Hawaii. In this population, there has been a sharp decrease in stroke mortality during the past 30 years. A detailed analysis indicates that the decline in stroke mortality has resulted from both a reduction in incidence and early case-fatality rates. The authors speculate that the favorable changes may be related to better blood pressure control and a decrease in cigarette smoking, but no one really knows. This study is a nice complement to the Minnesota study reported in Abstract 145-96-12–1.

Effect of Aspirin on Risk of Stroke or Death in Women Who Have Suffered Cerebral Ischemia
Jonas S, Zeleniuch-Jacquotte A (New York Univ)
Cerebrovasc Dis 4:157–162, 1994   145-96-12–3

Background.—Despite several studies, the question of whether aspirin fails to reduce the risk of stroke or death in women who have had a transient ischemic attack or stroke remains unsettled. A meta-analysis of recent clinical trials of the effect of aspirin on the occurrence of stroke or death in patients with a history of cerebral ischemia was reported.

Findings.—The analysis included 8 such trials with a total of 5,287 subjects. Overall, aspirin had a beneficial effect (odds ratio 0.82; 95% confidence interval, 0.72–0.94). The odds ratio was similar on separate analysis of the 3,691 men and the 1,596 women, although the benefit of aspirin was significant only for men. The confidence intervals were 0.70–0.96 for men and 0.63–1.05 for the smaller group of women.

Conclusion.—The lack of a valid biological hypothesis for a different treatment effect of aspirin by sex suggests that aspirin probably reduces the risk of stroke or death in women who have had cerebral ischemia. The recommendation to use aspirin for this purpose in both sexes is supported.

▶ The famous meta-analysis rears its head again. The favorable effect of aspirin on the occurrence of stroke or death in a patient cohort with prior cerebral ischemia is again confirmed. Analysis of outcomes in women shows a similar odds ratio, but the improvement in women did not reach statistical significance ($P = 0.12$). Remarkably, these meta-analysts conclude that the use of aspirin in men and women after prior episodes of cerebral ischemia is justified. What a scoop!

A Multifactorial Analysis of Risk Factors for Recurrence of Ischemic Stroke

Lai SM, Alter M, Friday G, Sobel E (Univ of Kansas, Wichita; Med College of Pennsylvania, Philadelphia; Univ of Southern California, Los Angeles)
Stroke 25:958–962, 1994   145-96-12–4

Background.—More recurrent strokes may be expected as elderly individuals become an increasing part of the population. The risk factors associated with recurrent stroke generally have been analyzed as isolated variables.

Methods.—A multivariate analysis was undertaken in 621 patients who had acute ischemic stroke to determine the contribution of 5 factors (hypertension, myocardial infarction, cardiac arrhythmia, diabetes, and transient ischemic attacks) to the occurrence of a second stroke. The patients were evaluated 4 months after the initial stroke and then approximately every 6 months.

Results.—More than half the patients had multiple risk factors. The most prevalent risk factors were hypertension and cardiac arrhythmia. During an average follow-up of 2 years, only a history of hypertension and ECG findings of atrial fibrillation were significantly and independently associated with an increased risk of a second stroke (table).

Conclusion.—In patients who have had an acute ischemic stroke, controlling high blood pressure and atrial fibrillation offers the most obvious way of minimizing the risk of a second stroke.

▶ A multivariate analysis of 5 variables that may be important as risk factors for stroke recurrence indicates that control of hypertension and atrial fibrillation offers the greatest likelihood of stroke risk reduction. These investi-

Significant Risk Factors for Stroke Recurrence

Variable	Coefficient*	Hazard Ratio*	95% CI	P
History of hypertension	.672	1.96	1.18–3.24	.01
Atrial fibrillation (by ECG)	.579	1.78	1.04–3.06	.04

* Coefficient and hazard ratio were estimated by adjusting for covariates, age, sex, and other significant risk factor(s) using the Cox proportional hazards model. Other insignificant factors included myocardial infarction by ECG, diabetes mellitus, transient ischemic attack, and cardiac arrhythmias other than atrial fibrillation.
Abbreviation: CI, confidence interval.
(Courtesy of Lai SM, Alter M, Friday G, et al: A multifactorial analysis of risk factors for recurrence of ischemic stroke. *Stroke* 25:958–962, 1994. Reproduced with permission. *Stroke* Copyright 1995, American Heart Association.)

gators noted an overall stroke recurrence rate of 13% over an average 24-month follow-up, and a prior report from Rochester, Minnesota (1), found an even higher rate of stroke recurrence—10% in the first year.

Reference

1. Broderick JP, Phillips SJ, O'Fallon WM, et al: Relationship of cardiac disease to stroke occurrence, recurrence, and mortality. *Stroke* 23:1250–1256, 1992.

Vascular Outcome in Men With Asymptomatic Retinal Cholesterol Emboli: A Cohort Study

Bruno A, Jones WL, Austin JK, Carter S, Qualls C (Veterans Affairs Med Ctr, Albuquerque, NM; Univ of New Mexico, Albuquerque)
Ann Intern Med 122:249–253, 1995   145-96-12-5

Objective.—A cohort study was done at a Veteran's Affairs medical center to learn whether an asymptomatic cholesterol embolism in the retina is a risk factor for future vascular events.

Methods.—Seventy consecutive patients who were found by dilated ocular examination to have asymptomatic retinal cholesterol emboli were compared with an equal number of control subjects matched for age,

Vascular Outcome Events in 70 Patients with Asymptomatic Retinal Cholesterol Emboli and in 70 Controls

Outcome	Patients		Controls		ARR (95% CI)	P Value
	Number	Rate, %/y	Number	Rate, %/y		
Cerebral infarction	17	8.5	2	0.8	9.9 (2.3–43.1)	0.002
Nonfatal MI or vascular death	17	7.7	12	4.9	1.4 (0.7–2.9)	0.39
All MIs	6	2.7	7	2.9	0.8 (0.3–2.5)	0.73
Vascular death	13	5.7	10	4.1	1.2 (0.5–2.8)	0.65
All deaths	20	8.8	15	6.2	1.3 (0.6–2.5)	0.49

Note: The P values were calculated using Cox proportional hazards analysis controlling for stroke history and smoking history.
Abbreviations: ARR, adjusted relative risk; *MI*, myocardial infarction; *CI*, confidence interval.
(Courtesy of Bruno A, Jones WL, Austin JK, et al: Vascular outcome in men with asymptomatic retinal cholesterol emboli: A cohort study. *Ann Intern Med* 122:249–253, 1995.)

sex, serum cholesterol, smoking history, and the occurrence of diabetes, hypertension, and ischemic heart disease. The patients had a median age of 69 years, and controls had a median age of 68 years.

Results.—The annual rate of stroke during a mean follow-up of 3.4 years was 8.5% in the patients with a retinal embolism and 0.8% in controls, for an adjusted relative risk of 9.9 (table). No patient died of

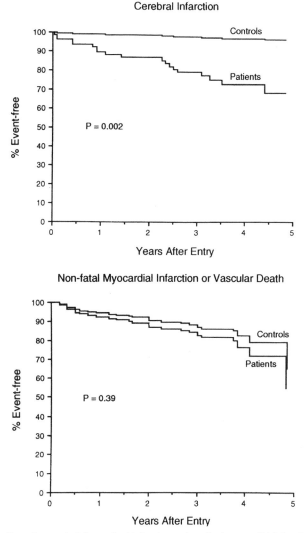

Fig 12–4.—Event-free survival for cerebral infarction and nonfatal myocardial infarction or vascular death in 70 men with asymptomatic retinal cholesterol emboli and 70 matched controls. Calculated using Cox proportional hazards analysis controlling for stroke history and smoking history. (Courtesy of Bruno A, Jones WL, Austin JK, et al: Vascular outcome in men with asymptomatic retinal cholesterol emboli: A cohort study. *Ann Intern Med* 122:249–253, 1995.)

stroke. Twelve of 17 strokes in study patients were in the carotid artery distribution on the side of the qualifying embolus. The patients had a relative risk of 1.4 for nonfatal myocardial infarction or vascular death (Fig 12–4).

Conclusion.—An asymptomatic retinal cholesterol embolism is a significant risk factor for stroke, apart from other commonly acknowledged vascular risk factors.

▶ For 30 years, we have all recognized cholesterol emboli in the retinal circulation as a serious finding, presumably associated with a significantly increased risk of stroke. In recent years, the late Dr. Gene Bernstein and others have told us that perhaps retinal emboli may not portend as much ill as previously suspected.

The authors of this interesting study followed 70 patients with retinal cholesterol emboli and 70 control patients for a mean of 3.4 years, and they found a remarkable annual stroke rate of 8.5% among patients and 0.8% among controls, for an adjusted relative risk of 9.9. Most of the strokes in the patient group occurred in the carotid territory ipsilateral to the qualifying retinal cholesterol embolus. Interestingly, ocular infarction did not occur in the patient group

These authors conclude—correctly, I am certain—that asymptomatic retinal cholesterol embolism is an important risk factor for cerebral infarction. I believe this is the only safe conclusion. Despite the observation reported by others that amaurosis may be a less important risk factor for stroke than cerebral transient ischemic attack, for all practical purposes, the only conclusion I can reach is to regard them as equally important. Certainly detailed cervical carotid duplex studies are indicated in these patients.

Compensatory Carotid Artery Dilatation in Early Atherosclerosis
Steinke W, Els T, Hennerici M (Univ of Heidelberg, Germany)
Circulation 89:2578–2581, 1994   145-96-12–6

Background.—Previous pathologic studies have shown that the development of progressive plaque in the coronary arteries may be accompanied by a compensatory increase in arterial diameter. There are few data on the dynamics of this process and on whether it is a general pathomechanism in the human arteries. Whether similar compensatory dilation occurs in atherosclerotic carotid arteries was studied.

Methods.—Thirty-two patients with nonstenotic carotid artery plaques were studied as part of a larger study of carotid atherosclerosis. At 6- to 12-month intervals, high-resolution duplex scanning and subsequent 3-dimensional plaque reconstructions were done to evaluate the effects of carotid plaque development on the vascular geometry of the involved arteries (Fig 12–5).

Results.—Forty-one percent of the follow-up studies showed plaque progression. Of these, three fourths were associated with a 0.4- to 1.2-mm

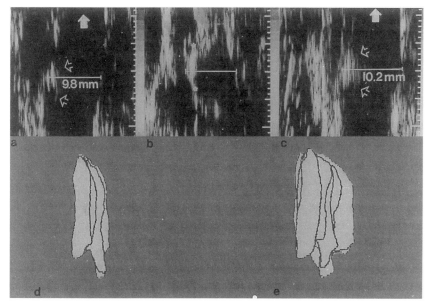

Fig 12–5.—Long-axis (a) and corresponding short-axis (b) high-resolution B-mode echotomograms showing a small nonstenotic plaque at the anterior wall (*open arrows* and *asterisks* indicate extent of plaque) if the carotid bifurcation (*filled arrow* indicates direction of flow). Follow-up study 6 months later (c) shows plaque progression and enlargement of the arterial diameter (10.2 mm compared with 9.8 mm). Three-dimensional plaque reconstructions (d and e) confirm the increased plaque volume. (Courtesy of Steinke W, Els T, Hennerici M, et al: Compensatory carotid artery dilatation in early atherosclerosis. *Circulation* 89:2578–2581, 1994. Reproduced with permission. *Stroke* Copyright 1994, American Heart Association.)

increase in the carotid artery diameter. In contrast, the arterial diameter increased in only 28% of studies that showed no plaque progression.

Conclusion.—As the volume of carotid artery plaque increases, the involved segments tend to enlarge in diameter. This dilation compensates for the arterial narrowing in early atherosclerosis.

▶ We now know that such dilation may be under the influence of very complicated shear stress receptors leading to the local elaboration of endothelial-derived nitric oxide. It has been presumed that this process was also applicable to other arteries, but detailed studies have been lacking. In this article, the highly experienced investigators from Heidelberg convincingly demonstrate that the progressive development of atherosclerosis in the carotid arteries is associated with similar arterial dilation, compensating, at least in part, for arterial narrowing in the early stages of the disease. Although this is what one would have predicted, I find this confirmation interesting, as well as important.

Carotid Surgery

Prevention of Functional Impairment by Endarterectomy for Symptomatic High-Grade Carotid Stenosis

Haynes RB, for the North American Symptomatic Carotid Endarterectomy Trial Collaborators (McMaster Univ, Hamilton, Ont, Canada)
JAMA 271:1256–1259, 1994   145-96-12–7

Background.—Although carotid endarterectomy has been shown to decrease the incidence of subsequent strokes among patients with transient ischemic attacks or partial strokes and ipsilateral high-grade internal carotid stenosis, its effects on functional status and the activities of daily living have not been determined. Whether endarterectomy prevents a deterioration in functional status among patients with transient ischemic attacks or nondisabling strokes and ipsilateral carotid stenosis of 70% to 99% was investigated.

Methods.—Six hundred fifty-nine patients with recent transient attacks or nondisabling stroke and ipsilateral atherosclerotic carotid stenosis of 70% to 99% were enrolled in a study involving 50 North American centers. By random assignment, 328 patients were treated with carotid endarterectomy and continuing medical care, and 331 were treated with medical care alone, including antiplatelet therapy.

Findings.—Patients assigned to carotid endarterectomy had an absolute risk reduction in functional status impairment of 5.6% for vision, 4.6% for language comprehension, and 8.3% for speech fluency. In addition, their risk reduction for swallowing was 4.3%; for lower extremity function, 6%; upper extremity function, 9.3%; for shopping, 7.4%; and for visiting outside their residence, 10.5%. Patients who were treated surgically had slower declines in functional status (Fig 12–6).

Conclusion.—Carotid endarterectomy reduces the risk of functional impairment among patients with recent symptomatic cerebral ischemia and ipsilateral high-grade carotid stenosis. As previously reported, this procedure also decreases the risk for ipsilateral stroke in such cases.

▶ Another thin slice rolls off the enormous North American Symptomatic Carotid Endarterectomy Trial (NASCET) salami roll. I swear, these investigators are going to publish 1,000 papers from this database. In this thin slice, the investigators attempt to determine whether carotid endarterectomy decreases functional impairment in patients with transient ischemic attacks or nondisabling strokes and very high-grade ipsilateral carotid stenosis. Using a debatable measuring system, they conclude that carotid endarterectomy reduced functional impairment as well as stroke among patients with ipsilateral high-grade carotid stenosis. These touchy-feely functional analyses do not impress me very much. Nonetheless, I am pleased that the NASCET Collaborators, in their infinite wisdom, have concluded that carotid surgery in selected patients is beneficial.

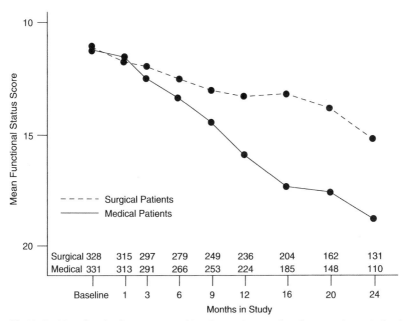

Fig 12–6.—Mean functional status scores of impairment. Larger values (lower on the vertical scale) imply worse functional status. The possible range is 10 (no impairment) to 70 (impaired in all domains), with death given a score of 71. The number of surgical patients and medical patients is listed by corresponding months in study. (Courtesy of Haynes RB, for the North American Symptomatic Carotid Endarterectomy Trial Collaborators: Prevention of functional impairment by endarterectomy for symptomatic high-grade carotid stenosis. *JAMA* 271:1256–1259, 1994. Copyright 1994, American Medical Association.)

Early Endarterectomy for Severe Carotid Artery Stenosis After a Nondisabling Stroke: Results From the North American Symptomatic Carotid Endarterectomy Trial
Gasecki AP, Ferguson GG, Eliasziw M, Clagett GP, Fox AJ, Hachinski V, Barnett HJM (Univ of Western Ontario, London, Canada; Univ of Texas, Dallas; Univ Hosp, London, Ont, Canada)
J Vasc Surg 20:288–295, 1994   145-96-12–8

Background.—The optimal time for performing carotid endarterectomy in patients with a recent stroke who are not disabled remains uncertain. Delaying the procedure may place these patients at risk of a recurrent major stroke.

Methods.—The results of early and delayed carotid endarterectomy were reviewed in 100 patients who had carotid stenosis of 70% or greater and had had a nondisabling hemispheric stroke or hemispheric/retinal infarction. Clinical evidence of ischemia had persisted for longer than 24 hours, but the patients were not significantly impaired in their daily activities. Forty-two endarterectomies were done within 30 days of the stroke, and 58 were delayed for 1 to 4 months.

Results.—The 2 groups were clinically comparable at baseline, but those having delayed surgery had more lesions on the symptomatic side on preoperative CT scanning. Strokes occurred within 30 days after carotid endarterectomy in 5% of patients in each group. There were no postoperative deaths. At 18 months, the combined rate of stroke and death was 12% in patients having early surgery and 10% in the delayed surgery group. In the early surgery group, abnormal baseline CT findings did not correlate with the later risk of stroke.

Conclusion.—There is no increase in operative risk for patients with symptomatic high-grade carotid stenosis who undergo carotid endarterectomy within 30 days of a nondisabling ischemic stroke.

▶ The great meat slicer of Drs. Barnett, Gasecki, et al. has produced yet another thin slice from the giant North American Symptomatic Carotid Endarterectomy Trial (NASCET) salami roll. The topic of the current NASCET study is the role of early endarterectomy for severe carotid artery stenosis after a nondisabling stroke. The authors conclude, remarkably, that carotid endarterectomy between 3 and 30 days after a nondisabling stroke works just as well as a delayed endarterectomy, done at 33–117 days. We are indebted to Dr. Barnett for another seminal observation.

Morbidity and Mortality Associated With Carotid Endarterectomy: Effect of Adjunctive Coronary Revascularization
Coyle KA, Gray BC, Smith RB III, Salam AA, Dodson TF, Chaikof EL, Lumsden AB (Emory Univ, Atlanta, Ga)
Ann Vasc Surg 9:21–27, 1995   145-96-12–9

Background.—When a patient who requires coronary revascularization is found to have significant carotid artery disease as well, it raises the question of whether simultaneous or staged operations should be done.

Objective.—Appropriate therapy was determined in a retrospective review. The operative results of 110 patients undergoing carotid endarterectomy and coronary artery bypass surgery at the same session, or during the same hospitalization, and 907 patients having only carotid endarterectomy in the same period (1983–1992) were compared.

Results.—The combined 30-day rate of postoperative stroke and mortality was 18.2% for patients having the operations concomitantly. The risk of postoperative stroke and mortality was 26.2% when the operations were done simultaneously and only 6.6% when coronary bypass surgery

Thirty-Day Morbidity and Mortality After Carotid Endarterectomy (CEA)
and Concomitant or Delayed Coronary Artery Bypass Graft (CABG)

	CEA + CABG Same (n = 65)	CEA + CABG Delayed (n = 45)
Stroke	15.4% (10)	4.4% (2)
Ipsilateral stroke	9.2% (6)	2.2% (1)
Death	10.8% (7)	2.2% (1)
Stroke + death	26.2% (17)	6.6% (3)

(Courtesy of Coyle KA, Gray BC, Smith RB III, et al: Morbidity and mortality associated with carotid endarterectomy: Effect of adjunctive coronary revascularization. *Ann Vasc Surg* 9:21–27, 1995.)

was delayed (table). Patients having only carotid endarterectomy had a combined 30-day risk of stroke or death of 2.1%.

Conclusion.—Performing both carotid endarterectomy and coronary bypass surgery at the same operative session substantially increases the risks of perioperative stroke and postoperative death. Apart from patients at very high risk, it is best to delay coronary bypass surgery for several days.

▶ I share the opinion of this group from Emory University that it is difficult to formulate optimal management plans for patients who require coronary revascularization and also have significant carotid artery disease. However, I am confused by their terminology. One tenth of their 1,017 patients with carotid artery disease underwent carotid endarterectomy during the same hospitalization or simultaneously with coronary artery bypass. I do believe it makes a difference, but nowhere in this article can I find information on how many patients actually underwent combined procedures. Nonetheless, the authors encountered a very worrisome stroke and death rate of 18.2% for the 110 patients undergoing concomitant procedures. They appropriately conclude that they much prefer to not combine the procedures. Who could argue with this conclusion? We combine carotid and coronary procedures in the same operation only 2 or 3 times per year, usually only for those patients having extremely frequent transient ischemic attacks with very high-grade stenosis associated with unstable angina pectoris.

Routine Completion Study During Carotid Endarterectomy Is Not Necessary

Jain KM, Simoni EJ, Munn JS (Michigan State Univ, Kalamazoo)
Am J Surg 168:163–167, 1994   145-96-12–10

Objective.—Many investigators have recently cited the need for a routine operative completion study during carotid endarterectomy, but there is no consensus on this issue. The incidence and clinical importance of residual stenoses are unclear. An 8-year experience with not performing routine completion studies during carotid endarterectomy was reviewed.

Methods.—The review included 417 patients who underwent 455 carotid endarterectomies. The patients' demographic characteristics, risk factors, ipsilateral neurologic events in the month after surgery, and mortality data were analyzed.

Results.—Fourteen patients had neurologic events and 4 died. Of the 14 patients with neurologic events, no technical defects were found in 13 patients. The remaining patient did not undergo exploratory surgery after an occlusion. At long-term follow-up, 10 of the 14 arteries were open. Of the remaining 4 patients, 2 were lost to follow-up, 1 died, and 1 did not have exploration of the artery.

Conclusion.—Routine completion studies need not be performed during carotid endarterectomy. With careful surgical technique, the postoperative neurologic complication rate is acceptable. Most postoperative neurologic deficits appear to result from processes that would not be detected by angiography or duplex scanning. The results suggest that technical advances may be more important in preventing residual stenoses than previously thought.

▶ These investigators report a 3.9% combined stroke/death rate in 455 carotid endarterectomies performed without routine completion arteriography. They find no persuasive indication for completion arteriography, a position with which I totally agree. I continue to be fascinated by the observation that the individuals who perform completion arteriography routinely identify around 10% of patients who are reopened to correct defects identified by arteriography. The rest of us, who never perform completion arteriography and never reopen, seem to achieve exactly the same clinical results as those who do. The only conclusion I can reach is that many of these reopenings and repairs must be unnecessary.

Continuous Transcranial Doppler Ultrasonography and Electroencephalography During Carotid Endarterectomy: A Multimodal Monitoring System to Detect Intraoperative Ischemia
Jansen C, Moll FL, Vermeulen FEE, van Haelst JMPl, Ackerstaff RGA (St Antonius Hosp, Nieuwegein, The Netherlands)
Ann Vasc Surg 7:95–101, 1993   145-96-12–11

Background.—Transcranial Doppler ultrasound monitoring (TCD) has been used during carotid endarterectomy to follow blood flow velocity in the ipsilateral middle cerebral artery, and electroencephalographic (EEG) monitoring has been used to display the electrical activity of the cortex. A TCD unit was added to EEG monitoring in an attempt to avoid the need for a shunt, which poses a risk of cerebral embolism and critical impairment of blood flow during cross-clamping.

Methods.—The outcome of carotid endarterectomy was examined in a prospective series of 130 operations done with both TCD and EEG monitoring.

Results.—The presence of an asymmetric EEG pattern was correlated with reduced flow velocity in the middle cerebral artery during cross-clamping of the carotid artery. Microemboli were detected during surgery in 80 patients. They correlated with signs and symptoms of ischemia, but not to a significant degree. There was only 1 intraoperative stroke (0.8%), which was not disabling.

Conclusion.—In addition to EEG monitoring, TCD measurements of flow velocity during carotid endarterectomy may limit the risk and the severity of stroke.

▶ Certain conclusions appear inescapable. When you clamp the carotid artery, the ipsilateral TCD will show a decrease in middle cerebral flow velocity. Microemboli may be frequently detected during, and especially immediately after, carotid endarterectomy if, indeed, the blips on the TCD tracing truly represent microemboli (about which I have some reservation). Increased numbers of microemboli tend to be associated with neurologic dysfunction, although the relationship is imprecise. These physicians predictably conclude that TCD monitoring provides important instant information to the surgeon. I am not persuaded that this is correct. Those who routinely use TCD and EEG monitoring seem to get the same results as the rest of us who do not.

Isolated Symptomatic Midcervical Stenosis of the Internal Carotid Artery

Ranval TJ, Solis MM, Barnes RW, Vitti MJ, Gagne PJ, Eidt JF, Barone GW, Harshfield DL, Schaefer RF, Read RC (John L McClellan Mem Veterans Hosp, Little Rock, Ark; Univ of Arkansas, Little Rock)
Am J Surg 168:171–174, 1994   145-96-12–12

Objective.—More than 1,500 carotid arteriograms performed in 819 patients in the years 1986–1991 were reviewed to determine the prevalence of isolated lesions in the midcervical part of the internal carotid artery.

Results.—Sixteen cases of midcervical internal carotid stenosis were found (Fig 12–7). Either atherosclerotic plaque or fibrous dysplasia was responsible for these stenoses. In 3 instances, stenosis was related to the hypoglossal nerve at exploration. In 2 other cases, the stenosis was found just distal to a short solitary cervical nerve contributing to the ansa cervicalis that crossed the carotid. One patient's transient ischemic attacks were relieved by dividing the stylohyoid ligament.

Conclusion.—Stenosis limited to the midcervical region of the internal carotid artery and unrelated to disease at the bifurcation may result from turbulent blood flow secondary to a tethering neural or myofascial band.

▶ Over 5 years, 16 patients with curious midcervical internal carotid stenoses were identified. In several cases, this was thought to be related to the normal hypoglossal nerve and, in at least 1 case, to the stylohyoid

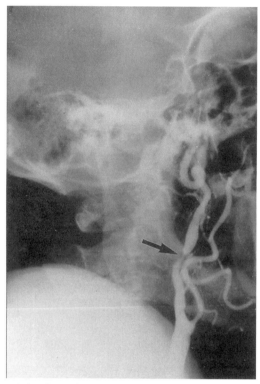

Fig 12–7.—The typical midcervical internal carotid artery lesion with post-stenotic dilation as demonstrated on a preoperative angiogram. Notice that there is little evidence of atherosclerosis at the usual sites, the bifurcation of the common carotid artery and the sipon. (Courtesy of Ranval TJ, Solis MM, Barnes RW, et al: Isolated symptomatic midcervical stenosis of the internal carotid artery. *Am J Surg* 168:171–174, 1994. Reprinted with permission from *American Journal of Surgery.*)

ligament. In other cases, an anomalous hypoglossal nerve appeared to be causing the stenosis. I must say I had not previously focused on this curious group of patients. I find this presentation interesting and shall look for these patients in the future.

Immediate and Long-Term Results of Carotid Endarterectomy for Asymptomatic High-Grade Stenosis
Riles TS, Fisher FS, Lamparello PJ, Giangola G, Gibstein L, Mintzer R, Su WT (New York Univ)
Ann Vasc Surg 8:144–149, 1994   145-96-12–13

Objective.—The long-term outcome of carotid endarterectomy was examined in a series of asymptomatic patients who underwent surgery for severe stenotic carotid bifurcation disease in the years 1983–1988. One hundred consecutive asymptomatic patients, from a total of 514 having endarterectomy, were entered into the study. Sixteen of the 100 study patients had staged bilateral endarterectomies.

Methods.—The degree of stenosis was determined by duplex scanning and confirmed angiographically. In all cases, the saphenous vein was used for patch closure of the arteriotomy. The average follow-up was 46 months. Approximately three fourths of the operations used cervical block anesthesia.

Results.—None of the 100 asymptomatic patients had a stroke or died during follow-up. The overall stroke-free rate at 5 years was 96%, and the ipsilateral stroke-free rate was 98%.

Conclusion.—Carotid endarterectomy on a prophylactic basis is warranted for asymptomatic patients with high-grade stenosis.

▶ This interesting patient subgroup was followed for a mean of 46 months. The stroke-free survival rate at 5 years was 96.3%, with an overall 5-year survival rate of 78.2%. These are superb results from a well-known carotid center.

Critical Carotid Artery Stenosis: Diagnosis, Timing of Surgery, and Outcome
Berman SS, Bernhard VM, Erly WK, McIntyre KE, Erdoes LS, Hunter GC
(Univ of Arizona, Tucson; Univ of Texas, Galveston)
J Vasc Surg 20:499–510, 1994   145-96-12–14

Background.—Critical carotid stenosis points to a high risk of carotid occlusion and is considered an indication for urgent or emergency endarterectomy. How the severity of stenosis, including atheromatous pseudo-occlusion (APO), influences the management and outcome of patients undergoing carotid endarterectomy was studied.

Methods.—The results of 203 consecutive carotid endarterectomies, performed in 197 patients, were reviewed. Ninety-one internal carotid arteries, including those exhibiting APO (Fig 12–8), were considered to be critically stenosed.

Results.—The 2 groups did not differ significantly with respect to demographic or risk factors, the symptomatic presentation, mean back pressure, or the use of a shunt or patch. The interval from angiography to surgery was 8–10 days for both groups. No vessel became occluded before endarterectomy was undertaken. Two patients with critical stenosis (2%) and 4 in the other group (3.6%) had a stroke perioperatively.

Conclusion.—The presence of critical carotid stenosis, including APO, does not mandate emergency intervention to prevent thrombosis. The lower limit of stenosis for which endarterectomy has clear advantages over nonoperative management must still be determined.

▶ The inescapable conclusion is that extremely high-grade carotid artery stenoses do not have to be operated upon immediately after arteriography. We routinely administer heparin to symptomatic patients with high-grade

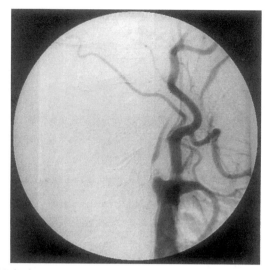

Fig 12–8.—Digital subtraction carotid arteriogram demonstrates atheromatous pseudocclusion with segmental occlusion of the internal carotid artery at bifurcation with reconstitution of hypoplastic-appearing internal carotid artery. At endarterectomy, there was high-grade stenosis with normal-caliber internal carotid artery distally. (Courtesy of Berman SS, Bernhard VM, Erly WK, et al: Critical carotid artery stenosis: Diagnosis, timing of surgery, and outcome. *J Vasc Surg* 20:499–510, 1994.)

stenosis, and we operate on them at the next elective operating schedule, usually the next day or within several days. I find no persuasive indication for taking the patient for emergency carotid endarterectomy, usually at night, with tired surgeons, unselected anesthesiologists, and suboptimal results. Our almost identical experience has been previously published (1).

Reference

1. 1995 YEAR BOOK OF VASCULAR SURGERY, p 337.

A Comparative Study of Saphenous Vein, Internal Jugular Vein, and Knitted Dacron Patches for Carotid Artery Endarterectomy

Goldman KA, Su WT, Riles TS, Adelman MA, Landis R (New York Univ)
Ann Vasc Surg 9:71–79, 1995
145-96-12–15

Introduction.—There is ongoing controversy as to which patch material should be used for patch closure after carotid endarterectomy. The possible influence of patch material on the immediate operative results of carotid endarterectomy, the early follow-up results, or the incidence of early restenosis was assessed in a retrospective study.

Patients.—The review included 275 consecutive primary carotid endarterectomies performed by 2 vascular surgeons over 2 years. Fifty-eight percent of the endarterectomies were closed with saphenous vein (SV), 9% with double-thickness internal jugular vein (JV), and 33% with knitted Dacron (KD). None of the arteries were closed primarily.

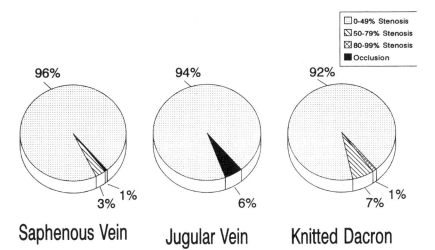

Fig 12–9.—Comparison of follow-up duplex results for carotid artery endarterectomy with different patch materials. No statistically significant differences exist among the 3 groups. (Courtesy of Goldman KA, Su WT, Riles TS, et al: A comparative study of saphenous vein, internal jugular vein, and knitted Dacron patches for carotid artery endarterectomy. *Ann Vasc Surg* 9:71–79, 1995.)

Findings.—The perioperative mortality rate was 1.1%, and the major and minor morbidity rate was 4.4%. Perioperative stroke occurred in 1.5% of patients, including 1.3% of the SV group, 4.0% of the JV group, and 1.1% of the KD group. Ninety-four percent of the patients were followed postoperatively for a mean of 14 months, and 80% were evaluated with duplex scanning. At follow-up, restenosis of greater than 50% was detected in 3.6% of the SV group, 0% of the JV group, and 8.4% of the KD group. Complete occlusion developed in 0.9% of the SV group, 5.6% of the JV group, and 0% of the KD group (Fig 12–9). There were no significant differences between groups in terms of perioperative morbidity or mortality or early postoperative restenosis.

Conclusion.—Various materials used for patch closure after carotid endarterectomy yield similar perioperative and early postoperative results. Possible differences between synthetic and autologous patching in terms of late restenosis or aneurysmal dilation must be assessed in studies with longer follow-up.

▶ This old saw continues to resurface with predictable regularity. In this large study, closure of the carotid endarterectomy site with SV, JV, or KD produced similar results through a mean follow-up of 14 months. In our practice, we are now closing most carotids with patches, and our preference is KD, most recently the impervious variant. It seems to be working well.

Carotid Endarterectomy With Primary Closure Does Not Adversely Affect the Rate of Recurrent Stenosis

Gelabert HA, El-Massry S, Moore WS (Univ of California, Los Angeles)
Arch Surg 129:648–654, 1994   145-96-12–16

Background.—Carotid endarterectomy demonstrably reduces the risk of subsequent stroke, but its efficacy depends on maintaining long-term patency. Recurrent carotid stenosis is, in most cases, ascribed to intimal hyperplasia that develops at the endarterectomy site.

Methods.—The results of carotid endarterectomy using primary closure were reviewed in 232 patients having 268 procedures in a 3-year period. The indications for endarterectomy were transient ischemic attacks in 119 instances and stroke in 41; 108 patients had asymptomatic carotid stenosis. Of the 232 patients who had surgery, 157 were followed for 2 years on average after 184 endarterectomies. Serial duplex scans were obtained to identify recurrent stenosis, defined as a reduction of more than 50% in luminal diameter.

Results.—Recurrent carotid stenosis was detected after 6.5% of endarterectomies. Eight of the 12 patients affected (4.3% of operations) had a normal completion angiogram or duplex scan within 3 months of surgery, thereby qualifying as having true recurrent stenosis. Recurrences were more frequent in women, hypertensive patients, and those who smoked, but none of these associations was significant.

Conclusion.—The low risk of recurrent stenosis after carotid endarterectomy with primary closure warrants continued use of this technique. Possibly, patch angioplasty is indicated in women and patients who smoke.

▶ I find it rather amazing that only 5% of this large group of patients had greater than 50% recurrent stenosis during a follow-up of 24 months. In fact, I believe this is the lowest incidence of recurrent stenosis I have ever encountered; it is especially noteworthy in the absence of any patching. On balance, these are amazing results.

Carotid Exploration for Acute Postoperative Thrombosis

Peer RM, Shah RM, Upson JF, Ricotta JJ (State Univ of New York, Buffalo)
Am J Surg 168:168–170, 1994   145-96-12–17

Background.—Carotid endarterectomy is one of the most frequent and best tolerated procedures performed in vascular surgery. However, its benefits are often negated by a high rate of complications, including postoperative hemorrhage and perioperative stroke. The incidence of reoperative surgery for perioperative stroke and hemorrhage was investigated to determine the pathogenesis and to define an algorithm for managing these problems.

Method.—The records of patients requiring reoperation after less than 24 hours during a 10-year period were assessed for operative findings, clinical outcome, and arterial patency.

Results.—Carotid endarterectomy was done on 920 patients during the study. Of them, there were 27 strokes and 10 deaths. Early reexploration was required for 27 patients (3%), 6 with expanding hematoma and 21 with suspected thrombosis associated with a new neurologic deficit. Two patients bled from the arteriotomy site and 4 from surrounding tissues. Reexploration for new postoperative neurologic events in the 21 patients revealed 19 (91%) with thrombosis of the internal carotid segment. Two patients who showed patent arteries and normal operative arteriograms were considered to have distal embolization, and the arteriotomy was not reopened. The causes of thrombosis were intimal flap in 6 patients, closure stenosis in 11, and no apparent reason in 2. Follow-up studies available for 16 patients showed patent arteries at 12 months. Among the patients explored for hemorrhage, 1 died of myocardial infarction, but no neurologic events or late infections were seen. Of the 21 patients who underwent a second procedure for neurologic deficits, 2 died, 8 were unchanged, 2 had minor residual deficit, and 9 had completely resolved deficits. Severe contralateral disease was more frequent in patients with residual deficits than in patients with no residual deficits.

Conclusion.—Carotid reexploration surgery for hemorrhage or for new-onset perioperative stroke carries a high risk of morbidity and mortality. However, the procedure can save lives and provides significant neurologic improvement or complete deficit resolution for a large number of patients who would otherwise be severely disabled.

▶ Nineteen of 21 patients reexplored after carotid endarterectomy because of neurologic deficit and presumed thrombosis were actually found to have an operative-site thrombosis. All arteries were reopened and repaired over a shunt with a patch. Two of these 21 patients died, 8 were unchanged, 2 had minor residual deficit, and 9 had completely resolved deficits. Although this experience, like so many before it, proves nothing, it does suggest that immediate reexploration is indicated for a new-onset neurologic deficit within hours after carotid endarterectomy. Despite a condition of genuine equipoise, I suspect this is a condition for which a prospective, randomized study will never be conducted.

Comparison of Measurement of Stump Pressure and Transcranial Measurement of Flow Velocity in the Middle Cerebral Artery in Carotid Surgery
Kalra M, Al-Khaffaf H, Farrell A, Wallbank WA, Charlesworth D (Univ Hosp of South Manchester, Manchester, England)
Ann Vasc Surg 8:225–231, 1994   145-96-12–18

Background.—It remains uncertain how best to assess the collateral circulation to the brain so as to determine the need for shunt placement

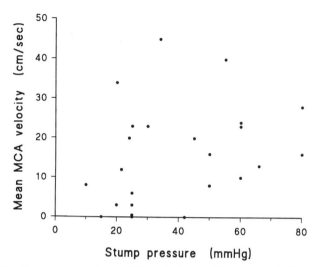

Fig 12–10.—The mean velocity in the middle cerebral artery (*MCA*) compared with stump pressure when both were measured simultaneously. There is no correlation between the 2 values. (Courtesy of Kalra M, Al-Khaffaf H, Farrell A, et al: Comparison of measurement of stump pressure and transcranial measurement of flow velocity in the middle cerebral artery in carotid surgery. *Ann Vasc Surg* 8:225–231, 1994.)

during carotid endarterectomy. Neither intraoperative electroencephalographic monitoring nor estimates of stump pressure in the internal carotid artery have proved totally reliable.

Methods.—The velocity of blood flow in the middle cerebral artery (MCA) was measured by transcranial Doppler ultrasound monitoring (TCD) in 24 consecutive patients having carotid endarterectomy. Baseline estimates were obtained preoperatively at rest, and the study was repeated after clamping of the carotid artery and continuously during the operation. Stump pressures were measured in the internal carotid artery, and back flow was assessed subjectively.

Results.—No correlation was observed between blood flow velocity in the MCA and carotid stump pressure after carotid clamping (Fig 12–10). Both peak and mean MCA flow velocities were significantly lower in patients whose stump pressures were less than 30 mm Hg and in those with poor back flow.

Conclusion.—Flow velocity in the MCA during carotid endarterectomy, as estimated by TCD, correlates with subjective assessments of carotid artery back flow but not with stump pressure in the internal carotid artery.

▶ I am surprised that no relationship was found between MCA velocity and stump pressure. Although low stump pressure predictably correlated with low MCA TCD flow velocity, there was no correlation across the board. I shall contemplate this interesting finding.

Cerebral Oxygen Saturation, Transcranial Doppler Ultrasonography and Stump Pressure in Carotid Surgery

Williams IM, Vohra R, Farrell A, Picton AJ, Mortimer AJ, McCollum CN (Univ Hosp of South Manchester, Manchester, England)
Br J Surg 81:960–964, 1994   145-96-12–19

Background.—Carotid endarterectomy is of definite benefit in preventing strokes, but no totally reliable means has been found of predicting which patients are at risk of perioperative stroke.

Methods.—Three methods were used to monitor cerebral perfusion in 33 patients undergoing elective carotid endarterectomy: transcranial Doppler ultrasonography (TCD) of the middle cerebral artery (MCA); light-reflective cerebral oximetry (Fig 12–11); and pressure monitoring in the internal carotid artery stump.

Results.—The median cerebral oxygen saturation was 70% before the carotid artery was cross-clamped, and it decreased to 63%. The TCD-estimated mean blood velocity decreased from 42 to 16 cm/sec when the clamps were applied. Carotid stump pressure was closely correlated with blood velocity in the MCA after 30 seconds of cross-clamping but not with the cerebral oxygen saturation. A decrease of 60% or greater in mean MCA velocity predicted a decrease of at least 5% in cerebral oxygen saturation. Changes in oxygen saturation also correlated with systolic

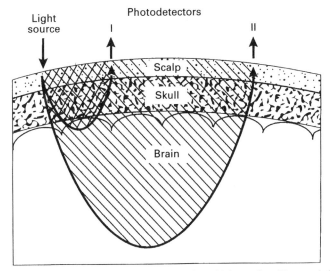

Fig 12–11.—Principle of the cerebral oximeter. Near-infra-red light is reflected in a parabolic fashion. The photodetectors are placed to measure oxyhaemoglobin in either the scalp-skull (I) or the scalp skull and brain (II). The oximeter calculates the oxygen saturation of the blood in the brain by subtracting that in the scalp and skull. (Courtesy of Williams IM, Vohra R, Farrell A, et al: Cerebral oxygen saturation, transcranial Doppler ultrasonography and stump pressure in carotid surgery. *Br J Surg* 81:960–964, 1994. Reprinted with permission of Blackwell Science Ltd.)

blood pressure throughout the perioperative period. Low pressure in the carotid stump did not predict significantly impaired cerebral oxygenation. *Conclusion.*—Cerebral oximetry has the potential to prevent many unneeded shunt placements in patients having carotid endarterectomy.

▶ These authors introduce the interesting procedure of light-reflective cerebral oximetry. The interesting findings in this study include the observation that stump pressure *did* correlate with MCA blood velocity, contrary to the results presented in the previous paper (Abstract 145-96-12–18). Unfortunately, the cerebral oxygen saturation did not correlate with much of anything except systolic blood pressure, although there was some correlation with a decrease in MCA TCD velocity. Decreased cerebral oxygenation was not predicted by low stump pressure. Because we choose to use a carotid artery shunt in all carotid endarterectomies, this sort of information is not likely to have much effect on our practice.

Carotid Endarterectomy in the Octogenarian
Coyle KA, Smith RB III, Salam AA, Dodson TF, Chaikof EL, Lumsden AB
(Emory Univ, Atlanta, Ga)
Ann Vasc Surg 8:417–420, 1994   145-96-12–20

Background.—The number of octogenarians is steadily increasing, and stroke is a prominent cause of death in both men and women of this age. Preventive endarterectomy should have a positive impact on the quality of older persons' lives.

Patients.—Seventy-nine patients who were 80 years of age and older underwent carotid endarterectomy during a recent 10-year period. They represented 7.4% of all patients having endarterectomy during this time. Among the 56% of patients who were symptomatic, transient ischemic attacks were the most common indication for endarterectomy (table). Ipsilateral stenoses averaged 76.8%. More than half the patients were hypertensive, more than 40% had coronary artery disease, and 10% had diabetes.

Results.—Three fourths of the procedures were done using local anesthesia. An intraluminal shunt was used in all but 2 cases. There was a

	Indications for Carotid Endarterectomy	
Indications	Octogenarians (%) ($n = 79$)	Nonoctogenarians (%) ($n = 992$)
Asymptomatic	44.3 (35)	45.8 (454)
Transient ischemic attacks	30.3 (24)	27.8 (276)
Stroke	15.2 (12)	15.2 (151)
Amaurosis fugax	8.9 (7)	10.8 (107)
Vascular tinnitus	1.3 (1)	0.4 (4)

(Courtesy of Coyle KA, Smith RB III, Salam AA, et al: Carotid endarterectomy in the octogenarian. *Ann Vasc Surg* 8:417–420, 1994.)

single postoperative death, from myocardial infarction, and 1 patient had a transient ischemic attack. There were no ipsilateral strokes during an average postoperative follow-up of nearly 3 years.

Conclusion.—Octogenarians may undergo carotid endarterectomy with no greater risk of mortality or morbidity than exists for younger patients.

▶ I agree that you can safely perform carotid endarterectomy safely in older individuals, but I wonder whether we should do it very often. When you consider that the average life span of a patient 80 years or older is 3 or 4 years and that the annual risk of stroke—even in highly stenotic arteries—is in the range of 5% to 6%, it is difficult to imagine that you are going to derive much benefit from this surgery when you factor in the inevitable surgical complication rate. The very admirable stroke death rate of 1.3% reported by these authors is not going to be routinely obtained in ths population. Surprisingly, I note that 44% of these carotid endarterectomies in patients older than age 80 years were performed for prophylaxis. This does, indeed, seem to be pushing the envelope a bit.

Risk of Stroke in the Distribution of an Asymptomatic Carotid Artery
Rothwell PM, for the European Carotid Surgery Trialists Collaborative Group (Western Gen Hosp, Edinburgh, Scotland)
Lancet 345:209–212, 1995   145-96-12–21

Background.—Carotid endarterectomy has been recommended for patients with asymptomatic carotid stenosis, but the risk of stroke in the absence of treatment remains uncertain. A substantial risk is needed to justify performing an operation because of the 1% mortality risk in symptomatic patients who undergo surgery and because of a 5% to 10% risk of stroke.

Objective.—The risk of stroke in the distribution of the asymptomatic carotid artery was examined in 2,295 patients randomized in the European Carotid Surgery Trial who had had a transient ischemic attack, minor or nondisabling major ischemic stroke, or retinal infarction in the carotid distribution within the previous 6 months. The average follow-up was 4.5 years.

Results.—Of 69 carotid territory strokes occurring during follow-up (table), 9 were fatal. The 3-year risk value for stroke was 2.1%, and the value for fatal stroke was 0.3%. The 127 patients who had 70% or greater carotid stenosis had a 5.7% chance of having a stroke (Fig 12–12).

Conclusion.—The potential benefit from endarterectomy in patients with asymptomatic carotid stenosis would appear to be limited, and population screening is not warranted. Only in the context of a randomized controlled trial is such surgery justified.

▶ Interestingly, these investigators looked at the behavior of the asymptomatic opposite carotid in the 2,300 patients randomized in the European Carotid Surgery Trial. During a mean follow-up of 4.5 years, there were 69

Details of All Strokes Lasting More Than 7 Days in Distribution of Asymptomatic Carotid Artery

	Degree of symptomless stenosis(%)				Total
	0–29	30–69	70–99	Occlusion	
Patients	1,270	843	127	55	2,295
Strokes	28	26	13	2	69
Kaplan-Meier 3-year risk	1.8%	2.1%	5.7%	3.7%	2.1%
(95% CI)	(1.1–2.6)	(1.1–3.2)	(1.5–9.8)	(0–8.9)	(1.5–2.8)
CT scan appearance					
Infarction	17	15	8	0	40
Haemorrhage	2	1	0	0	3
No CT scan available	9	10	5	2	26
Strokes after endarterectomy					
Symptomatic side surgery	3	0	2	0	5
Asymptomatic side surgery	1	2	4	0	7
Status after 6 months post-stroke					
Rankin 0–2	16	15	4	1	36
Rankin >2	5	4	4	1	14
Not known	5	3	2	0	10
Dead	2	4	3	0	9

(Courtesy of Rothwell PM, for the European Carotid Surgery Trialists Collaborative Group: Risk of stroke in the distribution of an asymptomatic carotid artery. *Lancet* 345:209–212, 1995. Copyright 1995, The Lancet Ltd.)

carotid territory strokes on the opposite side, giving a 3-year Kaplan-Meier stroke risk of 2.1%. The risk of stroke in the patients with a severe stenosis (> 70%) was 5.7%. These investigators conclude that there is very limited indication for surgery for asymptomatic carotid stenosis. They go on to the monumental conclusion that population screening is not justified. Clearly, this paper was written before the ACAS study results were published, and these results must be reinterpreted in light of those results.

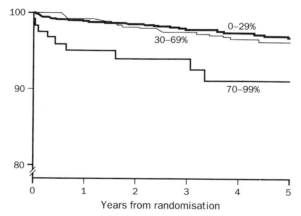

Fig 12–12.—Actuarial analysis of survival free from stroke lasting longer than 7 days in the distribution of an asymptomatic artery. (Courtesy of Rothwell PM, for the European Carotid Surgery Trialists Collaborative Group: Risk of stroke in the distribution of an asymptomatic carotid artery. *Lancet* 345:209–212, 1995. Copyright 1995, The Lancet Ltd.)

Do Neck Incisions Influence Nerve Deficits After Carotid Endarterectomy?

Skillman JJ, Kent KC, Anninos E (Beth Israel Hosp, Boston)
Arch Surg 129:748–752, 1994   145-96-12–22

Background.—The nerves at risk of being injured during surgery on the area of the carotid bifurcation are shown in Figure 12–13. The risks associated with transverse and vertical neck incisions for carotid endarterectomy were compared in a prospective, unrandomized study of 80 consecutive patients who had 85 operations. Forty-four endarterectomies were done via a vertical incision, and 41 were done through a transverse incision.

Results.—Seventh cranial nerve palsy developed in 32% of patients with a transverse incision and 25% of those with a vertical incision. The respective rates of twelfth cranial nerve palsy were 15% and 20%. More than 70% of deficits resolved within 3–6 months after operation. For cosmetic reasons, the patients clearly preferred a transverse incision.

Conclusion.—Neither incision is clearly advantageous with respect to safety. Patients favor a transverse incision, and adequate exposure is consistently achieved with this approach.

▶ Almost without exception, everyone who looks for cranial nerve deficits after carotid endarterectomy finds a disturbing number. I am amazed at the

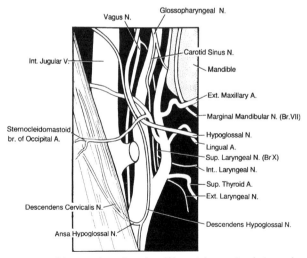

Fig 12–13.—Anatomy of the seventh, tenth, and twelfth cranial nerves in relation to the area of carotid bifurcation. (Courtesy of Skillman JJ, Kent KC, Anninos E: Do neck incisions influence nerve deficits after carotid endarterectomy? *Arch Surg* 129:748–752, 1994. Copyright 1994/95, American Medical Association.)

32% incidence of seventh nerve palsy and the 15% incidence of twelfth nerve palsy for tranverse incisions. I do not have this much, but, on the other hand, I do not look for it very carefully, pursuing the well-described ostrich philosophy that there are some things you would prefer not to know. At any rate, these authors conclude that transverse and oblique incisions produce the same incidence of cranial nerve complications. I am sure they are right.

Fate of the Non-Operated Carotid Artery After Contralateral Endarterectomy
Naylor AR, John T, Howlett J, Gillespie I, Allan P, Ruckley CV (Royal Infirmary, Edinburgh, Scotland)
Br J Surg 82:44–48, 1995   145-96-12–23

Introduction.—The value of long-term follow-up with serial postoperative imaging of the nonoperated internal carotid artery after contralateral endarterectomy has not been established. A group of 219 patients who underwent carotid endarterectomy was followed to evaluate clinical outcome and to determine whether noninvasive surveillance can identify those at risk for stroke.

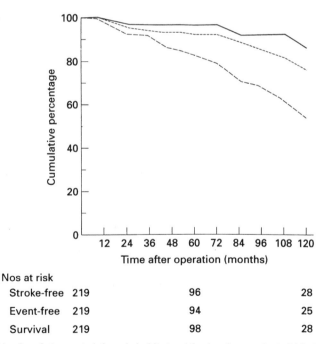

Nos at risk			
Stroke-free	219	96	28
Event-free	219	94	25
Survival	219	98	28

Fig 12–14.—Cumulative survival (*long dashed line*) and freedom from stroke (*solid line*) and/or any cerebral ischemic event (*short dashed line*) in the nonoperated hemisphere. (Courtesy of Naylor AR, John T, Howlett J, et al: Fate of the non-operated carotid artery after contralateral endarterectomy. *Br J Surg* 82:44–48, 1995. Reprinted with permission of Blackwell Science, Ltd.)

Patients and Methods.—The carotid endarterectomies were performed between 1975 and 1990. Demographic data, clinical features at diagnosis, concurrent diseases, and risk factors were recorded, and the results of preoperative angiography were examined. Patients were assessed at 4 weeks, 6 months, and then annually for 10 years. Imaging was part of the follow-up after 1983, and 151 patients were studied with either IV digital subtraction angiography or duplex ultrasound and Doppler waveform analysis.

Results.—There were 44 deaths during follow-up, including 22 resulting from mycocardial infarction. The cumulative survival rate was 97% at 1 year, 82% at 5 years, and 53% at 10 years. Only 10 patients had a stroke in the nonoperated hemisphere during follow-up, giving a mean incidence of stroke of 1% per year. Cumulative freedom from stroke in the nonoperated hemisphere was 99% at 1 year, 96% at 5 years, and 86% at 10 years (Fig 12–14.) Only 1 of the 10 strokes was preceded by a transient ischemic attack and none were associated with severe (70% or greater) stenosis of the internal carotid artery (Fig 12–15). Ten patients with an initial internal carotid artery stenosis of less than 70% were found to have significant disease progression during the surveillance period. Only 3 be-

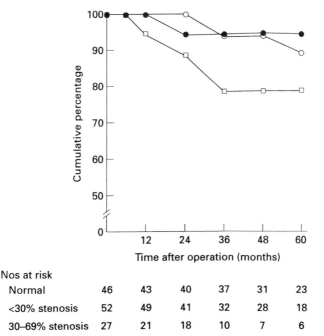

Nos at risk

Normal	46	43	40	37	31	23
<30% stenosis	52	49	41	32	28	18
30–69% stenosis	27	21	18	10	7	6

Fig 12–15.—Cumulative freedom fron any cerebral ischemic event (stroke, transient ischemic attack, amaurosis fugax) in the nonoperated hemisphere, with reference to the extent of internal carotid artery disease at the outset: *open circle*, normal; *filled circle*, less than 30% stenosis; *square*, 30% to 69% stenosis. (Courtesy of Naylor AR, John T, Howlett J, et al: Fate of the non-operated carotid artery after contralateral endarterectomy. *Br J Surg* 82:44–48, 1995. Reprinted with permission of Blackwell Science, Ltd.)

came symptomatic, however, and in each case, the onset of symptoms preceded recognition of significant disease progression.

Conclusion.—The long-term risk of stroke in the nonoperated internal carotid artery territory was found to be very small in this series of patients. Not one of the high-risk patients was identified in 530 studies, and none of the observed strokes could have been prevented by the form of surveillance used. Thus, the follow-up program is not recommended for cost effectiveness or benefit to the patient.

▶ These results should be compared with the information presented in Abstract 145-96-12–21. The cumulative freedom from stroke in the nonoperated hemisphere was 96% at 5 years, giving a mean incidence of stroke of 1% per year. These authors conclude, as have many before them, that the long-term risk of stroke in the nonoperated internal carotid artery territory is small. They find no convincing benefit for postoperative surveillance of the opposite side. We shall have to await a subgroup analysis of outcomes in the opposite side in the ACAS group, if, indeed, ACAS plans to engage in the traditional salami slicing demonstrated so brilliantly by the North American Symptomatic Carotid Endarterectomy Trial Collaborators (1).

Reference

1. North American Symptomatic Carotid Endarterectomy Trial Collaborators: Beneficial effect of carotid endarterectomy in symptomatic patients with high-grade carotid stenosis. *N Engl J Med* 325:445–453, 1991.

Carotid Artery Resection for Cancer of the Head and Neck
Meleca RJ, Marks SC (Wayne State Univ, Detroit)
Arch Otolaryngol Head Neck Surg 120:974–978, 1994   145-96-12–24

Background.—Advanced squamous cell cancer of the head and neck may involve the carotid artery. Carotid artery resection, one treatment option, is, in turn, associated with a high neurologic morbidity and mortality. Debate continues regarding the decision to ligate or replace the resected artery. The morbidity and mortality associated with ligation compared with reconstruction of the carotid artery after resection were examined.

Methods.—A retrospective record review of 1,784 patients who underwent surgery for head and neck cancer at the reporting institutions from January 1985 through June 1992 was conducted. Chi-square analysis was performed comparing the morbidity of those who underwent carotid resection and ligation with those who had replacement of the resected artery.

Results.—A total of 20 patients underwent carotid artery resection, with 12 undergoing ligation and 8 interposition grafting. Neurologic complications occurred in 7 of the 12 patients with carotid artery ligation (58%), whereas only 1 of the 8 patients with grafts (13%) had such complications (table). After surgery, 3 of 19 patients survived disease-free for 1 year, and 1 survived disease-free for 8 months. Median disease-free survival postoperatively was 6.3 months. Fourteen of 19 patients overall and 7 of 11

Morbidity and Mortality for Carotid Artery Resection		
	No. (%) of Patients	
	Ligation	Replacement
Morbidity	7/12 (58)	1/8 (13)*
Cerebrovascular accident	5/12 (42)	1/8 (13)*
Transient ischemic attack	2/12 (17)	0/8
Mortality	1/12 (8)	0/8

* *P* < 0.005.
(Courtesy of Meleca RJ, Marks SC: Carotid artery resection for cancer of the head and neck. *Arch Otolayrngol Head Neck Surg* 120:974–978, 1994. Copyright 1994, American Medical Association.)

who survived at least 5 months after surgery had locoregional control at the time of their death or at their most recent follow-up.

Conclusion.—Nonsurgical therapy is preferred for treating patients with advanced squamous cell carcinoma of the head and neck involving the carotid artery because of the poor prognosis and high morbidity associated with surgery. In individuals who have received radiation therapy and who have limited disease adherent to the carotid artery, resection can provide locoregional control and a chance for prolonged disease-free survival. Interposition grafting should be used to minimize the risk of neurologic morbidity when carotid artery resection is performed.

▶ This study purports to compare carotid ligation with carotid interposition grafting in patients requiring carotid excision in association with surgery for head and neck cancer. The decision to ligate or replace the carotid was based on intraoperative internal carotid artery stump pressure of 50 mm or greater or an angiogram demonstrating cerebral cross-filling. Unfortunately, these are primitive measures of the need for carotid replacement. Numerous investigators have described the use of balloon test occlusion preoperatively or, preferably, single-photon emission CT perfusion studies (1). Remarkably, 58% of 12 patients undergoing ligation experienced neurologic sequelae compared with 1 patient (13%) undergoing interposition grafting. I suggest that the authors use more appropriate methods to determine the need for carotid reconstruction in the future. The wisest procedure is simply to perform carotid interposition grafting in all patients in whom the procedure is feasible.

Reference

1. 1995 YEAR BOOK OF VASCULAR SURGERY, p 320.

Plaque Characteristics

Ultrasonic Carotid Artery Plaque Structure and the Risk of Cerebral Infarction on Computed Tomography

Geroulakos G, Domjan J, Nicolaides A, Stevens J, Labropoulos N, Ramaswami G, Belcaro G, Mansfield A (St Mary's Hosp Med School, London)
J Vasc Surg 20:263–266, 1994   145-96-12–25

Background.—The North American and the European Symptomatic Carotid Endarterectomy Trials have claimed conclusive benefit for patients with 70% to 99% stenosis of the internal carotid artery who undergo endarterectomy. It has been proposed, however, that plaque structure may be a more important factor in producing stroke than the degree of stenosis. The ultrasonic characteristics of carotid plaques were studied in relation to symptoms and the presence of cerebral infarcts on CT.

Methods.—A total of 105 carotid plaques that caused internal carotid artery stenosis greater than 70% in 83 consecutive patients were characterized ultrasonographically. All patients also had cranial CT scanning. Plaques were classified as uniformly echolucent (type 1), predominantly echolucent with less than 50% echogenic areas (type 2), predominantly echogenic (type 3), uniformly echogenic (type 4), or plaques that could not be classified (type 5).

Results.—Type 1 plaques were significantly associated with a lack of symptoms from the ipsilateral hemisphere. Infarcts were identified by CT in 26 hemispheres. The incidence of brain infarcts was 37% in patients with type I plaques and 18% in those with other types of plaque.

Conclusion.—Echogenic plaques in the internal carotid artery are more often associated with both symptoms and cerebral infarcts than other types of plaque. Presumably, they are less stable and, therefore, prone to embolization.

▶ This group from St. Mary's Hospital Medical School has done a retrospective study of sonographically determined plaque characteristics, and has related these to both clinical symptoms and to CT-documented cerebral infarctions. The investigators studied only severe lesions and divided plaques into 5 categories based on echolucency/echogenicity. Their analysis suggests that echolucent plaques are more likely to produce infarction than those that are echogenic (i.e., fibrous), an hypothesis that has been advanced by numerous prior investigators (1, 2).

The goal of this line of inquiry is to develop discriminators of carotid lesions other than diameter stenosis. This is important, because the majority of medically managed patients in both the symptomatic and asymptomatic endarterectomy trials did *not* experience stroke, even with severely stenosing lesions. Unfortunately, the quest for the grail must continue.

Although the authors found significant increases in symptoms and infarction in completely echolucent ("soft") plaques compared with other categories, significance was lost when predominantly echolucent and predominantly echogenic plaques were compared. Furthermore, symptoms were present in more than half of the patients with any echolucent components, and only truly fibrous plaques were studied. Infarction on CT was seen in 20% of even the most sonographically benign plaques. This is of practical concern in view of the safety of well-performed carotid endarterectomy demonstrated in many modern series.

Finally, one must note that an unspecified number of plaques could not be easily classified because of heavy calcification with shadowing. A more sophisticated analysis of plaque characteristics would clearly improve our discriminant ability in selecting patients for endarterectomy. Sonographic plaque characteristics, diameter stenosis, and lumen character (ulceration) are all likely candidates. The ultimate solution may involve a weighted risk system including all 3. Because sonography was not part of the North American Symptomatic Carotid Endarterectomy Trial, we will need to await a multifactorial analysis of ACAS subjects or other prospective studies for an answer.—J. Ricotta, M.D.

References

1. 1995 YEAR BOOK OF VASCULAR SURGERY, p 109.
2. Nicolaides A: ISCVS Program, 1995, p 78.

The Relationship Between Carotid Plaque Composition, Plaque Morphology, and Neurologic Symptoms
Seeger JM, Barratt E, Lawson GA, Klingman N (Univ of Florida, Gainesville; VA Med Ctr, Gainesville, Fla)
J Surg Res 58:330–336, 1995   145-96-12–26

Background.—It is possible that the composition of atherosclerotic plaques influences the risk of such complications as ulceration, subintimal hemorrhage, and embolization as well as the progression of plaque and, therefore, the risk of ischemic neurologic events.

Methods.—The morphological findings were reviewed in 78 carotid endarterectomy specimens from 74 patients, 38 of whom had been symptomatic. The plaques were examined for surface ulceration and subintimal hemorrhage, and the plaque content of lipid, cholesterol, collagen, and calcium was determined.

Results.—Plaques from symptomatic patients contained more lipid and cholesterol than those from asymptomatic patients. The most stenotic regions of the plaque contained relatively large amounts of cholesterol and calcium and relatively less collagen. Plaque sections exhibiting surface ulceration or subintimal hemorrhage contained relatively more cholesterol and less collagen, regardless of whether symptoms were present.

Conclusion.—Lipid-rich carotid plaque with relatively little collagen is prone to complications and is associated with ischemic symptoms.

▶ Detailed plaque analysis revealed that symptomatic patients had more lipid and cholesterol in their carotid plaques than did asymptomatic patients, and subtle differences were also noted in calcium and collagen content. Plaque sections found to have surface ulceration and subintimal hemorrhage contained more cholesterol and less collagen than did plaques without these changes. Although the authors suggest that these compositional changes may correlate with plaque symptomatology, I have my doubts.

Angiographic Detection of Carotid Plaque Ulceration: Comparison With Surgical Observations in a Multicenter Study

Barnett HJM, for the North American Symptomatic Carotid Endarterectomy
Trial (John P Robarts Research Inst, London, Ont, Canada)

Stroke 25:1130–1132, 1994   145-96-12–27

Introduction.—In selecting patients for carotid endarterectomy, the presence of carotid plaque ulceration is often considered. However, the importance of this finding is debated, largely because of inaccuracy in its preoperative diagnosis. The agreement between angiography and surgical observation in the detection of plaque ulceration was assessed.

Methods.—The study sample comprised the first 500 patients entered into the North American Symptomatic Carotid Endarterectomy Trial, a multicenter study of the role of this operation in symptomatic patients with moderate-to-severe stenosis of the ipsilateral carotid bifurcation. All patients underwent biplanar selective carotid angiography to assess the degree of stenosis and plaque appearance. The plaque appearance was categorized on blinded neuroradiologic review as ulcerated, irregular plaque/uncertain ulceration, or smooth/no ulceration. After randomization, half of the patients had carotid endarterectomy. The angiographic and surgical findings were then compared.

Results.—Fifty-eight percent of patients were found to have ulcerated plaques at surgery. Angiography had a sensitivity of 5.9% and a specificity of 74.1% in detecting such plaques. The positive predictive value was 71.8%. The results were similar after analysis by receiver operating characteristic (ROC) methods; the estimated area under the ROC curve was .61.

Conclusion.—Angiography and surgical observation show little agreement in the detection of carotid plaque ulceration in the first multicenter study of this issue. Nevertheless, angiography remains the only practical preoperative investigation of the presence of carotid plaque ulceration. The likely surgical findings cannot be reliably predicted by any available preoperative imaging study.

▶ *Warning:* Another paper-thin slice is rolling off the North American Symptomatic Carotid Endarterectomy Trial salami roll. In this article, Dr. Barnett informs us that there is little agreement between angiography and plaque examination in detecting carotid plaque ulceration. Again, we are indebted to Dr. Barnett for his thoughtful comments.

13 Grafts and Graft Complications

Vein Graft

Is Infrapopliteal Bypass Compromised by Distal Origin of the Proximal Anastomosis?

Brothers TE, Robison JG, Elliott BM, Arens C (Med Univ of South Carolina, Charleston; Veterans Affairs Med Ctr, Charleston, SC)

Ann Vasc Surg 9:172–178, 1995   145-96-13–1

Background.—Some patients with severe infrapopliteal arterial occlusive disease will have relative sparing of the superficial femoral and popliteal arteries. For these patients, distal organization of the proximal anastomosis (DOPA) beyond the adductor hiatus can be used to minimize the graft length required and maximize the use of available autogenous conduit. The results of DOPA bypass were evaluated and compared with those of grafts originating more proximally (POPA).

Methods.—From 1986 to 1993, the investigators performed 62 DOPA infrapopliteal revascularizations using autogenous vein for limb salvage and 203 POPA infrapopliteal bypasses. The 2 groups were compared for limb salvage and patency results by life-table analysis.

Results.—At 54 months, primary patency rates were 57% with DOPA and 50% with POPA bypass, secondary patency rates were 67% and 65%, and limb salvage rates were 53% and 66%. None of these differences were significant. In both groups, patients with tissue necrosis had worse limb salvage results than those without this characteristic, 52% vs. 70%. Tissue necrosis was seen in 71% of the DOPA group vs. 49% of the POPA group.

Conclusions.—The distal organization of the proximal anastomosis approach to infrapopliteal bypass appears to affect long-term patency to a limited degree. However, atherosclerotic disease that involves the popliteal and tibial vessels while sparing the superficial femoral artery behaves in a particularly virulent way. These patients are more likely to have tissue necrosis, which is associated with a worse prognosis for limb salvage.

▶ In our present experience with lower-extremity bypass, less than 50% of all bypasses originate from the common femoral artery. We clearly believe that the most distal possible origin of a leg bypass graft is desirable, a position shared by these investigators. See also Abstract 145-96-10–7.

Long-Term Results of Femoropopliteal Bypass With Stabilized Human Umbilical Vein

Jarrett F, Mahood BA (Univ of Pittsburgh, Pa; Shadyside Hosp, Pittsburgh)
Am J Surg 168:111–114, 1994   145-96-13–2

Background.—For patients in whom the saphenous vein is absent or inadequate or for whom a shortened anesthesia time is desired, a stabilized human umbilical vein (SHUV) graft is an acceptable alternative graft material. However, there have been few data on the long-term results of SHUV grafting. The findings of a long-term follow-up study of the results of femoropopliteal bypass with SHUV were reported.

Methods.—The analysis included 171 patients undergoing 211 consecutive femoropopliteal bypass grafts with SHUV since 1977. The 112 men and 59 women had a mean age of 69 years. The patients have been followed up at regular intervals for as long as 10 years. The results were assessed in terms of the operative indications, the patients' diabetic status, and the number of runoff vessels.

Results.—The cumulative patency rate, as calculated by the life-table method, was 70% at 1 year, 45% at 5 years, and 26% at 10 years (Fig 13–1). The patency rate was better for grafts performed because of claudication rather than for extremity salvage, although this difference was significant only at 1 and 3 years. The nondiabetic patients had better early patency rates than patients with diabetes, but the difference was not significant. The infection and aneurysm rates were 3%.

Conclusions.—For patients in whom saphenous vein is unavailable or inadequate for grafting, an SHUV provides an acceptable alternative material for femoropopliteal bypass. The chances of long-term patency are excellent for grafts that remain patent for the first 6 months.

▶ These authors have had the remarkable experience of implanting 211 umbilical vein femoropopliteal bypasses. Patency was 45% at 5 years, with

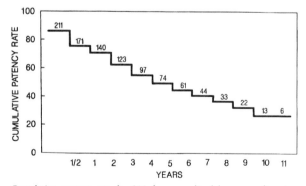

Fig 13–1.—Cumulative patency rate for 211 femoropopliteal bypass grafts using umbilical vein. (Courtesy of Jarrett F, Mahood BA: Long-term results of femoropopliteal bypass with stabilized human umbilical vein. *Am J Surg* 168:111–114, 1994. Reprinted with permission from *American Journal of Surgery.*)

an overall incidence of infection of 3% and a 3% rate of aneurysm formation. It appears that, on balance, the SHUV graft provides about the same results as any other prosthetic (1).

Reference

1. 1993 YEAR BOOK OF VASCULAR SURGERY, pp 316, 318.

Randomized Prospective Study of Angioscopically Assisted In Situ Saphenous Vein Grafting

Clair DG, Golden MA, Mannick JA, Whittemore AD, Donaldson MC (Brigham and Women's Hosp, Boston; Univ of Pennsylvania, Philadelphia)
J Vasc Surg 19:992–1000, 1994   145-96-13–3

Background.—Angioscopy has been studied as an adjunctive technique to improve the surgical outcomes of infrainguinal in situ vein bypass grafting. One hypothesis is that angioscopically assisted valve lysis and vein branch identification during in situ saphenous vein bypass would decrease graft failure caused by technical reasons, local operative morbidity, and hospital stay. This hypothesis was tested in a randomized, prospective study.

Methods.—The study included 59 patients who were undergoing primary bypass to an infrageniculate artery. They were randomly assigned to receive in situ saphenous vein bypass with valvulotomy and branch identification with either angioscopic visualization and the use of short, intermittent incisions—the scope group, 32 patients—or direct visualization with the use of a continuous incision—the no-scope group, 27 patients. The 2 groups were compared for their operative findings, morbidity, length of hospital stay, and graft patency.

Results.—The 2 groups were similar in their incidence of diabetes, claudication vs. critical ischemia as the indication for surgery, or popliteal vs. infrapopliteal location of distal anastomoses. There were no significant differences in rates of wound complications, (9.3% in the scope group vs. 3.7% in the no-scope group); early graft occlusion, (6.2% vs. 7.4%); mean postoperative hospital stay (8.0 days vs. 8.6 days). Cumulative secondary patency rates at 48 months were also similar: 79% in the scope group vs. 91% in the no-scope group (table).

Conclusions.—Angioscopically assisted preparation of the in situ vein for infrageniculate grafting appears to offer no significant advantages over conventional vein graft preparation. There are no significant differences in local operative morbidity, length of hospital stay, or mid-term graft patency rate.

▶ There are many reports from Brigham and Women's Hospital on small groups of well-studied patients; these reports are admired by many and often quoted. Some give useful information and some do not. This one, which expresses the strong bias of the senior author, does not. It represents

Cumulative Primary Revised Patency Rates Comparing Scope and No-Scope Groups

Interval	Grafts at Risk	Number of Grafts Failing	Number of Grafts Withdrawn	Interval Patency (%)	Cumulative Patency (%)	SE
0–3 months						
Overall	59	6	8	89.2	89.2	4.3
Scope	32	3	4	90.3	90.3	5.3
No scope	27	3	4	88.0	88.0	6.6
3–6 months						
Overall	45	1	6	97.6	87.0	4.6
Scope	25	1	2	95.8	86.5	6.3
No scope	20	0	4	100	88.0	6.6
6–12 months						
Overall	38	0	9	100	87.0	4.6
Scope	22	0	5	100	86.5	6.3
No scope	16	0	4	100	88.0	6.6
12–24 months						
Overall	29	1	13	95.6	83.2	5.6
Scope	17	1	7	92.6	80.1	8.5
No scope	12	0	6	100	88.0	6.6
24–36 months						
Overall	15	0	9	100	83.2	5.6
Scope	9	0	5	100	80.1	8.5
No scope	6	0	4	100	88.0	6.6
36–48 months						
Overall	6	0	6	100	83.2	5.6
Scope	4	0	4	100	80.1	8.5
No scope	2	0	2	100	88.0	6.6

(Courtesy of Clair DG, Golden MA, Mannick JA, et al: Randomized prospective study of angioscopically assisted in situ saphenous vein grafting. *J Vasc Surg* 19:992–1000, 1994.)

a classic example of a beta error (low incidence of adverse events and too few patients to show a "statistically" significant difference). The real value of angioscopy (if any) remains to be elucidated. However, it is my view that angioscopy is useful in determining the suitability of a "remote" vein for use as a bypass and for in situ vein graft preparation. That will be difficult to "prove." However, is that necessary?—W. Abbott, M.D.

▶ It is.—J.M. Porter, M.D.

The Use of Spliced Vein Bypasses for Infrainguinal Arterial Reconstruction

Chang BB, Darling RC III, Bock DEM, Shah DM, Leather RP (Albany Med College, NY)
J Vasc Surg 21:403–412, 1995   145-96-13–4

Background.—Autogenous veins, both in situ and excised, are widely used in arterial bypass surgery, but this type of surgery usually requires a segment of high-quality vein that is adequate in diameter. Two or more vein segments may be spliced together when necessary to complete a reconstruction, but the effect of splicing on long-term patency remains uncertain.

Methods.—During a 14-year span, when 1,806 in situ and 150 excised vein bypass procedures were done, 184 bypasses necessitated splicing together vein segments. These included 111 in situ bypasses involving the splicing of 1 or more pieces of excised vein (partial in situ bypass). An additional 73 bypasses were completed using multiple pieces of spliced excised vein. The most frequent sources of excised, spliced vein segments were the distal part of the ipsilateral greater saphenous vein and the lesser saphenous vein.

Results.—The overall primary patency rates at 1 and 4 years for patients given autogenous spliced vein grafts were 72% and 45%. The respective secondary patency rates were 79% and 61%. The partial in situ bypasses had 1- and 4-year secondary patency rates of 80% and 70%, respectively. The comparable rates for in situ bypasses completed without a spliced segment were 91% and 83%. Secondary patency rates for patients having spliced excised vein bypasses were 78% and 67%, compared with 85% and 75%, respectively, for those given a single excised vein bypass. Limb salvage rates at 4 years were 96% for in situ bypass, 85% for partial in situ bypass, 95% for single excised vein bypasses, and 90% for spliced excised vein bypasses.

Conclusions.—Bypass patency may be compromised when excised vein segments are used to complete partial in situ bypasses. When spliced excised vein segments of good quality are used, acceptable patency may be expected. Spliced autogenous vein bypasses are clearly superior to prosthetic bypass for infrageniculate arterial reconstruction.

▶ While the spliced vein results are interesting, I am absolutely floored by a 4-year *primary* patency rate of all in situ vein grafts of 83%. This has got to be the highest primary patency ever reported, and I tip my hat with humility to Dr. Leather and his superb associates. I wonder whether they really meant primary assisted?

Vein Adaptation to the Hemodynamic Environment of Infrainguinal Grafts

Fillinger MF, Cronenwett JL, Besso S, Walsh DB, Zwolak RM (Dartmouth-Hitchcock Med Ctr, Lebanon, NH)
J Vasc Surg 19:970–979, 1994   145-96-13–5

Introduction.—Changes in shear stress and other hemodynamic parameters appear to induce a remodeling response in arteries. However, there are few data on the effects of the hemodynamic environment on functioning human vein grafts. Duplex ultrasonography was used to assess changes in the diameter of human saphenous vein grafts after infrainguinal bypass.

Methods.—Duplex ultrasonography was performed to assess 48 in situ saphenous vein grafts during the first year after infrainguinal arterial bypass. The hemodynamic variables measured were volumetric flow rate, average velocity, peak systolic velocity, and vein diameter in the proximal and distal thirds of the grafts. Measurements were made at 1 week and 3,

6, and 12 months after the operation. On the basis of their size in the below-knee segment 1 week after bypass, the grafts were divided into 3 groups: small, less than 3.55 mm in diameter; medium, 3.5 to 4 mm in diameter; and large, greater than 4 mm in diameter.

Results.—From 1 week to 12 months, the mean distal vein diameters increased from 2.9 to 3.6 mm in the small group, whereas they decreased from 4.3 to 3.9 mm in the large group. The values in the medium group were 3.7 and 3.8 mm. Linear regression of the percentage change in diameter vs. the initial vein graft diameter confirmed that the large veins decreased and the small veins increased in diameter. Values for volumetric flow rate, peak systolic velocity, and shear stress tended toward uniformity with time. Shear stress was the best predictor of vein diameter change. Initial shear stress was 29 dynes/cm^2 in veins that increased in diameter by more than 10%, compared with 13 dynes/cm^2 in veins that decreased in diameter by the same percentage. There was no significant difference in initial volumetric flow rates between these 2 groups with 135 and 130 mL/min, respectively.

Conclusions.—In patients who have undergone infrainguinal bypass, the in situ vein graft diameter, volume flow rate, peak systolic velocity, and shear stress all tend to stabilize at uniform values with time, regardless of the initial diameter of the vein graft. Shear stress is the hemodynamic variable most closely related to the change in vein graft diameter. Thus, functioning saphenous vein grafts appear to adapt to their hemodynamic environment by modulating diameter to normalize shear stress.

▶ Interestingly, these authors conclude that in situ vein grafts tend to stabilize at a uniform graft diameter, volume flow rate, peak systolic velocity, and shear stress, regardless of the initial vein diameter. Their study shows another example of vascular size adaptation to normalize shear stress. This is becoming a recurring theme, and it is undoubtedly an important one. See also the comment after Abstract 145-96-12–6.

Cryopreserved Saphenous Vein Allografts for Below-Knee Lower Extremity Revascularization
Martin RS III, Edwards WH, Mulherin JL Jr, Edwards WH Jr, Jenkins JM, Hoff SJ (Vanderbilt Univ Med Ctr, Nashville, Tenn; St Thomas Hosp, Nashville, Tenn)
Ann Surg 219:664–672, 1994   145-96-13–6

Background.—Aneurysmal degeneration and poor patency have led to unsatisfactory results with arterial and venous allografting. The mechanisms of allograft failure may involve endothelial loss and host rejection. Recent, modern methods of cryopreservation—including rate-controlled freezing, dimethyl sulfoxide, and other cryopreservants—have led to renewed interest in the possibilities of venous allografting. For patients requiring bypass in ischemic limbs, cryopreserved saphenous vein allografts may be a useful alternative conduit. The results of this conduit for arterial bypass to the distal popliteal and tibial arteries were assessed.

Methods.—From 1987 to 1993, 115 cryopreserved vein allografts were placed in 87 limbs of patients with no available autologous vein. The allografts were placed in the distal popliteal artery in 14 cases and the tibial artery in 101. The patients were 47 men and 35 women (mean age, 71 years). Bypass was performed because of rest pain in 49% of cases, gangrene in 31%, and claudication in 18%. For 2 patients, the indication was aneurysmal allograft replacement (table). The patients were followed up for a mean of 25 months.

Results.—Patency was unaffected by the site of proximal or distal anastomosis; the patency of runoff vessels; the use of anticoagulation; patient age or sex; the presence of diabetes, hypertension, or smoking; the surgical indication; the source of the graft; or the use of multiple segments. Aneurysmal dilation necessitated revision surgery in 6 grafts. Specimens of allografts explanted from 4 patients showed no histologic evidence of an immune response. The patients did not receive immunosuppressive drug treatment. The primary graft patency rate at 4 years was only 3% (Fig 13–2), although the 4-year limb salvage rate was 62%.

Conclusions.—Cryopreserved vein allografts can achieve satisfactory limb salvage when used for revascularization of the lower extremities. However, the long-term patency rates are not as good as with autogenous vein, and the allografts are more expensive than prosthetic grafts. Cryopreserved vein allografts should be used only when sufficient autogenous vein is unavailable and when the risk for prosthetic graft–related infection is high.

► This large, well–followed-up series of 115 cryopreserved allografts implanted in 87 limbs demonstrates no added benefits compared with the much less costly prosthetic graft for below-knee arterial reconstructions. The patency rates at 24 months are uniformly poor for both types of conduits.—E.S. Weinstein, M.D.

► I currently find absolutely no indication for the use of cryopreserved saphenous vein allografts, which, in addition to producing very poor results, are unmercifully expensive (1–3).—J.M. Porter, M.D.

Sites of Proximal and Distal Anastomosis for 115 Lower Extremity Cryopreserved Vein Allografts

Proximal	No.	(%)	Distal	No.	(%)
Common femoral	70	60.9	Peroneal	42	36.5
Aortofemoral graft	18	15.7	Anterior tibial	28	24.3
Deep femoral	9	7.8	Posterior tibial	23	20.0
Superficial femoral	7	6.1	Popliteal	14	12.2
Femoral popliteal graft	6	5.2	Tibioperoneal trunk	7	6.1
Femoral femoral graft	5	4.3	Dorsalis pedis	1	0.9
Totals	115			115	

(Courtesy of Martin RS III, Edwards WH, Mulherin JL Jr, et al: Cryopreserved saphenous vein allografts for below-knee lower extremity revascularization. *Ann Surg* 219:664–672, 1994.)

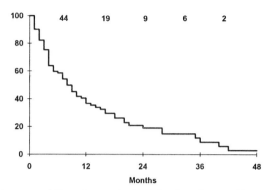

Fig 13–2.—Primary cumulative patency rates for below-knee bypass with cryopreserved vein allografts. (Courtesy of Martin RS III, Edwards WH, Mulherin JL Jr, et al: Cryopreserved saphenous vein allografts for below-knee lower extremity revascularization. *Ann Surg* 219:664–672, 1994.)

References

1. 1995 YEAR BOOK OF VASCULAR SURGERY, pp 343, 344.
2. 1994 YEAR BOOK OF VASCULAR SURGERY, p 365.
3. 1993 YEAR BOOK OF VASCULAR SURGERY, p 320.

Prosthetic Grafts

Failure of Glow-Discharge Polymerization Onto Woven Dacron to Improve Performance of Hemodialysis Grafts

Farmer DL, Goldstone J, Lim RC, Reilly LM (Univ of California, San Francisco)
J Vasc Surg 18:570–576, 1993   145-96-13–7

Background.—Both autogenous fistulas and prosthetic grafts such as those of expanded polytetrafluoroethylene (e-PTFE) remain patent after 1 year in 60% to 80% of cases when used for hemodialysis access. The 2- to 6-week delay involved is a disadvantage. An alternative is the Plasma-TFE vascular graft, a thin-walled graft of woven Dacron bonded by glow-discharge polymerization to an ultrathin layer of tetrafluoroethylene. The internal surface of the graft is presumed to have low thrombogenicity. Good patency rates are reported even when dialysis begins within a week of graft placement.

Methods.—Plasma-TFE grafts were used in 19 fistulas—12 in the forearm and 7 in the arm—and the results were compared with those achieved with 28 PTFE grafts. The groups were similar with regard to age, diabetes, and other comorbid conditions. A majority of patients in both groups had previously had dialysis access procedures.

Results.—The Plasma-TFE grafts could be used shortly after placement, but primary and secondary patency rates were less than 50% after 1 year. Ten of the 19 grafts had to be replaced, 5 of them within the first month.

Either failed graft thrombectomy or marked intimal hyperplasia precluded the revision of these fistulas. Only 4 of the 28 PTFE grafts failed.

Conclusion.—Although it allows early hemodialysis access, the Plasma-TFE graft cannot be recommended for this or other indications because of its poor long-term secondary patency rate.

▶ I know nothing about this new Dacron graft surrounded by glowing PTFE. In the experience of the San Francisco group, this new graft did not give a satisfactory performance as a dialysis fistula, and it has been abandoned by the authors. On the basis of these results, I do not plan to use this graft for dialysis access.

Influence of a Vein Cuff on Polytetrafluoroethylene Grafts for Primary Femoropopliteal Bypass
Raptis S, Miller JH (Univ of Adelaide, South Australia)
Br J Surg 82:487–491, 1995   145-96-13–8

Background.—Polytetrafluoroethylene (PTFE) can be directly anastomosed to a recipient artery, but several techniques for incorporating vein tissue into the distal anastomosis have been proposed in the hope of improving long-term patency. The vein cuff was initially intended for use in the tibial vessels because of size mismatches between grafts and recipient vessels. It was later adopted for use in popliteal anastomoses both above and below the knee.

Methods.—The potential benefit of using a vein cuff at the distal anastomosis of a primary PTFE femoropopliteal bypass graft was studied in a series of 559 primary PTFE bypasses. Most proximal anastomoses were done by direct suture. The distal anastomosis was made by directly suturing PTFE to the arteriotomy, by using a vein patch, or by constructing a vein cuff from a segment at least twice the length of the arteriotomy (Fig 13–3).

Results.—Sixty-two percent of the bypasses remained patent after 3 years. Patency rates in the above-knee position were 69% with a cuff and 68% without. In the below-knee position, grafts bearing a vein cuff had a substantially better 3-year patency rate (57% vs. 29%). Removing thrombis from occluded cuffed PTFE grafts improved the cumulative 3-year patency rate to 74%. The limb salvage rate at 3 years was 97% for patients who had claudication at the time of surgery and 89% for those who had a threatened extremity when cuffed PTFE bypasses were performed. Outflow continued in half of the cuffed PTFE bypasses that became occluded, making possible either thrombectomy or construction of a new bypass. Available vein tissue was rarely used to salvage an occluded PTFE graft. When it was, the risks for occlusion and amputation were high.

Conclusion.—When autologous vein bypass is not feasible, the use of PTFE with a vein cuff interposed at the distal anastomosis is preferable to the use of PTFE alone.

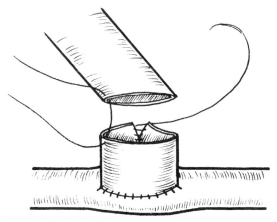

Fig 13–3.—Construction of a vein cuff. (Courtesy of Raptis S, Miller JH: Influence of a vein cuff on polytetrafluoroethylene grafts for primary femoropopliteal bypass. *Br J Surg* 82:487–491, 1995. Reprinted by permission of Blackwell Science Ltd.)

▶ The idea of a vein cuff at the end of a PTFE graft was first proposed by the late Dr. Justin Miller of Australia, one of the co-authors of this paper. The concept was expanded by Dr. John Wolfe and his group at St. Mary's, and a slightly new concept was put forth by Dr. Robert Taylor, who is currently at St. George's Hospital, London. Each concept has been attractive and seems to be associated with increased patency compared with the PTFE graft without the interposed vein portion. In this large clinical follow-up from the originating house, considerably improved patency was noted with the cuff compared with grafts that do not have the cuff. Because the series was not randomized, the amount of new information contributed is actually small.

Endothelial Seeding of Polytetrafluoroethylene Femoral Popliteal Bypasses: The Failure of Low-Density Seeding to Improve Patency
Herring M, Smith J, Dalsing M, Glover J, Compton R, Etchberger K, Zollinger T (St Vincent Hosp, Indianapolis, Ind; Methodist Hosp, Omaha, Neb; Indiana Univ Hosp, Indianapolis; et al)
J Vasc Surg 20:650–655, 1994   145-96-13–9

Background.—Endothelialization might increase the patency rate of synthetic vascular grafts, but it generally does not occur spontaneously in humans. Endothelial seeding may enhance the patency of femoropopliteal bypass grafts.

Methods.—Nine surgeons at 4 hospitals randomly assigned patients to receive either an endothelially seeded polytetrafluoroethylene (PTFE) femoropopliteal bypass graft or an autologous vein graft. A seeded graft was used if no satisfactory vein was available. Sixty-six seeded PTFE grafts and 53 autologous vein grafts were compared.

VESSEL PATENCY

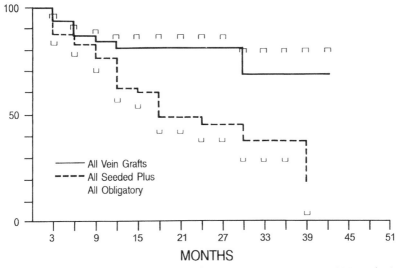

Fig 13–4.—Actuarial life-table of graft patency for 2 treatment categories ($P = 0.006$), randomized vein grafts, and a pooled group of randomized and obligatory seeded grafts. (Courtesy of Herring M, Smith J, Dalsing M, et al: Endothelial seeding of polytetrafluoroethylene femoral popliteal bypasses: The failure of low-density seeding to improve patency. *J Vasc Surg* 20:650–655, 1994.)

Results.—Scanning electron microscopic study of the seeded grafts showed that endothelium attached satisfactorily to the discarded graft ends. At 30 months, patency was superior for vein grafts (Fig 13–4). Ninety-two percent of vein grafts and only 38% of seeded PTFE grafts were patent at this time. Anastomotic hyperplasia was observed in the failed grafts.

Conclusion.—Endothelial seeding does not enhance the patency of femoropopliteal PTFE bypass grafts, even those placed below the knee. Autogenous vein grafts are much more likely to remain patent at this site.

▶ This is a very important paper by one of the originators of the PTFE endothelial seeding concept. One hundred nineteen patients were randomly assigned to receive vein grafts and PTFE seeded grafts. At 30 months, the vein graft patency was 91.6%, compared with the seeded PTFE patency of only 37.8%. Each of the contributing institutions reported similar results. We can only conclude from this work that endothelial seeding of PTFE grafts does not improve clinical patency. Too bad.

Proof of Fallout Endothelialization of Impervious Dacron Grafts in the Aorta and Inferior Vena Cava of the Dog

Shi Q, Hong-De Wu M, Hayashida N, Wechezak AR, Clowes AW, Sauvage LR (Univ of Washington, Seattle; The Hope Heart Inst, Seattle)
J Vasc Surg 20:546–557, 1994   145-96-13–10

Background.—Possible mechanisms by which porous synthetic vascular grafts become endothelialized include ingrowth of pannus from the host intima across the anastomoses, ingrowth of microvessels from the perigraft tissues, and deposition of circulating cells onto the luminal surface of the graft (so-called fallout).

Methods.—To determine whether blood cells contribute to the endothelialization of isolated Dacron vascular grafts, a multicomponent graft was placed in the canine descending thoracic aorta. The 18-cm graft consisted of 2 parallel central Dacron limbs, one preclotted and the other made impervious by silicone rubber, and 30-μm polytetrafluoroethylene grafts anastomosed at either end. An 8-cm graft totally coated with silicone rubber was also placed in the abdominal aorta and inferior vena cava. Grafts were in place for 4 to 12 weeks. The flow surfaces were examined stereomicroscopically after being stained with silver nitrate and were also examined by scanning and transmission electron microscopy. The flow surface was stained immunocytochemically to demonstrate endothelial and smooth-muscle cells.

Results.—Both pannus formation and transmural ingrowth of microvessels were effectively prevented in the impervious central grafts. Nevertheless, islands of endothelial cells were present on the flow surfaces at all implant sites 4 weeks after graft placement. In descending thoracic aortic grafts, cells positive for α-actin and microvessels were shown beneath some endothelial islands (Fig 13–5).

Conclusion.—Dacron grafts in both the arterial and venous systems of the dog are endothelialized by fallout of circulating cells.

▶ The inescapable conclusion is that fallout endothelialization of vascular grafts does occur in the dog model. Similar results have been shown by Scott et al. from Asheville (1).

Reference

1. Scott SM, Barth MG, Gaddy LR, et al: The role of circulating cells in the healing of vascular prostheses. *J Vasc Surg* 19:585–593, 1994.

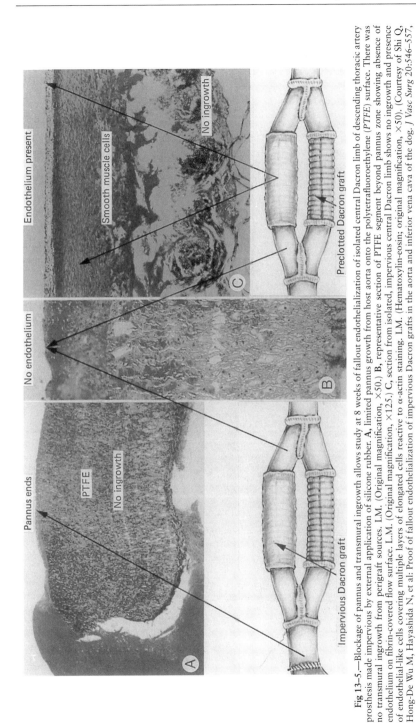

Fig 13–5.—Blockage of pannus and transmural ingrowth allows study at 8 weeks of fallout endothelialization of isolated central Dacron limb of descending thoracic artery prosthesis made impervious by external application of silicone rubber. **A,** limited pannus growth from host aorta onto the polytetrafluoroethylene *(PTFE)* surface. There was no transmural ingrowth from perigraft sources. LM. (Original magnification, ×50.) **B,** representative section of PTFE segment beyond pannus zone showing absence of endothelium on fibrin-covered flow surface. L.M. (Original magnification, ×125.) **C,** section from isolated, impervious central Dacron limb shows no ingrowth and presence of endothelial-like cells covering multiple layers of elongated cells reactive to α-actin staining. LM. (Hematoxylin-eosin; original magnification, ×50.) (Courtesy of Shi Q, Hong-De Wu M, Hayashida N, et al: Proof of fallout endothelialization of impervious Dacron grafts in the aorta and inferior vena cava of the dog. *J Vasc Surg* 20:546–557, 1994.)

Dilation of Woven and Knitted Aortic Prosthetic Grafts: CT Scan Evaluation

Alimi Y, Juhan C, Morati N, Girard N, Cohen S (Hôpital Nord, Marseille, France)

Ann Vasc Surg 8:238–242, 1994   145-96-13–11

Background.—A lack of studies on the short- and medium-term outcome of woven and knitted aortic prosthetic grafts prompted a CT study of 58 asymptomatic patients having reconstruction of the infrarenal aorta.

Methods.—Contrast-enhanced CT studies were made, centering on the proximal anastomosis, the body of the prosthesis, and the prosthetic limbs an average of 19 days after surgery and again 19 months after reconstruction.

Results.—The early and late CT studies showed that in end-to-side aortoprosthetic anastomoses, the anteroposterior diameter increased by 1.9% for woven grafts and 8.8% for knitted grafts (Table 1). In end-to-end aortoprosthetic anastomoses, the prosthetic body increased in diameter by 12.6% on early CT stans for woven grafts and by 28% for knitted grafts. Late studies showed further dilation of 2.2% for woven grafts and 6.2% for knitted prosthetic grafts. The prosthetic graft limbs increased by 22% for woven grafts and by 35% for knitted prosthetic grafts on early scans compared with the manufacturers' values. Secondary increases were 3% and 8%, respectively.

Conclusion.—The results of previous studies are summarized in Table 2. In most instances, an aortic prosthesis dilates shortly after placement, probably soon after it is declamped. Subsequent dilation proceeds more slowly and is more evident in knitted than in woven aortic prostheses.

▶ Knitted Dacron grafts dilate more than woven grafts, but both undergo significant dilatation. Some of this undoubtedly reflects the lack of precise initial sizing by the manufacturer, resulting in the actual graft being larger than the size predicted immediately after implantation. I thought we already knew all this.

TABLE 1.—Mean Values of Primary and Secondary Dilations of the Diameters of Aortoprosthetic End-to-Side Anastomoses, the Bodies, and the Limbs of the 4 Types of Prosthetic Grafts Used

Type of graft	No. of grafts studied	Aortoprosthetic anastomosis		Graft body			Graft limbs		
		N	PD (%)	N	PD (%)	SD (%)	N	PD (%)	SD (%)
Gelseal (Vascutek)	12	5	4.2	7	19.6	6.1	18	27.6	7.1
Gelsoft (Vascutek)	26	13	10.5	13	32.4	6.2	50	37.2	7.9
USCI (Bard)	8	2	0	6	9.3	0	6	35.7	5.0
Hemashield (Meadox)	12	5	2.7	7	15.4	4.2	22	19.9	2.9

Abbreviations: PD, primary dilation (differences between diameter provided by the manufacturer and that seen with the early CT scan); *SD*, secondary dilation (difference between diameters measured on early and late CT scan).

(Courtesy of Alimi Y, Juhan C, Morati N, et al: Dilation of woven and knitted aortic prosthetic grafts: CT scan evaluation. *Ann Vasc Surg* 8:238–242, 1994.)

TABLE 2.—Review of the Literature on Late Dilation of Woven and Knitted Prosthetic Grafts

Reference	N	Prosthesis Type	Scan type	Follow-Up (mo)	Dilation (%)	False Aneurysm (%)
Blumenberg et al.	106	Knitted	Duplex	5–38	23	—
Nunn et al.	95	Knitted	Duplex	33	17.6	—
Nunn et al.	33	Knitted	CT	175	67	31
Mikati et al.	52	Knitted	CT	76	58	15
Present series	58	Woven	CT	19	14.8	—
		Knitted			34.2	—

(Courtesy of Alimi Y, Juhan C, Morati N, et al: Dilation of woven and knitted aortic prosthetic grafts: CT scan evaluation. *Ann Vasc Surg* 8:238–242, 1994.)

Experimental Grafts

Clinical Use of Low Porosity Woven Ultrafine Polyester Fiber Grafts
Satoh S, Niu S, Kanda K, Hirai J, Nakazima S, Wada Y, Oka T, Noishiki Y
(Kyoto Prefectural Univ of Medicine, Japan; Yokohama City Univ, Japan)
Artif Organs 19:57–63, 1995   145-96-13–12

Objective.—Ultrafine polyester fibers (UFPF) of approximately 3 μm in thickness have higher affinity with cells. Compared with conventional polyester fibers of about 12 μm in diameter, UFPF induce pronounced proliferation of fibroblasts on their surfaces. On the basis of these findings, a vascular graft made with woven UFPF—the Toray graft—has been developed. The Toray graft is durable enough for aortic reconstruction. Its water permeability is low—100 mL/min/cm^2:120 mm Hg H$_2$O—and pretreatment is generally not needed to seal the fabric interstices so that profuse hemorrhage is avoided. One group has been using the Toray graft clinically since 1990. Their experience with 81 cases was reported.

Experience.—The investigators have clinically applied the Toray graft in 81 patients: 28 with thoracic artery aneurysms, 6 with thoracoabdominal aneurysms, 42 with abdominal aortic aneurysms, and 5 with atherosclerotic obstructions of the peripheral arteries. Eight patients died after surgery, all of whom died of causes unrelated to the Toray graft. The remaining 73 patients were in good condition after surgery. The graft was presealed with human albumin when the operation required extracorporeal circulation. When used for repair of abdominal aortic aneurysms, the graft was preclotted in situ with nonheparinized autologous blood, after the proximal anastomosis was completed. This preclotting procedure took only about 2 minutes. When used in the reconstruction of peripheral arteries for intra-aortic balloon pumping, the graft was not sealed.

The Toray graft proved easy to handle; fraying of cut edges was not a problem with any direction of cutting. The graft was soft and pliable enough for easy adaptation and anastomosis, even after presealing. There

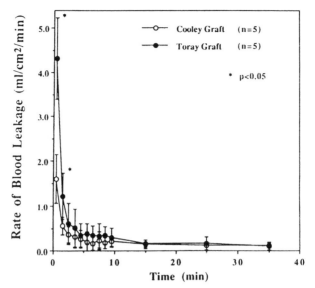

Fig 13–6.—Time-dependent change of the totally heparinized human blood leakage from the graft walls with no presealing, which was measured using an in vitro circuit system, is shown. (Courtesy of Satoh S, Niu S, Kanda K, et al: Clinical use of low porosity woven ultrafine polyester fiber grafts. *Artif Organs* 19:57–63, 1995. Reprinted by permission of Blackwell Science, Inc.)

was minimal bleeding from the graft wall, anastomotic sites, and suture pores immediately after graft implantation, and the bleeding that did occur stopped spontaneously (Fig 13–6).

Conclusions.—The Toray graft is easy to handle despite its low porosity. It can be safely applied in the reconstruction of arterial systems, even when totally heparinized for extracorporeal reconstruction.

► An experimental ultrafine polyester graft with fibers about one fourth the thickness of conventional Dacron fibers was constructed. This graft theoretically attracts fibroblasts and induces a pronounced proliferation on the surface. The graft was tightly woven and manufactured in a velour configuration. Early clinical results were encouraging, although I am unable to identify any unique benefits of this graft. The authors state that the graft is quite easy to handle, has minimal blood leakage, and has no cut-edge fraying. Perhaps we will hear more about this graft in the future.

Thrombogenicity of an Elastomer-Coated Aortofemoral Dacron Prosthetic Graft in Humans
Becquemin J-P, Haiduc F, Cavillon A (Hôpital Henri Mondor, Créteil, France)
Ann Vasc Surg 8:443–451, 1994   145-96-13–13

Objective.—A new elastomer-coated prosthetic graft (Polygraph, Intervascular Co.) was evaluated in 30 patients who had either occlusive arterial disease or an aneurysm of the infrarenal abdominal aorta.

Methods.—The Polygraph is a Dacron prosthesis impregnated with silicon polymer. Thirty other patients had vascular reconstruction with a Meadox knitted double-velour prosthesis, and 30 received the Bard-USCI knitted prosthesis. Patients were randomly assigned to receive 1 of the 3 prostheses just before placement. Patients were followed for an average of 1 year.

Results.—Blood loss was greatest in patients given the Polygraph, but not significantly so. Surgery times were similar in all groups. The actuarially calculated primary patency rate at 3 years was 71.5% for patients given the Polygraph, lower than the rate in the other groups. Secondary patency was achieved in 74% of patients in the Polygraph group and in all patients in the 2 comparison groups.

Conclusion.—Patients who require aortoiliac or aortofemoral reconstruction should not receive a silicon elastomer–impregnated prosthesis because it carries a high risk for thrombosis.

▶ An experimental new graft consisting of Dacron with an inert external covering of silicone was implanted in 30 patients. I am unable to perceive any hypothetical benefit of the silicone-covered graft other than the authors' statement that such silicone coating is associated with satisfactory healing and little thrombogenicity, as well as a reduced periprosthetic inflammatory reaction. At any rate, the new prosthesis was compared in a random trial with 2 different knitted Dacron prostheses. The 36-month patency was distinctly inferior for the new graft, leading these authors to conclude that the thrombogenicity of the elastomer-coated prosthetic graft was significantly higher than that of the plain Dacron grafts. The authors then recommend that prosthetic grafts impregnated with silicone elastomer not be used in patients having aortic surgery. On the basis of their results, I agree.

An Integrated Approach to the Design and Engineering of Hybrid Arterial Prostheses

Miwa H, Matsuda T (National Cardiovascular Ctr Research Inst, Osaka, Japan; Shinshu Univ, Nagano, Japan)
J Vasc Surg 19:658–667, 1994   145-96-13–14

Objective.—Small-caliber vascular grafts seeded with endothelial cells (ECs) have shown reduced thrombogenicity in the experimental setting. A new hybrid graft has been developed that consists of a microporous polyurethane graft, an artificial basement membrane made of a complex gel of type I collagen and dermatan sulfate, and a monolayer of autogenous ECs. The graft is 5 cm long and has an inner diameter of 3 mm. In vitro studies have shown reduced adhesion of platelets to the EC layer.

Methods.—Twenty EC-seeded grafts were placed into the carotid arteries of dogs, using no anticoagulation. The implants were in place for as long as 26 weeks.

Results.—Three fourths of the seeded grafts remained patent. After 12 weeks, the entire inner graft surface was covered by ECs, and circumferentially oriented smooth-muscle cells were seen at this time. The grafts averaged 80 μm in intimal thickness at 12 weeks and showed little further increase at 26 weeks.

Conclusion.—This small-caliber vascular graft is completely endothelialized, highly antithrombogenic, and biomechanically compatible. Hyperplasia is minimal.

▶ These authors have ingeniously devised a homemade graft, half prosthetic and half autogenous, consisting of a polyurethane wall, an artificial basement membrane of complex type I collagen and dermatan sulfate, and an autogenous endothelial cell monolayer. This was made in a small-graft format with an inside diameter of 3 mm. The grafts were implanted into the carotid arteries of dogs without anticoagulation and followed for as long as 26 weeks; the overall patency for seeded grafts of 75%. It is quite possible that combining biomechanical and cellular engineering designs in a small-diameter graft may finally lead to improved results. Stay tuned. I am absolutely certain there will be more to follow.

Graft Infection

Treatment of Vascular Graft Infection By In Situ Replacement With a Rifampin-Bonded Gelatin-Sealed Dacron Graft
Goëau-Brissonnière O, Mercier F, Nicolas MH, Bacourt F, Coggia M, Lebrault C, Pechère JC (Ambroise Paré Hospital, Paris; René Descartes Univ, Paris; American Hosp of Paris; et al)
J Vasc Surg 19:739–744, 1994   145-96-13–15

Purpose.—Once a prosthetic vascular graft has been infected, graft excision and extra-anatomical reconstruction are nearly always required. Infection-resistant vascular prostheses might play a useful role in the treatment of these patients. The ability of rifampin bonding to inhibit infection after in situ replacement of an infected vascular prosthesis was studied in dogs.

Methods.—Gelatin-sealed grafts were contaminated with Staphylococcus epidermidis and then used to replace the infrarenal aorta of 18 dogs. One group of dogs received no further surgery. In the other 2 groups, the infected grafts were removed and replaced with either an untreated gelatin-sealed graft or a rifampin-bonded graft. The latter grafts were soaked for 15 minutes in a 60-mg/mL saline solution of rifampin at 37°C. No systemic adjunct antibiotics were given in any of the 3 groups. The grafts were removed for bacteriologic analysis 4 weeks after initial implantation.

Results.—All of the initially implanted grafts and all of the untreated replacement grafts showed gross infection at the time of removal. In contrast, all of the rifampin-bonded replacement grafts showed normal incorporation. Bacteria did not grow from any of the rifampin-bonded replacement grafts, but all of the initially implanted and untreated replacement grafts were infected. Bacterial counts were similar in control grafts, in initially implanted grafts, and in untreated replacement grafts. Blood, liver, spleen, kidney, and lung culture results were negative.

Conclusions.—When used to replace infected vascular prostheses in dogs, rifampin-bonded, gelatin-sealed Dacron grafts appear to be resistant to infection. In low-grade graft infections, in which the responsible pathogen is susceptible to rifampin, antibiotic-bonded grafts may be useful in treating vascular prosthetic infections.

▶ These results indicate that a rifampin-bonded, gelatin-sealed graft may be directly implanted into a field infected with *S. epidermidis* in dogs, with expectation of at least 4 weeks of satisfactory function. I have absolutely no interest in in situ implantation of grafts in an infected field. The surgical principle of remote grafting through a clean field has stood the test of time, and I have never understood the interest of so many to ignore this important surgical principle. I remain unconvinced that grafts with antibiotics bound to their surface are going to be of any real clinical utility.

Accuracy of Disincorporation for Identification of Vascular Graft Infection
Padberg FT Jr, Smith SM, Eng RHK (Univ of Medicine and Dentistry of New Jersey, Newark)
Arch Surg 130:183–187, 1995   145-96-13–16

Purpose.—In vascular prosthetic grafting, disincorporation is associated with graft infection. However, graft infection is not always present when tissue incorporation does not occur. Enhanced microbiological culture techniques were used to compare the presence or absence of tissue incorporation in vascular prosthetic grafts with the bacterial culture results.

Methods.—Samples of vascular prostheses removed from 113 aortofemoral, extra-anatomical, infrainguinal, and hemoaccess sites at vascular reoperative surgery in 59 patients were studied. All grafts underwent gentle sonication followed by quantitative culture. The culture results were predicted from the incorporation or disincorporation status of the prostheses, as assessed at surgery. Any bacterial growth was considered to represent graft infection.

Results.—Thirty-one sites yielded cultures positive for bacteria. There were 31 disincorporated sites, 23 of which were culture positive and 8 of which yielded no growth. The other 82 sites showed good incorporation; 74 were culture negative, but 8 yielded bacterial growth. The rate of incorrect prediction was 14%. Sensitivity—defined as concurrence of disincorporation and a culture positive for bacteria, relative to all culture-positive grafts—was 74%. Specificity—defined as concurrence of incorporation and cultures negative for bacteria relative to all culture negative grafts—varied with the length of graft implantation. Specificity was 90% in prostheses implanted for more than 2 weeks and 97% for those implanted for longer than 12 weeks (table).

Accuracy of Tissue Incorporation or Disincorporation in the Identification of Vascular
Prosthetic Infection

Graft Sites	No. of Sites	Sensitivity*	Specificity†	Percentage Positive Predictive Value‡	Percentage Negative Predictive Value§	Accuracy‖
Vascular reconstructions at						
2 wk	56	70	96	78	94	91
12 wk	45	75	97	86	95	93
Hemoaccess grafts at						
2 wk	57	76	83	73	86	81
12 wk	40	69	96	92	82	88
All sites at						
2 wk	113	74	90	74	90	86
12 wk	85	71	97	89	89	89

* Determined by dividing the number of disincorporated grafts with cultures positive for bacteria by the total number of culture-positive grafts (at 2 weeks. 23/31; at 12 weeks, 17/24).

† Determined by dividing the number of incorporated grafts with cultures negative for bacteria by the total number of culture-negative grafts (at 2 weeks, 74/82; at 12 weeks, 59/61).

‡Determined by dividing the number of disincorporated grafts with cultures positive for bacteria by the total number of disincorporated grafts (at 2 weeks, 23/31; at 12 weeks, 17/19).

§Determined by dividing the number of incorporated grafts with cultures negative for bacteria by the total number of incorporated grafts (at 2 weeks, 74/82; at 12 weeks, 59/66).

‖ Determined by dividing the sum of disincorporated grafts with cultures positive for bacteria and incorporated grafts with cultures negative for bacteria by the total number of graft samples (at 2 weeks. [23 + 71]/113; at 12 weeks, [17 + 59]/85).

(Courtesy of Padberg FT Jr, Smith SM, Eng RHK: Accuracy of disincorporation for identification of vascular graft infection. *Arch Surg* 130:183–187, 1995. Copyright 1994/95, American Heart Association.)

Conclusions.—In vascular graft prostheses, the surgical finding of incorporation or disincorporation accurately predicts the bacterial culture
results in 89% of sites. The finding of disincorporation is associated with
the presence of bacteria in 71% of cases. When incorporation is present,
the presence of bacteria is reliably excluded in 97% of cases.

▶ This experienced clinical surgeon makes the interesting observation that
the presence of a positive bacterial growth around a graft being remotely
removed from patients can be predicted by whether the graft is well incorporated into surrounding tissue. Bacteria grew in 23 of 31 disincorporated
grafts and in 8 of 82 well-incorporated grafts. Thus, the surgical finding of
graft disincorporation accurately predicts culture report in 89% of patients.
I find this report fascinating and doubtless true. It is noted that most positive
cultures grew *Staphylococcus*.

Selective Preservation of Infected Prosthetic Arterial Grafts: Analysis of a 20-Year Experience With 120 Extracavitary-Infected Grafts

Calligaro KD, Veith FJ, Schwartz ML, Goldsmith J, Savarese RP, Dougherty
MJ, DeLaurentis DA (Montefiore Med Ctr/Albert Einstein School of Medi-
cine, New York; Thomas Jefferson Univ, Philadelphia)
Ann Surg 220:461–471, 1994   145-96-13-17

Objective.—Experience with infected prosthetic arterial grafts was reviewed in 120 patients seen over 20 years, during which time an attempt

was made—where appropriate—to salvage all or at least part of the graft. Ninety-five patients had polytetrafluoroethylene grafts, and 25 had Dacron grafts.

Management.—In 20 patients with arterial bleeding and 6 with systemic sepsis, grafts were immediately removed. In 43 patients whose infected grafts were occluded, the graft was subtotally excised, leaving a 2- to 3-mm remnant that was oversewn. In 51 cases an attempt was made to preserve all the graft. Wounds were débrided aggressively and as often as necessary for the wound to heal. When revascularization was necessary, the preferred approach was to tunnel a secondary bypass through uninfected tissue, often routing it laterally. The average follow-up was 3 years.

Results.—The hospital mortality rate was 12%, and amputation was necessary in 13% of surviving patients. Only 4% of patients in whom complete graft preservation was possible required amputation, and the long-term success rate in these patients was 71%. The only wound isolate that significantly compromised the results was *Pseudomonas*. Partial graft preservation was successful in 85% of surviving patients whose grafts were occluded.

Conclusion.—In patients with infected prosthetic arterial grafts, a policy of selective partial or complete graft preservation is preferable to routinely removing all the graft.

▶ The controversial aspect of this paper involves the 51 patients in whom total graft preservation was attempted with local wound care. These patients initially were seen with simply an exposed graft, no sepsis, and anastomoses intact with no bleeding. Even with this relatively favorable clinical presentation, a bad outcome (death, amputation, bleeding, nonhealing wound, or recurrent infection) occurred in approximately 40% of patients. I fail to understand how the authors can conclude that this is a "better method" of management.—R. Yeager, M.D.

▶ Amen.—J.M. Porter, M.D.

Call Mosby Document Express at **1 (800) 55-MOSBY** to obtain copies of the original source documents of articles featured or referenced in the YEAR BOOK series.

14 Vascular Trauma

Carotid

The Spectrum of Blunt Injury to the Carotid Artery: A Multicenter Perspective

Cogbill TH, Moore EE, Meissner M, Fischer RP, Hoyt DB, Morris JA, Shackford SR, Wallace JR, Ross SE, Ochsner MG, Sugerman HJ, Lambert PJ, Moore FA, Jurkovich GJ, Cocanour CS, Potenza B, Chang MC, Trevasani GT, Aprahamian C, Frankel HL (Gundersen/Lutheran Med Ctr, La Crosse, Wis; Denver General Hosp; Univ of Colorado, Denver; et al)
J Trauma 37:473–479, 1994   145-96-14-1

Introduction.—Blunt trauma to the carotid artery frequently results in death or permanent neurologic impairment. Because this injury is rare, few comprehensive studies have been done on its clinical presentation, treatment, and outcome. Patients were stratified by type of arterial injury, and guidelines for evaluation and management were established.

Methods.—Inpatient hospital records from 11 institutions across the country were retrospectively reviewed for carotid artery injuries from blunt trauma that occurred from January 1987 through December 1992. Available outpatient records were also examined for long-term follow-up. Neurologic function was classified as good, moderate impairment, or severe impairment.

Results.—Sixty carotid artery injuries were identified in 49 patients during the 6-year study. The median age of the group was 33 years; 63% of patients were male. Motor vehicle crashes caused injury in 72% of the

TABLE 1.—Outcome Stratified by Type of Arterial Injury

	Number of Patients	Mortality	Number with Good Neurological Outcome
Arterial Dissection*	25	2 (8%)	16 (64%)
Arterial Thrombosis	20	8 (40%)	6 (30%)
Pseudoaneurysm*	11	1 (9%)	7 (64%)
Disruption	7	7 (100%)	0 (0%)
Carotid-Cavernous Fistula	3	0 (0%)	3 (100%)

* Pseudoaneurysm with concomitant arterial dissection occurred in 6 instances.
(Courtesy of Cogbill TH, Moore EE, Meissner M, et al: The spectrum of blunt injury to the carotid artery: A multicenter perspective. *J Trauma* 37:473–479, 1994.)

TABLE 2.—Treatment Modalities Used to Manage 60 Carotid Artery Injuries From Blunt Mechanisms

	Arterial Thrombosis	Arterial Dissection	Dissection with Pseudoaneurysm	Pseudoaneurysm	Arterial Disruption	Carotid-Cavernous Fistula	Total
Anticoagulation	5	9	2	0	0	0	16
Surgical Repair/Graft	1	3	4	2	0	0	10
Surgical Ligation	2	0	0	1	0	0	3
Balloon Occlusion	1	1	0	0	0	3	5
None	11	6	0	2	7	0	26
Total	20	19	6	5	7	3	60

(Courtesy of Cogbill TH, Moore EE, Meissner M, et al: The spectrum of blunt injury to the carotid artery: A multicenter perspective. *J Trauma* 37:473–479, 1994.)

patients. Associated injuries were common and included craniocerebral trauma in 24 patients and facial fractures in 17. The admission Glasgow Coma Score was greater than or equal to 13 in 24 patients and less than or equal to 7 in 18. Twenty-four patients had a normal initial neurologic examination, but 14 showed significant neurologic deficits more than 12 hours after admission. Angiography confirmed the diagnosis in 42 patients. The most common types of arterial injury were arterial dissection and arterial thrombosis (Table 1). All but 4 patients had CT of the head at admission; results were normal in 39%. Various treatments were used: anticoagulation, surgical repair/graft, surgical ligation, and balloon occlusion (Table 2). Sixteen patients died, 13 as a direct result of the carotid artery injury. Only 6 of 12 surviving patients in the arterial thrombosis group achieved a good neurologic outcome. Six patients with complete arterial disruption died before any treatment could be administered. Among the 33 survivors, 22 had good functional neurologic outcome; 7 had moderate neurologic deficits, including monoplegia and hemiplegia; and 4 had to be institutionalized because of severe neurologic disability.

Conclusion.—Blunt injury to the carotid artery has diverse manifestations. Early diagnosis and stratification of injuries by type, location, and neurologic presentation are essential to the development of a successful treatment strategy. Anticoagulation can be used effectively in cases of dissection without complete occlusion and balloon occlusion for carotid-cavernous fistulas. A high level of suspicion for carotid injury is required because neurologic symptoms may be delayed.

▶ During a 6-year period, only 60 blunt injuries to the carotid arteries in 49 patients were recognized at 11 major trauma institutions. As one may suspect, most involved motor vehicle accidents. Both arteriography and duplex ultrasound appeared equally accurate in diagnosis. Arterial injuries included thrombosis, arterial dissection, pseudoaneurysm, arterial disruption, and arteriovenous fistula. Both thrombosis and dissection were primarily managed with supportive therapy only without surgery. The overall mortality rate was 33%, with a good neurologic outcome in only 45% of patients. On balance, although there is nothing new in this article, it does describe a current experience and again emphasizes that in blunt carotid injury, neurologic symptoms may develop in a delayed fashion, typically within 12 hours. The authors suggest that in asymptomatic patients, we should have a high index of clinical suspicion based on a careful reconstruction of injury mechanisms. This suggestion appears a bit gratuitous to me, although a more liberal use of carotid duplex in neurologically normal patients after blunt injuries should be considered. I find nothing in this article that is going to change practice patterns.

Physical Examination Alone is Safe and Accurate for Evaluation of Vascular Injuries in Penetrating Zone II Neck Trauma
Atteberry LR, Dennis JW, Menawat SS, Frykberg ER (Univ of Florida Health Science Ctr, Jacksonville)
J Am Coll Surg 179:657–662, 1994   145-96-14–2

Background.—Evidence from past studies suggests that in patients with penetrating injuries of zone II of the neck, physical examination by itself may detect significant vascular injuries as accurately as angiography. This prospective study attempted to validate physical examination for planning management in 66 patients with penetrating neck injuries seen consecutively in a 22-month period.

Methods.—Angiography was not done if an injury was in zone II and definite signs of vascular damage (active bleeding, an expanding hematoma or one larger than 10 cm, a bruit or thrill, neurologic deficit) were lacking. Patients were observed for at least 23 hours. In the first year, the carotid artery was examined ultrasonographically within 48 hours of admission.

Results.—Two of the 36 patients entering the study had débridement and closure of a large laceration. Six other patients had arteriography because (1) the area of the vertebral arteries was injured; (2) zone I or zone III was involved; or (3) suggestive but not definite signs of vascular injury were present. All studies were negative. None of the remaining 28 patients had any evidence of vascular injury during an average follow-up of 1.8 months. None of the 18 carotid ultrasound studies showed an injury necessitating surgical repair.

Conclusion.—Patients with penetrating zone II neck injuries who have no definite signs of vascular injury may be safely managed without arteriography or even ultrasound imaging.

▶ In many trauma centers, there is a major move away from routine arteriography because of proximity injury. Definite signs of a cervical vascular injury include bleeding, expanding hematoma, large hematoma, thrill, or neurologic deficit. According to the authors, patients with penetrating injury in zone II and no sign of vascular injury can be safely managed without either arteriography or ultrasonography. The Jacksonville Trauma Center has a policy of a similar management for extremity injuries that appears to work well (1).

Reference

1. 1993 YEAR BOOK OF VASCULAR SURGERY, p 338.

Carotid Artery Trauma: A Review of Contemporary Trauma Center Experiences

Ramadan F, Rutledge R, Oller D, Howell P, Baker C, Keagy B (Univ of North Carolina, Chapel Hill)
J Vasc Surg 21:46–56, 1995   145-96-14-3

Objective.—In an attempt to resolve some of the issues regarding the optimal management of carotid artery injuries and their outcome, 82 patients with an injured common or internal carotid artery were reviewed. *Results.*—Mortality was 17% in this series, and 28% of the patients had a stroke. Half the patients who were admitted in a comatose state and 41% of those in shock died. Twenty-one percent of patients with internal carotid injuries and 11% of those with common carotid injuries died. The respective stroke rates were 41% and 11%. Patients with blunt injuries were much more likely to have a stroke than those with penetrating injuries (56% vs. 15%) but they were less likely to die (7% vs. 22%). Neither a compromised airway nor the presence of other injuries worsened the prognosis. Surgical repair and percutaneous balloon occlusion were associated with the best survival rate and the best functional outcomes (table). *Conclusion.*—Injured carotid arteries should be reconstructed when possible. Ligation is indicated only as a last resort to save a patient's life. Repair may be feasible even in the presence of shock and neurologic impairment.

▶ In this paper, a statewide computerized trauma registry was used to identify 82 patients with carotid artery injuries over almost 6 years. Overall, this paper presents a somber picture of the outcome of carotid artery trauma. The authors recommend operative repair, but the database is weak.

Outcome Based on Admission Neurologic Status and Therapeutic Intervention

Treatment group	Neuro status	No.	Alive & well No.	Alive & well %	Permanent deficit No.	Permanent deficit %	Dead No.	Dead %
No operation	Coma	6	1	17	1	17	4	66
	Neuro deficit	4	0	0	4	100	0	0
	Intact	17	7	41	7	41	3	18
Ligation	Coma	7	3	43	0	0	4	57
	Neuro deficit	1	0	0	0	0	1	100
	Intact	6	3	50	3	50	0	0
Repair	Coma	6	2	34	2	33	2	33
	Neuro deficit	5	2	40	3	60	0	0
	Intact	24	22	92	2	8	0	0
Balloon	Coma	1	0	0	1	100	0	0
	Neuro deficit	0	0	0	0	0	0	0
	Intact	5	5	100	0	0	0	0
Total patients		82	45	55	23	28	14	17

(Courtesy of Ramadan F, Rutledge R, Oller D, et al: Carotid artery trauma: A review of contemporary trauma center experiences. *J Vasc Surg* 21:46–56, 1995.)

Blunt Trauma Injuries of the Internal Carotid Artery
Ortega AE, Yellin AE, Weaver FA (Univ of Southern Calif, Los Angeles)
Contemp Surg 46:26–29, 1995   145-96-14–4

Background.—Blunt trauma of the internal carotid artery (ICA) typically results from nonspecific injury to the head or neck. Often, no distinctive neurologic findings are seen at the outset. Such findings may appear acutely months after the injury, and many physicians have questioned whether arterial reconstruction is advisable in this setting.

Clinical Experience.—In the years 1976–1993, 5 patients were seen with ICA injury after blunt trauma. In 3 patients, the initial neurologic findings were normal but a deficit later developed (table). All patients were managed without surgery, but only 1 was given anticoagulants. Three of the 5 patients were discharged with a marked residual neurologic deficit.

Case Report.—Man, 26 (patient 3), received a blow to the back of his head and awoke the next morning with numbness on his left side. Assessment elsewhere revealed hypertension and hemiparesis. A cranial CT study reportedly was negative. Left hemiparesis was accompanied by left-sided facial weakness. Angiography showed bilateral ICA dissections starting at the bifurcation. Prograde blood flow continued in a narrowed stringlike lumen. Heparin was given intravenously. The patient improved somewhat, but in the following days, permanent hemiplegia developed. He could walk when seen 2 years later but required a brace on his left leg and had only minimal use of his left arm.

Conclusion.—Most blunt injuries of the ICA are best managed without surgery. Surgery may be considered if the ICA is patent but narrowed and an unstable neurologic deficit is present. Arterial reconstruction occasionally may be the only hope if the ICA is occluded and there is a profound deficit.

▶ Three of 5 patients with blunt trauma causing injury to the carotid artery were neurologically intact immediately after injury. Carotid dissection after intimal disruption as a direct result of trauma was the most frequent injury mechanism encountered. These physicians believe that mandibular fracture should alert one to the possibility of ICA injury. Anticoagulation is favored in selected patients. On balance, this group of papers (Abstracts 145-96-14–1 to 145-96-14–4) leads me to conclude that we are not very good at early diagnosis of blunt injuries to the carotid artery. A significant number of patients with severe carotid injury caused by blunt trauma have periods of neurologic normality, which divert suspicion, and when symptoms do occur, the role of surgery is unclear. I wish I knew more about this condition. See also the commentary for Abstract 145-96-14–1.

Blunt Trauma Injuries of the Internal Carotid Artery (ICA)

Patient	Age	Sex	Injury	Neurologic Status — Initial	Normal Interval Hours	Late	Diagnostic Test — CT	Angiogram	Treatment	Outcome
1	23	M	MVA	Confusion Dysconjugate gaze	0	Intact	—	ICA DIS	Nonop	Intact
2	20	F	MVA	Intact	33	HPS	NL	ICA DIS / ICA PT	Nonop	Intact
3	26	M	Blow	Intact	24	HPS	NL	ICA DIS, BIL / ICA PT	Nonop ACG	HPS
4	53	M	MVA	Intact	5	HPG	NL	ICA DIS / ICA PT	Nonop	HPG
5	28	F	MVA	Comatose	24	HPS	INF	ICA DIS / ICA PT	Nonop	HPS

Abbreviations: MVA, motor vehicle accident; DIS, dissection; PT, patent; BIL, bilateral; HPS, hemiparesis; HPG, hemiplegia; *nonop*, nonoperative; ACG, anticoagulation; NL, normal; INF, infarct.

(Courtesy of Ortega AE, Yellin AE, Weaver FA: Blunt trauma injuries of the internal carotid artery. *Contemp Surg* 46:26–29, 1995.)

Upper Extremity Trauma

Blunt Injury to the Subclavian or Axillary Artery

Prêtre R, Hoffmeyer P, Bednarkiewicz M, Kursteiner K, Faidutti B (Hôpital Cantonal Univ, Geneva)
J Am Coll Surg 179:295–298, 1994   145-96-14–5

Objective.—Management and outcome were analyzed in a series of 15 consecutive patients seen from 1988 to 1992 with blunt injuries of the subclavian or axillary artery.

Patients.—Twelve men and 3 women aged 17 to 85 years were seen. Ten of them had multiple injuries, and 6 were in shock when admitted. Arterial bleeding was a significant component of shock in 3 patients. Ten patients had obvious ischemic changes in the upper extremity.

Management and Outcome.—Two patients died of associated injuries. Two patients who had extensive tissue destruction underwent immediate amputation. Five patients lived but had a denervated extremity as a consequence of brachial plexus damage. Only 1 of these patients had a potentially reversible lesion. In 3 patients, the arterial injuries were sutured; 7 had grafting (6 by autologous vein and 1 by prosthesis); and 2 had intimal flap resection. In 3 patients with extensive damage, the artery was ligated. Ten of 11 repaired arteries remained patent after a median follow-up of 30 months. Only 1 of 7 patients who required amputation or had a denervated limb could resume working at the same job.

Conclusions.—Blunt injuries of the subclavian and axillary arteries entail significant morbidity and may be fatal. For patients who survive, brachial plexus lesions frequently result in severe disability.

▶ There is little that is new in this pedestrian review, but it again confirms that a significant number of patients with blunt injury to the arteries of the upper extremity have severe associated brachial plexus injury. In my opinion, severe neurologic injury should lead to serious consideration of immediate arm amputation, despite the obvious repairability of the arterial injury. For many of these unfortunate patients, the painful denervated extremity becomes the total focus of their lives and deprives them of the opportunity for real rehabilitation. Early amputation and vigorous rehabilitation in these patients, in my opinion, gives them the greatest opportunity of continued function, although with significant disability.

Brachial Artery Compression by the Lacertus Fibrosus

Bassett FH III, Spinner RJ, Schroeter TA (Duke Univ, Durham, NC)
Clin Orthop 307:110–116, 1994   145-96-14–6

Series.—Five patients had classic findings of compression of the brachial artery at the level of the elbow by the lacertus fibrosus, or bicipital aponeurosis. The patients, all males, were 17–36 years of age.

Clinical Findings.—All patients had findings of intermittent claudication, including pallor of the hand, paresthesias in the fingertips, crampy pain in the foream and anteromedial aspect of the elbow, and easy fatigability. The symptoms were worsened by raising the hand overhead or pronating the forearm. No patient had a history of trauma. The forearm muscles appeared hypertrophic. Resisted elbow flexion or pronation of the forearm obliterated the radial pulse and also reproduced the symptoms. The pulse deficit was confirmed by Doppler study. Two patients also had findings of ulnar neuropathy at the elbow.

Management.—Surgery was performed after conservative measures had failed. Four patients had surgery with the use of local anesthesia. An incision in the antecubital fossa revealed a tight lacertus fibrosus indenting the brachial artery. The structure was fully released and partially excised. In 1 patient with co-existing ulnar neuropathy, the nerve was transposed subcutaneously.

Results.—Four of the patients were dramatically relieved of symptoms and could resume their normal work and athletic activities within 3 weeks. One patient subsequently had ulnar nerve decompression but continued to have symptoms of brachial artery compression. One patient had symptoms of musculocutaneous nerve entrapment and did well after decompression.

Conclusion.—Hypertrophy of the elbow muscles and lacertus fibrosus from excessive use may produce vascular, neural, or combined neurovascular lesions.

▶ I always have a healthy suspicion of newly described syndromes in my field that I have never before encountered. Dr. Bassett is an eminent orthopedic surgeon but, like other orthopedic surgeons, probably knows little about arterial disease. He describes 5 male patients with a diagnosis of what he terms intermittent claudication of the upper extremity, from which I presume he means these patients must routinely walk on their hands. The exacerbation of symptoms by elevating the arms over the head is especially worrisome because this is known to normally occlude the subclavian artery in many patients. Both elbow flexion and forearm pronation obliterated the radial pulse in these patients. Confusingly, several of these patients had co-existent ulnar neuropathy at the elbow. In am disturbed to find no report of any arteriography in any patient. Resection of the lacertus fibrosus with variable repair of the ulnar nerve produced a dramatic result in all patients. I await confirmation of this syndrome before accepting it as gospel.

Trauma and Deep Venous Thrombosis

Prevention of Venous Thromboembolism in Trauma Patients
Knudson MM, Lewis FR, Clinton A, Atkinson K, Megerman J (Univ of California, San Francisco; Henry Ford Hosp, Detroit; Kendall Healthcare Products Co, Mansfield, Mass)
J Trauma 37:480–487, 1994   145-96-14–7

Objective.—Thromboembolic complications are common among patients with trauma. There are no established methods for preventing venous thromboembolism for this heterogeneous group of patients. Two standard methods of prophylaxis against deep venous thrombosis (DVT) were prospectively compared in a group of patients with trauma.

Methods.—Four hundred patients with trauma were classified into 3 groups according to their injuries. Patients in each group were then randomly assigned to a method of treatment. Those in group I received either sequential gradient pneumatic leg compression (SCD), low-dose subcutaneous heparin, or control treatment; those in group II received either heparin or control treatment; and those in group III received either SCD or control treatment. At admission and every week thereafter, the patients underwent venous duplex ultrasound scanning.

Results.—Two hundred fifty-one patients completed the study. Venous thrombosis of the lower extremity occurred in 15 patients, for a rate of 6%. Another 2 patients had pulmonary embolism, 1 of whom died. Immobilization for more than 3 days, age of 30 years or older, and the presence of pelvic or lower extremity fractures were all significant risk factors for the development of thromboembolism. Within group III— which comprised patients with neurotrauma who could not receive heparin—SCD was more effective than control treatment in the prevention of DVT. For the other groups, protection was not conferred by either heparin or SCD; however, ultrasound surveillance permitted prompt recognition and treatment of occult DVT.

Conclusions.—Risk factors that increase the risk for thromboembolic complications in patients with trauma have been identified. Serial venous duplex ultrasound scanning is useful in high-risk patients because it can identify clinically silent DVT. However, no method of prophylaxis is established as ideal for each individual patient with trauma.

▶ Just how important is venous thrombosis in patients with trauma? Certainly it occurs, but does it do so at a rate more like 6% or 60%? The literature on this subject is confusing. In this very nice study from San Francisco, 251 patients with trauma were randomly assigned to various prophylactic measures and were screened with routine venous duplex examinations. Fifteen patients (6% of total) had DVT develop with the usual risk factors. Interestingly, perhaps because of the small number of positive results, neither heparin nor sequential compression appeared to offer protection against DVT in most patients. I hope the results represent a type II error based on a small number of positive patients. On the other hand, the finding that only 6% of patients had DVT develop is quite important by itself.

Surgical Prophylaxis for Pulmonary Embolism
Leach TA, Pastena JA, Swan KG, Tikellis JI, Blackwood JM, Odom JW (Univ of Medicine and Dentistry of New Jersey, Newark)
Am Surg 60:292–295, 1994   145-96-14–8

Background.—Patients who have multiple trauma are at particular risk for developing fatal pulmonary embolism. Eleven such deaths occurred in a single year at 1 center. It usually is not feasible to give patients with trauma prophylactic anticoagulation, and injuries such as long bone fractures may preclude pneumatic compression.

Objective.—A protocol was developed so that trauma victims considered to be at high risk for pulmonary embolism could undergo placement of an inferior vena cava filter on a prophylactic basis.

Results.—A total of 205 Greenfield filters have been inserted in 201 patients since 1986, all but 5 of them prophylactically. No patients died after placement, and morbidity was slight. No patient with a filter in place died of pulmonary embolism, but 4 patients died of this cause before a filter could be inserted (table).

Conclusion.—Patients with trauma who are at risk for pulmonary embolism should have a vena caval filter inserted prophylactically as soon as possible after being admitted.

▶ Based on the observation of a large number of fatal pulmonary emboli on a level I trauma service, these investigators developed a protocol for prophylactic inferior vena cava filter placement in high-risk patients with trauma. During the past 9 years they have installed 205 prophylactic Greenfield filters with no mortality and minimal morbidity. No patient with a Greenfield filter sustained a fatal pulmonary embolism, leading the authors to tout the merits of prophylactic filtration. I do not agree with this. The vagaries of filter insertion appear to afford many patients suboptimal protection, and filter complications, including cardiac migration, continue to occur. It is a shame these authors did not conduct a randomized study. As it is, this is only anecdotal and, in my opinion, sends the wrong message.

Prospectus for Pulmonary Emboli (PE) and Associated Fatal Complications During the Periods in the Study

Year	1985–1986	1986–1992
Admissions	1257	10,948
At risk for P.E.	350	3130
High risk for P.E.	28	201*
Fatal P.E.	11	4†

* Greenfield filters were inserted into these special high-risk patients.
† These patients died before Greenfield filters could be inserted.
(Courtesy of Leach TA, Pastena JA, Swan KG, et al: Surgical prophylaxis for pulmonary embolism. *Am Surg* 60:292–295, 1994.)

Surveillance Venous Scans for Deep Venous Thrombosis in Multiple Trauma Patients

Meyer CS, Blebea J, Davis K Jr, Fowl RJ, Kempczinski RF (Univ of Cincinnati, Ohio)

Ann Vasc Surg 9:109–114, 1995   145-96-14–9

Background.—About 40% of patients with multisystemic trauma reportedly develop deep venous thrombosis (DVT) in the lower extremity. The estimated risk for associated pulmonary embolism is approximately 10%.

Methods.—The findings on surveillance venous duplex scanning of the lower extremities were reviewed in 183 patients with multiple injuries, 122 men and 61 women (average age, 38 years), who were admitted to the ICU and had a total of 261 scans. All patients received prophylaxis against DVT by either pneumatic compression of the lower extremities or subcutaneous heparin.

Results.—Most patients had blunt injuries. Nearly two thirds of them lacked symptoms suggestive of DVT. Six percent of the 261 venous scans were positive for DVT in the proximal region of the lower extremity, and 2% showed a thrombus in the calf veins (table). In one third of the cases, the thrombus extended to more than 1 anatomical site. Symptomatic patients were more likely than those without symptoms to have proximal thrombosis, as were patients with spinal injury.

Cost-Effectiveness.—The per-case cost of identifying proximal DVT was $6,688. Routine surveillance scanning of all patients with trauma admitted to the surgical ICU would cost $300 million annually on a national basis. A prospective trial is needed to document the safety and cost of examining only symptomatic or high-risk patients.

▶ These authors state that DVT afflicts patients with trauma at a rate of 42%. I wish those interested in DVT and trauma could agree on a database. All patients admitted to this trauma study underwent DVT prophylaxis and routine venous scans. Six percent of the scans were positive for proximal lower extremity DVT, and 2% showed a thrombus limited to the calf. Patients with spinal injuries had a proximal DVT incidence of only 18%. Interestingly, these investigators conclude that routine DVT surveillance is too expensive to be applied to all patients with trauma. This study suffers from

Deep Venous Thrombosis Location			
	Side		
Venous location	Right	Left	Total
Common femoral	6	6	12
Superficial femoral	5	5	10
Popliteal	1	3	4
Calf	5	6	11
	17	20	

(Courtesy of Meyer CS, Blebea J, Davis K Jr, et al: Surveillance venous scans for deep venous thrombosis in multiple trauma patients. *Ann Vasc Surg* 9:109–114, 1995.)

being retrospective. I find it interesting, but because of its retrospective nature, I attribute little importance to it.

Venous Injury: To Repair or Ligate, the Dilemma Revisited
Timberlake GA, Kerstein MD (Tulane Univ School of Medicine, New Orleans, La)
Am Surg 61:139–145, 1995   145-96-14–10

Objective.—The best method to manage injuries of major veins remains uncertain. Accordingly, management was reviewed in 322 patients with such injuries.

Management.—Eighty-three patients had isolated venous injuries, and two thirds of them had the injured vein ligated (table). Of 239 patients with combined arterial and venous injures, 71% underwent ligation. Vein injuries were repaired by either end-to-end anastomosis or lateral phleborrhaphy. Fasciotomy was performed as indicated. The average follow-up was 32 months.

Results.—No patient with isolated vein injury developed permanent sequelae, but approximately one third developed transient limb edema. Edema also occurred transiently in 36% of the patients with combined arterial and venous injuries and permanently in 4 patients (2%). Whether the injured vein was ligated or repaired did not influence the occurrence of edema. No limb loss followed ligation of an injured vein.

Conclusion.—Ideally, all venous injuries will be repaired but, in the civilian setting, ligation rarely leads to permanent sequelae. Vein ligation, therefore, is acceptable for hemodynamically unstable patients and those with extensive local injury or associated organ injury.

▶ This retrospective review of patients with trauma examines the relative merits of vein injury ligation compared with vein injury repair. These inves-

Method of Treatment and Results in 83 Patients With Isolated Venous Injury

Vein Injured	Treatment Modality*	Adjunctive Fasciotomy	None	Sequelae Transient Edema	Long Term Edema
Popliteal (18)	Ligation (10)	10	3	7	0
	Repair (8)	6	5	3	0
Femoral (45)	Ligation (29)	22	17	12	0
	Repair (16)	2	14	2	0
Iliac (17)	Ligation (12)	3	9	3	0
	Repair (5)	0	4	1	0
IVC (3)	Ligation (3)	0	2	1	0
	Repair (0)	0	0	0	0

* Ligation = 54; 35 with fasciotomy, 23 with transient edema. Repair = 29; 8 with fasciotomy; 3 with transient edema.
Abbreviation: IVC, inferior vena cava.
(Courtesy of Timberlake GA, Kerstein MD: Venous injury: To repair or ligate, the dilemma revisited. *Am Surg* 61:139–145, 1995.)

tigators conclude that vein injury ligation causes no ill effects in most patients. Anyone disagree?

Miscellaneous

Immediate Versus Delayed Fluid Resuscitation for Hypotensive Patients With Penetrating Torso Injuries

Bickell WH, Wall MJ Jr, Pepe PE, Martin RR, Ginger VF, Allen MK, Mattox KL (Saint Francis Hosp, Tulsa, Okla; Baylor College of Medicine, Houston; City of Houston Emergency Med Services; et al)

N Engl J Med 331:1105–1109, 1994   145-96-14–11

Introduction.—Hypotensive trauma victims have routinely received isotonic fluids intravenously before having surgery, but there has been concern that this practice may have adverse effects if applied before bleeding is controlled.

Objective.—The effects of delaying fluid resuscitation until surgery were studied in a prospective series of 598 patients aged 16 years and older who had penetrating torso injuries and a prehospital systolic blood pressure of 90 mm Hg or less. The patients underwent thoracotomy, laparotomy, neck exploration, or groin exploration.

Management.—Patients either received Ringer's acetate solution starting before admission to the hospital or were given no fluid other than that needed to keep the line open before surgery. After induction of anesthesia, all patients received crystalloid and packed red blood cells as needed to maintain a systolic arterial pressure of 100 mm Hg, a hematocrit of 25% or greater, and a urine output of at least 50 mL/hr.

Results.—In the prehospital phase, the 309 patients assigned to immediate fluid resuscitation received an average of 870 mL of isotonic solution, whereas the 289 in the delayed resuscitation group received 92 mL. The 2

Outcome of Patients With Penetrating Torso Injuries, According to Treatment Group

Variable	Immediate Resuscitation	Delayed Resuscitation	P Value
Survival to discharge — no. of patients/total patients (%)	193/309 (62)*	203/289 (70)†	0.04
Estimated intraoperative blood loss — mL‡	3127 ± 4937	2555 ± 3546	0.11
Length of hospital stay — days§	14 ± 24	11 ± 19	0.006
Length of ICU stay — days§	8 ± 16	7 ± 11	0.30

* Ninety-five percent confidence interval, 57% to 68%.
† Ninety-five percent confidence interval, 65% to 75%.
‡ The estimated intraoperative blood loss was calculated for patients who survived the operation: 268 in the immediate-resuscitation group and 260 in the delayed-resuscitation group.
§ The lengths of stay in the hospital and ICU were calculated for patients who survived the operation: 227 in the immediate-resuscitation group and 238 in the delayed-resuscitation group.
(Reprinted by permission of Bickell WH, Wall MJ Jr, Pepe PE, et al: Immediate versus delayed fluid resuscitation for hypotensive patients with penetrating torso injuries. *N Engl J Med* 331:1105–1109, 1994. Copyright 1994, Massachusetts Medical Society.)

groups received similar amounts of Ringer's acetate and hetastarch during surgery. The survival rate was 70% in the delayed resuscitation group and 62% in patients who were immediately resuscitated, a significant difference (table). The intraoperative blood losses were similar in the 2 groups, and the complication rates did not substantially differ. The difference in survival persisted after adjustment for prehospital and trauma-center intervals.

Implication.—These results call into question the traditional practice of aggressive preoperative fluid resuscitation in hypotensive trauma victims. It is not the value of the fluid resuscitation itself that is being questioned but, rather, the appropriate timing and extent of treatment.

▶ I think it is always great fun to see a successful challenge mounted to surgical dogma, or, as my friend Jack Collin would say, received wisdom. This prospective trial was conducted to determine the effects of delaying fluid resuscitation until the time of operative intervention in patients with hypotension with penetrating injuries to the trunk. Although one always has to be concerned that the 2 randomly assigned groups were truly comparable, the conclusions are clear: Delay of aggressive fluid resuscitation until operative intervention improves outcome. I consider this to be important new information that everyone caring for patients with trauma should carefully consider.

Contemporary Management Strategy for Major Inferior Vena Caval Injuries
Klein SR, Baumgartner FJ, Bongard FS (Harbor-Univ of California, Los Angeles, Torrance)
J Trauma 37:35–42, 1994   145-96-14-12

Background.—Injuries to the inferior vena cava (IVC) are potentially fatal and necessitate immediate and definitive management. An 8-year experience with IVC trauma was reviewed, with emphasis placed on identifying the factors related to survival.

Patients.—The experience included 38 patients. All but 4 were men, and the mean patient age was 30 years. Twenty-four patients were injured by penetrating trauma—16 gunshot wounds and 8 stab wounds—and 14 by blunt trauma. Twenty-one percent died. Although all patients were awake when they came to medical attention, 45% had a systolic blood pressure of less than 90 mm Hg. The mean Injury Severity Score was 27, and all patients were found at laparotomy to have active retroperitoneal bleeding or an expanding hematoma. Twelve patients had retrohepatic caval injuries, 3 of which involved the hepatic veins. Seven had a suprarenal injury, 9 had a pararenal injury, and 10 had an infrarenal injury (table).

Findings.—Five of the 8 patients who died had retrohepatic injuries, 2 had pararenal injuries, and 1 had an infrarenal injury. Thirty-three of the 38 patients had successful surgical repair, 26 by lateral venorrhaphy and 7 by polytetrafluoroethylene patch repair. In 8 of the 12 patients with retrohepatic injuries, a diaphragmatic division was used to gain entry to

Surgical Strategy for Extrahepatic Caval Injury ($n = 26$)

Intervention	Number
Approach	
Laparotomy	24
Laparotomy and right thoracotomy	2
Management	
Total isolation	6
Partial isolation	17
No isolation	3
Repair	
Ligation	1
Simple venorrhaphy	21
Prosthetic repair	4

(Courtesy of Klein SR, Baumgartner FJ, Bongard FS: Contemporary management strategy for major inferior vena caval injuries. *J Trauma* 37:35–42, 1994.)

the right chest. Atrial-caval shunts were used in 2 patients, both of whom lived. Of 20 patients who were reevaluated after at least 3 months, 3 had an occluded IVC and 1 had a disorder similar to the Budd-Chiari syndrome.

Conclusions.—Injuries to the IVC continue to be potentially deadly. They must be treated by prompt volume restoration, a stratified selective management strategy, and prevention of hypothermia. Some patients can be managed by prosthetic IVC reconstruction.

▶ The complexities and hazards of major vena caval injury are nicely reviewed in this paper from Harbor UCLA Medical Center. A survival rate of 79% in these patients is exemplary and points to a very high level of surgical trauma care at this institution. I am impressed by these results.

The Management of Open Fractures Associated With Arterial Injury Requiring Vascular Repair
Seligson D, Ostermann PAW, Henry SL, Wolley T (Univ of Louisville, Ky; Univ of Bochum, Germany)
J Trauma 37:938–940, 1994   145-96-14-13

Introduction.—Open fractures with arterial injury requiring vascular repair are associated with a high rate of amputations, up to 60% or more. The results of treatment of these fractures were evaluated, particularly in terms of the local use of aminoglycoside-laden polymethylmethacrylate (PMMA) bead chains to decrease the rate of infection.

Patients.—Between 1983 and 1992, 72 patients were treated for open fractures associated with arterial injury requiring vascular repair. The fractures involved the humerus in 4 patients, the forearm in 10, the femur in 8, the tibia in 31, the ankle in 10, and the foot in 9.

Treatment.—Fracture management included copious wound irrigation, radical débridement, and fasciotomy. Before vascular repair, fractures were stabilized with external skeletal fixation in 42 patients and with open reduction and internal fixation in 7. Twenty-three patients underwent primary amputation. Primary wound management consisted of open wound care in 26 cases, loose closure in 12, primary closure with free latissimus dorsi transfer in 3, and antibiotic-bead-pouch technique in 31. In addition to systemic antibiotics, 40 patients received implantation of tobramycin-PMMA beads in their wounds. Vascular repair was achieved with direct suture in 41 cases and a venous graft in 8.

Outcome.—Seven secondary amputations were done because of infection or poor revascularization, for an overall amputation rate of 41.6%. The wound infection rate was 13.9%, and the rate of osteomyelitis was 4.2%. The infection rate after primary free flaps was 66.6%. The wound infection rate in wounds implanted with the tobramycin-PMMA beads was significantly reduced to 5% compared with 25% in the wounds not treated with local antibiotic therapy. The rate of osteomyelitis tended to be lower in wounds treated with the bead chains (2.5%) than those without bead chains (6.3%).

Conclusion.—Open fractures with arterial injury requiring vascular repair are critical injuries. Management of these injuries requires a high level of expertise from a team of trauma specialists and should not be relegated to less experienced staff. To reduce the rate of infection, temporary wound coverage with the antibiotic-bead-pouch technique appears to be a better option until the wound can be closed in a sterile and viable environment.

▶ These results are awful. Thirty-two percent of patients underwent primary amputation, and 7 (10%) secondary amputations were done because of infection or poor revascularization; this resulted in an overall amputation rate of 41.6%. The wound infection rate was 14%, and osteomyelitis developed in 4% of patients. Although we have had a more modest experience with open fractures associated with arterial injury, I had not recognized the disastrous results reported in this paper.

Rural Vascular Trauma: A Twenty-Year Review
Humphrey PW, Nichols WK, Silver D (Univ of Missouri, Columbia)
Ann Vasc Surg 8:179–185, 1994   145-96-14–14

Objective.—Two hundred ten patients, mostly from rural areas, who were seen over 2 decades with 248 vascular injuries were reviewed.

Patients and Injuries.—In the years 1970–1983, the interval from injury to treatment averaged 6 hours. In 1983–1990, when nearly half the patients were transported by helicopter, the delay averaged 4 hours. The 41% of patients with blunt injuries were the most severely affected, accounting for 89% of amputations and 80% of deaths. Vessels in the upper extremity were injured in 47% of patients and in the lower limb in 26%. Arterial injury was present in 87% of cases, and major venous injury was present in 13%.

Management and Outcome.—Angiograms were obtained before surgery in 30% of patients. About half the injuries involved direct anastomosis or lateral suture repair (table). In the most recent 10-year period, 6 patients

Vessel Repair		
Type of repair	No.	%
Lateral suture repair/end to end	126	50.8
Autogenous vein graft	40	16.1
Synthetic graft	15	6.0
Ligation	47	19.0
Other (primary amputation, thrombectomy)	20	8.1
Total	248	100

(Courtesy of Humphrey PW, Nichols WK, Silver D: Rural vascular trauma: A twenty-year review. *Ann Vasc Surg* 8:179–185, 1994.)

had major peripheral venous injuries repaired at the same time, with 1 amputation resulting. Mortality was 4.8% overall and 9.3% in patients with blunt injuries. Survival has not improved since the advent of helicopter transport, but the rate of amputation has decreased from 18% to 7%.

▶ I am always suspicious of any paper that contains "in a community hospital" or "in a rural area" in the title. It overwhelmingly suggests to me that we are going to encounter another mundane report from these presumably disadvantaged service areas of results about as good as those from major centers. From the morass of information presented in this article, I can conclude that the limb amputation rate was around 10%, the mortality rate was 4.8%, and a fair number of complications occurred. Although the extraordinary detail presented in unfocused reviews like this one doubtless represents an honest effort on the part of the authors, it presents the reader with an almost impossible task. On balance, I take away absolutely nothing from this article, although I admire the authors' intent in presenting it.

Adverse Outcome of Nonoperative Management of Intimal Injuries Caused by Penetrating Trauma

Tufaro A, Arnold T, Rummel M, Matusmoto T, Kerstein MD (Johns Hopkins Univ, Baltimore; Hahnemann Univ, Philadelphia)
J Vasc Surg 20:656–659, 1994   145-96-14–15

Objective.—The outcome of nonoperative treatment was examined in a 5-year review of 118 patients admitted to 2 level I trauma centers who had "soft" signs of vascular injury. All had isolated penetrating injuries.

Methods.—Sixteen axillary arteries, 31 brachial arteries, 36 common femoral, 22 superficial femoral, and 13 deep femoral arteries were at risk. Angiography showed abnormalities in 23 extremities. Seven patients with presumably minor intimal flap injuries were merely observed, and the remaining patients were explored operatively.

Results.—All but 1 of the 7 observed patients returned with acute pain or paresthesia in the injured extremity. Angiography showed common femoral thrombosis in 2 cases and a superficial femoral artery to superficial femoral vein fistula in 2 others. One patient each had axillary artery thrombosis, a pseudoaneurysm of the brachial artery, and a pseudoaneurysm of the deep femoral artery. All these lesions were repaired surgically. *Conclusion.*—Intimal injuries secondary to penetrating trauma may be less benign than is often assumed, despite the absence of "hard" signs of vascular trauma. More aggressive exploration of these injuries would seem to be warranted.

▶ The detection and management of vascular injury resulting from vascular trauma continue to be debated. Kerstein, Tufaro, and colleagues reviewed 188 patients with "soft signs" of vascular trauma (i.e., "proximity injury") who underwent angiography. Positive results were obtained in about one fifth of cases. Seven patients with "minor" intimal flap were observed, 6 of whom returned with late signs of vascular injury (presumably at the original site) requiring operation. The authors suggest that reports in the trauma literature underestimate the risk for such "minor" injury because of a lack of long-term follow-up. Indeed, their patients had symptoms develop at a mean interval of 19 months after their initial injury. Although this article does not address the indications for angiography or the role of ultrasound in patients with penetrating injury, the results suggest a paraphrase of the adage "if it's broke, fix it!"—J. Ricotta, M.D.

▶ Although we have a numerator, we do not have a denominator. In my opinion, abundant prior publications indicate the safety of following minor intimal injuries. In my opinion, the isolated peculiar results reported in this article do not negate the large amount of published information to the contrary. I shall await further information before changing my mind. See a recent interesting letter about this article (1).—J.M. Porter, M.D.

Reference

1. Dennis JW, et al: *J Vasc Surg* 22:119–120, 1995.

Blunt Pediatric Vascular Trauma: Analysis of Forty-One Consecutive Patients Undergoing Operative Intervention
Fayiga YJ, Valentine RJ, Myers SI, Chervu A, Rossi PJ, Clagett GP (Univ of Texas Southwestern Med Ctr, Dallas)
J Vasc Surg 20:419–425, 1994   145-96-14-16

Background.—Half of all childhood deaths result from trauma, but the contribution of blunt vascular injuries to disability and death in children remains uncertain.

Methods.—Forty-one patients 17 years of age and younger, who were seen in the past 18 years, had surgery for a total of 48 blunt vascular injuries.

Findings.—Seven brachial artery injuries and 1 injury of the superficial femoral artery resulted from orthopedic trauma incurred in a fall. All patients had a pulse deficit and were readily given a diagnosis. All underwent vascular repair and were free of sequelae. The remaining patients included 17 who were injured in a motor vehicle crash, 12 injured in a motor vehicle

Distribution of the 23 Major Intra-Abdominal Vascular Injuries in Patients Sustaining Motor Vehicle Trauma

	MVC	MPC
Aorta	—	—
Inferior vena cava		
Retrohepatic	3	2
Infrarenal	—	4
Iliac		
Artery	1	—
Vein	—	—
Hepatic		
Artery	—	1
Vein	3	2
Portal vein	—	2
Renal vein	2	3
Total	9	14

(Courtesy of Fayiga YJ, Valentine RJ, Myers SI, et al: Blunt pediatric vascular trauma: Analysis of forty-one consecutive patients undergoing operative intervention. *J Vasc Surg* 20:419–425, 1994.)

or pedestrian accident, and 4 with severe crush injuries. Two thirds of these patients were in shock when admitted. Two thirds of the 17 patients with major abdominal vein injuries (table) died. These injuries went unrecognized before laparotomy. Only 3 patients had major abdominal arterial injuries. Three patients had major injuries of thoracic vessels, and 9 had associated injuries to extremity vessels secondary to orthopedic trauma.

Conclusion.—Serious vein injuries are more of a problem than arterial injuries in children who incur blunt abdominal trauma. These injuries are rarely recognized before surgery, and more than half of affected children die. In contrast, blunt arterial injuries secondary to long bone fracture are readily recognized and easily treated.

▶ I suppose we can accept the authors' definition of pediatric as age 17 years and younger, but when I think of some of the teenaged Texans who weigh 250 lb at age 16 years, it does seem to stretch the definition just a bit. The mean age of the patient group was 9.8 years, with 34% 5 years of age or under. Twenty-one major abdominal venous injuries resulted in a 65% mortality. On balance, these were serious injuries with a somber outcome. The authors present a convincing case that torso venous injuries are the most dangerous subdivision of vascular injuries in children.

Computed Tomography as a Screening Exam in Patients With Suspected Blunt Aortic Injury

Durham RM, Zuckerman D, Wolverson M, Heiberg E, Luchtefeld WB, Herr DJ, Shapiro MJ, Mazuski JE, Salimi Z, Sundaram M (St Louis Univ, Mo)
Ann Surg 220:699–704, 1994   145-96-14–17

TABLE 1.—Computed Tomography Signs of Aortic Injury

Discrepancy in size of ascending/descending aorta
False lumen
Thickening of aortic wall
Irregularity of aortic wall
Intraluminal lucency
Periaortic hematoma
Dilation of the aorta at origin of L subclavian
Focal hematoma not adjacent to the aorta
Diffuse mediastinal hematoma
Aortic diameter > 5 cm

(Courtesy of Durham RM, Zuckerman D, Wolverson M, et al: Computed tomography as a screening exam in patients with suspected blunt aortic injury. *Ann Surg* 220:699–704, 1994.)

Background.—As many as 15% of patients who die in motor vehicle accidents may have blunt aortic trauma. Perhaps a third of patients with such injuries reach the hospital, but their subsequent mortality is high. Whether blunt trauma victims should be screened for injury to the thoracic aorta by thoracic CT scanning remains controversial.

Methods.—Both CT and aortography were done in 155 patients who had incurred blunt trauma and were suspected of having aortic injury. The CT scans were reviewed independently by 4 attending radiologists who had no knowledge of the clinical or angiographic findings. Computed tomographic signs of aortic injury are listed in Table 1.

Results.—Eight patients had aortic injuries that necessitated surgical treatment. In 5 of these patients, all reviewers read the CT scans as positive. Excluding poor-quality studies, CT had a sensitivity of 88% and a specificity of 53% in detecting aortic injury (Table 2).

Conclusions.—Because the CT signs of aortic injury are often subtle and because the sensitivity of CT is observer-dependent, CT does not reliably rule out aortic injury. When CT studies are liberally interpreted, the number of aortograms required is not significantly decreased.

▶ The authors' conclusion that CT does not reliably exclude blunt thoracic aortic injury has been previously reported (1). I consider this matter established and am not in need of any additional confirmation.

TABLE 2.—Computed Tomography as a Screening Examination

Radiologist	Sensitivity	Specificity	Positive Predictive Value	Negative Predictive Value
1	100%	42%	9%	100%
2	88%	71%	15%	99%
3	88%	26%	6%	97%
4	63%	73%	12%	97%
Average	85%	53%	11%	98%

(Courtesy of Durham RM, Zuckerman D, Wolverson M, et al: Computed tomography as a screening exam in patients with suspected blunt aortic injury. *Ann Surg* 220:699–704, 1994.)

Reference

1. 1995 YEAR BOOK OF VASCULAR SURGERY, p 371.

Traumatic Rupture of the Thoracic Aorta: Should One Always Operate Immediately?
Maggisano R, Nathens A, Alexandrova NA, Cina C, Boulanger B, McKenzie R, Harrison AW (Univ of Toronto)
Ann Vasc Surg 9:44–52, 1995   145-96-14–18

Background.—The traditional approach to blunt traumatic rupture of the thoracic aorta (TRA) is to operate immediately, but a policy of selective delayed repair might make sense, especially for patients who also have head trauma or have cardiac dysfunction or respiratory failure.

Objective.—Selective repair was evaluated in a series of 59 consecutive patients admitted to a regional trauma unit with TRA at the aortic isthmus.

Management.—Twelve patients (group I) either arrived at the unit in extremis or rapidly became unstable while being triaged. Three patients (group II) had no contraindications to early repair and underwent repair after TRA was diagnosed. The remaining 44 patients (group III) required intensive care because of concomitant injuries (Table 1) or sepsis, and operative repair was delayed or not performed.

Results.—In group III cases, repair was delayed for 1 day to 7 months. Eight patients have not yet undergone repair and remain well after 1–4 years. Overall survival was 17% in group I, 100% in group II, and 82% in group III. Three deaths in group III were related to surgery. Only 2 group III patients (4.5%) died of aortic rupture within 3 days of admission.

Conclusions.—Most patients with TRA who survive to be admitted have multisystem injuries and may undergo repair on a delayed basis with a low risk for aortic rupture. Contraindications to immediate repair are listed in Table 2.

TABLE 1.—Associated Injuries in Group III

Injury	%
Pulmonary	75
Major orthopedic	72
Central nervous system	66
Rib fractures	52
Pneumothorax/hemothorax	30
Spleen	30
Liver	25
Myocardial contusion	25
Diaphragmatic rupture	14
Bladder rupture	5

(Courtesy of Maggisano R, Nathens A, Alexandrova NA, et al: Traumatic rupture of the thoracic aorta: Should one always operate immediately? *Ann Vasc Surg* 9:44–52, 1995.)

TABLE 2.—Contraindications to Surgical Repair,
Sunnybrook Health Science Centre, May 1993

Central nervous system
  Glasgow coma motor score of <6 within 10 days of
  injury
  CT scan of the head demonstrating hemorrhage
Respiratory
  Pao$_2$/Fio$_2$ < 200
  Inability to tolerate collapse of the left lung
Cardiovascular system
  Inotropic support required
Coagulation
  PT, PTT > 1.5 times normal despite factor replacement

Abbreviations: PT, prothrombin time; *PTT,* partial thromboplastin time;
Pao$_2$/Fio$_2$, partial pressure of oxygen in arterial blood/forced inspiratory
oxygen.
(Courtesy of Maggisano R, Nathens A, Alexandrova NA, et al: Traumatic
rupture of the thoracic aorta: Should one always operate immediately? *Ann
Vasc Surg* 9:44–52, 1995.)

▶ These authors conclude, as have others before them, that patients with contained traumatic rupture of the thoracic aorta and severe associated injuries do not necessarily require immediate aortic repair. They have delayed repair in 44 patients, with an overall survival in these delayed patients of 82%. Two of 44 patients in whom repair was delayed died as a result of ruptured aorta within 72 hours of admission. These authors conclude, and I suspect accurately, that contrary to received wisdom, traumatic rupture of the aorta does not always require immediate operative repair. Selective repair based on the patient's clinical status appears preferable.

Call Mosby Document Express at **1 (800) 55-MOSBY**
to obtain copies of the original source documents of
articles featured or referenced in the YEAR BOOK series.

15 Venous Thrombosis and Pulmonary Embolism

Venous Thrombosis

A Pilot Study of Subcutaneous Recombinant Hirudin (HBW 023) in the Treatment of Deep Vein Thrombosis

Schiele F, Vuillemenot A, Kramarz Ph, Kieffer Y, Soria J, Soria C, Camez A, Mirshahi MC, Bassand JP (Hôpital de l'Hôpital Dieu, Paris; Hôpital Lariboisère, Paris)

Thromb Haemost 71:558–562, 1994   145-96-15–1

Background.—Recombinant hirudin is a pure, specific antithrombin agent that effectively inactivates clot-bound thrombin in vitro and has proved effective in animal models of thrombosis. When used intravenously, however, its short half-life requires constant infusion to ensure stable plasma levels. Recombinant hirudin given subcutaneously twice daily was studied.

Methods.—Ten patients with a recent history of deep venous thrombosis received 0.75 mg of recombinant hirudin per kg of body weight twice daily for 5 days, after which standard heparin and acenocoumarol therapy began. Lower limb venography, pulmonary angiography, ventilation or perfusion lung scanning was done the day before hirudin treatment began and again on day 5. The plasma levels of hirudin and the activated partial thromboplastin time (aPTT) were estimated after the first and tenth injections.

Results.—One patient probably had recurrent pulmonary embolism on day 4 of hirudin treatment, but the other 9 patients remained well. No hemorrhagic complications or other adverse side effects developed. Plasma levels of hirudin peaked 3–4 hours after injection. The values of aPTT paralleled the hirudin level. Levels of thrombin and antithrombin complexes decreased insignificantly during hirudin treatment.

Conclusion.—Subcutaneous injection of hirudin twice daily for 5 days provides stable plasma levels and ensures effective anticoagulation.

▶ Multiple reports in recent editions of the YEAR BOOK have shown increasing interest in the use of hirudin as a specific antithrombin. In this pilot study of 10 patients with deep venous thrombosis treated with hirudin for 5 days, excellent results were obtained. As I have stated on many prior occasions, I suspect we will be using hirudin or some variant as our anticoagulant of choice in preference to heparin.

Femoral Deep Vein Thrombosis Associated With Central Venous Catheterization: Results From a Prospective, Randomized Trial
Trottier SJ, Veremakis C, O'Brien J, Auer AI (St John's Mercy Med Ctr, St Louis, Mo)
Crit Care Med 23:52–59, 1995   145-96-15–2

Objective.—Because critically ill patients often require a central venous catheter, the risk for catheter-induced deep venous thrombosis (DVT) was estimated in a randomized trial enrolling 45 medical or surgical patients in an ICU who required catheterization.

Methods.—The patients were randomly assigned to have a central venous catheter placed in either (1) the subclavian or internal jugular vein or (2) the femoral vein. The veins of the lower extremity were assessed by duplex ultrasound scanning before catheter placement, after the catheter was removed, and again 1 week later.

Results.—None of 21 patients assigned to have a catheter placed in upper access sites had positive ultrasound findings, whereas 25% of the 24 patients assigned to femoral access had DVT (Fig 15–1). Seven patients in the lower access group had nondiagnostic studies. The 2 study groups did not differ with respect to age, duration of catheterization, coagulation values, or measures taken to prevent DVT.

Conclusions.—One fourth of the critically ill patients who were given central venous catheters through the femoral route had DVT in the lower extremity. Duplex ultrasound study is warranted after a femoral vein catheter is removed.

▶ Twenty-five percent of patients with a central venous catheter placed through the femoral vein had lower extremity DVT develop, and an additional significant number had ultrasound abnormalities, possibly indicating DVT. The conclusion that the femoral vein is a poor site for long-term IV catheterization appears inescapable. If this route must be used in an emergency, it should be changed as soon as possible to a more conventional upper extremity setting.

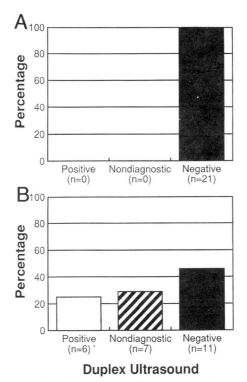

Duplex Ultrasound

Fig 15–1.—Catheter-related femoral deep vein thrombosis results for the upper access group (A) and the lower access group (B). *P = 0.02 by Fisher's exact test. (Courtesy of Trottier SJ, Veremakis C, O'Brien J, et al: Femoral deep vein thrombosis associated with central venous catheterization: Results from a prospective, randomized trial. *Crit Care Med* 23:52–59, 1995.)

Inferior Vena Cava Thrombosis as a Complication of Femoral Vein Catheterisation
Shefler A, Gillis J, Lam A, O'Connell AJ, Schell D, Lammi A (Children's Hosp, Camperdown, Australia)
Arch Dis Child 72:343–345, 1995   145-96-15–3

Background.—In the pediatric ICU, the femoral vein has become a major site for central venous catheterization. Although inferior vena cava (IVC) thrombosis is a known complication of femoral venous catheters, the incidence and evolution of this problem in the pediatric ICU is unknown. This issue was addressed in a prospective study using ultrasonography.

Methods and Results.—Ultrasound examinations of indwelling femoral venous catheters were performed in children in the ICU to assess the frequency and evolution of IVC thrombosis. The analysis included 56 catheters in 54 children. Six cases of IVC thrombosis were identified. Just 1 of the children with ultrasound evidence of IVC thrombosis had clinical signs of this complication. The femoral venous catheter had been in place for more than 6 days in every case of IVC thrombosis.

Conclusions.—Ultrasound identifies the presence of IVC thrombosis in 10% of children in an ICU who have femoral venous catheters. This problem can be avoided by routinely changing the catheters every 6 days or by performing twice-weekly ultrasound studies in patients whose catheters remain in situ for 6 or more days. When IVC thrombosis is detected, the catheter should be changed immediately.

▶ In this study, which is similar to that reported in Abstract 145-96-15–2, 54 children underwent 56 episodes of femoral vein catheterization. All catheters were used for 48 hours or more or were used for hemodialysis. Thrombosis of the IVC was identified sonographically in 6 patients (10.7% of patients with catheters). A general relationship between thrombus formation and duration of catheter use was noted. This information, combined with the information in Abstract 145-96-15–2, suggests that great caution should be used with indwelling femoral vein catheters.

Pulmonary Embolism

Pulmonary Embolism in Patients With Upper Extremity DVT Associated to Venous Central Lines—A Prospective Study

Monreal M, Raventos A, Lerma R, Ruiz J, Lafoz E, Alastrue A, Llamazares JF (Hosp Universitari Germans Trias i Pujol, Badalona, Spain)
Thromb Haemost 72:548–550, 1994   145-96-15–4

Objective.—The risk factors for pulmonary embolism (PE) were examined in a prospective series of 85 consecutive patients in whom deep venous thrombosis (DVT) of the upper extremity was related to the presence of a central venous catheter.

Methods.—All patients received IV heparin when DVT was diagnosed. A ventilation-perfusion lung scan was performed within 24 hours of diagnosis, regardless of whether respiratory symptoms were present.

Results.—Pulmonary embolism was detected in 13 patients. Sixty-six patients had normal lung scans, and 7 others were excluded—6 because of an indeterminate scan and 1 because femoropopliteal thrombosis was also present. Two patients with PE died with recurrent massive embolism despite adequate heparinization. Pulmonary embolism developed in 26% of 38 patients in whom a polyvinyl chloride or polyethylene catheter was present and in 7% of 41 patients with a polyurethane or siliconized catheter.

Conclusions.—Pulmonary embolism is not rare in patients with a central venous catheter who have DVT develop in the upper extremity, even if adequate heparin therapy is provided. One should not rely on clinical signs; only 4 of 13 patients with PE in this series had symptoms. The risk appears to be less with the newer soft catheters.

▶ In this remarkable study, 16.5% of patients with catheter-related upper extremity DVT had significant pulmonary embolism occurring within 48 hours of diagnosis of DVT. Two of these 13 patients died of massive PE. These authors conclude that upper extremity DVT associated with catheters represents a high risk for PE compared with DVT not related to catheters (1). Their second conclusion is that polyurethane or siliconized catheters appear safer than polyvinyl or polyethylene catheters. Currently, when we diagnose a catheter-related upper extremity DVT, we immediately remove the catheter and begin heparin therapy, which is the same treatment used by these authors. I suppose we had better expect about a 15% to 20% incidence of PE with a small incidence of death from PE in these patients. I did not realize PE occurrence was this great.

Reference

1. Monreal M, Ruiz J, Olazabal A, et al: Upper extremity deep venous thrombosis and pulmonary embolism: A prospective study. *Chest* 99:280–283, 1991.

Thrombosis and Embolism in Long-Term Central Venous Access for Parenteral Nutrition
Dollery CM, Sullivan ID, Bauraind O, Bull C, Milla PJ (Hosp for Sick Children, London)
Lancet 344:1043–1045, 1994   145-96-15–5

Introduction.—Silicone catheters are widely used for long-term central venous access for parenteral nutrition. Infection and line-tip thrombosis are well-known complications, but less is known about thromboembolic events. Long-term cyclical parenteral nutrition (CPN) is rare in pediatric practice. The extent of, and factors contributing to, thromboembolic complications in children receiving long-term CPN were studied.

Methods.—Thirty-four children, aged 1 week to 13 years, who received CPN for gut failure for 2 months to 9 years were studied. Eight patients received CPN prepared with heparin, 1 unit/mL. All but 1 patient underwent perfusion scanning with technetium-99, all had echocardiography, and 3 had pulmonary angiography.

Findings.—Ten pulmonary emboli, 5 right atrial thrombi, and 1 superior vena cava obstruction occurred in 12 patients; 4 patients died. At 5 years, the actuarial survival rate free from thrombosis was 53%, and the survival rate free from fatal pulmonary thromboembolic events was 74% (Fig 15–2). Three patients underwent open heart surgery to remove right atrial thrombi or pulmonary emboli. Neither the underlying diagnosis, sepsis, nor hemoconcentration was associated with thrombosis, although thromboembolism tended to occur more frequently in patients with autoimmune enteropathy compared with other diagnoses. The addition of small quantities of heparin to CPN and the osmolarity or lipid content of the CPN did not affect the occurrence of thrombosis.

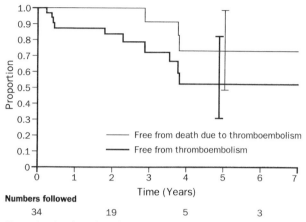

Numbers followed

34   19   5   3

Fig 15-2.—Proportion free from thromboembolism and death from thromboembolism. Estimates of 95% confidence intervals at 5 years are shown. (Courtesy of Dollery CM, Sullivan ID, Bauraind O, et al: Thrombosis and embolism in long-term central venous access for parenteral nutrition. *Lancet* 344:1043–1045, 1994. Copyright 1994, by The Lancet Ltd.)

Conclusion.—Major thrombotic complications in children receiving long-term CPN are more common than previously recognized, and the high prevalence of thrombosis and associated mortality and morbidity suggests the need to re-evaluate current practices of prophylactic anticoagulation. Surveillance for pulmonary embolism may be a useful guide for anticoagulation.

▶ Thirty-four children with gut failure received long-term parenteral nutrition ranging from 2 months to 9 years. Although not stated, I assume all these catheters were in the brachiocephalic veins. This retrospective study undoubtedly suffers from absent data points. Major thrombosis or pulmonary embolism, or both, was identified in 12 patients, 4 of whom died. Survival free from fatal pulmonary embolism was 74% at 5 years. Several patients required surgery to remove right atrial thrombi or pulmonary emboli. These authors conclude that major right atrial thrombosis and pulmonary embolism are frequent in children receiving long-term parenteral nutrition, and they recommend anticoagulation. A routine diagnostic surveillance program is recommended. I suspect these are reasonable considerations.

Diurnal Changes in Heparin Effect During Continuous Constant-Rate Infusion. A Study in Nine Patients With Venous Thromboembolism

Krulder JWM, Van Den Besselaar AMHP, Van Der Meer FJM, Meinders AE, Briët E (Univ Hosp, Leiden, The Netherlands)
J Intern Med 235:411–417, 1994   145-96-15-6

Background.—There are few data on diurnal rhythms in the results of blood coagulation testing in patients who are and are not receiving anticoagulant treatment. If there are significant diurnal variations in the anticoagulant effects of heparin, they may necessitate adjustments of the heparin dose. Diurnal variations in the effects of heparin and their impact on clinical care were evaluated in patients receiving full-dose heparin.

Methods.—Nine patients with acute venous thromboembolic disease were studied during a 24-hour period. All were receiving unfractionated heparin by continuous infusion. During the study day, the following values were determined: anti-IIa activity, anti-Xa activity, activated partial thromboplastin time (APTT) by Cephotest and automated APTT, antithrombin III, and cortisol.

Results.—The anticoagulant effect peaked from 4 to 6 AM and reached its minimum at noon. The differences in measured values between these times were 0.40 U mL^{-1} for anti-IIa activity (table), 0.36 U mL^{-1} for anti-Xa activity, 15 seconds for the Cephotest APTT, and 113 seconds for the automated APTT. The antithrombin III value decreased from 98% at the start to 83% at the end of the study day, whereas cortisol had a typical diurnal rhythm. Anti-IIa activity was maximal at 4 AM, both APTTs were maximal at 6 AM, and anti-Xa activity was maximal at 8 AM. All values were minimal at noon. There was a 26% difference in anti-IIa activity, a nonsignificant difference in anti-Xa activity, a 22% difference in the Cephotest APTT, and a 44% difference in the automated APTT.

Conclusions.—For patients receiving continuous IV infusion of unfractionated heparin, the anticoagulant effect is maximal from 4 AM to 8AM

					Anti-IIa Activity					
	Subject									
Time	1	2	3	4	5	6	7	8	9	Average ± SD
06:00	1.55									1.55 ± 0.00
08:00	1.85	1.40		1.05						1.43 ± 0.33
10:00	1.80	1.50	0.72	0.95						1.24 ± 0.43
12:00	1.65	1.60	0.55	0.92		0.99	1.03		0.78	1.07 ± 0.38*
14:00	1.85	1.70	0.56	1.07		1.11	0.96		0.72	1.14 ± 0.44
16:00	1.90		0.55	0.81		1.14	0.96		0.87	1.04 ± 0.42
18:00	2.00	1.70	0.58	0.83	0.23	1.29	1.04	1.41	0.99	1.12 ± 0.52
20:00	2.00	1.70	0.52	1.13	0.26	1.41	1.01	1.32	1.11	1.16 ± 0.51
22:00	2.10	2.05	0.50	1.03	0.19	1.65	0.95	1.41	1.17	1.23 ± 0.61
00:00	2.25	2.25	0.48	0.91	0.25	1.47	0.75	1.50	0.99	1.21 ± 0.68†
02:00	2.35	2.10	0.49	0.97	0.26	1.35	0.44	1.20	0.81	1.11 ± 0.69
04:00	2.30	2.65	0.55	0.98	0.27	1.98	0.90	1.53		1.39 ± 0.80
06:00	2.45	2.40	0.61	1.09	0.24	1.71	0.82	1.35	1.26	1.33 ± 0.71
08:00		2.50	0.54	1.09	0.24	1.68	0.72	1.23	1.08	1.13 ± 0.66
10:00			0.65		0.27	1.50		1.41	0.87	0.94 ± 0.46
12:00					0.27	1.38		1.29	0.96	0.97 ± 0.44
14:00					0.03			1.59		0.81 ± 0.78
16:00					0.12			1.68		0.90 ± 0.78
18:00					0.20			1.47		0.83 ± 0.63

Note: Anti-IIa activity in U mL^{-1}. Results at 12.00, 18.00, and 00.00 hours were tested for statistically significant differences from result at 06.00 with Student's *t*-test:
* $P < 0.05$.
† $P < 0.03$.
(Courtesy of Krulder JWM, Van Den Besselaar AMHP, Van Der Meer FJM, et al: Diurnal changes in heparin effect during continuous constant-rate infusion: A study in nine patients with venous thromboembolism. *J Intern Med* 235: 411–417, 1994. Reprinted with permission from Blackwell Science Ltd.)

and minimal at noon. However, the difference between the minimal and maximal values varies widely among individual patients. Because the changes are most dramatic from 6 AM to 8 AM, it may be best to perform laboratory control at standard times, such as 10 AM and 10 PM.

▶ I had no idea that constant-dose continuous IV heparin infusion in patients treated for DVT results in an important diurnal anticoagulant effect, with a maximum effect occurring between 4 and 8 AM and minimal effect at noon. This study recommends that laboratory control be performed at fixed times daily, usually around 10 AM and 10 PM. However, for individual patients, the time of maximum and minimum anticoagulant effect varies widely. I suspect that the optimal laboratory control of heparin dosage requires considerably more attention than we routinely devote to it.

Silent Pulmonary Embolism in Patients With Deep Venous Thrombosis: Incidence and Fate in a Randomized, Controlled Trial of Anticoagulation Versus No Anticoagulation
Nielsen HK, Husted SE, Krusell LR, Fasting H, Charles P, Hansen HH (County Hosp of Århus, Denmark; Municipal Hosp of Århus, Denmark)
J Intern Med 235:457–461, 1994   145-96-15–7

Introduction.—Patients with deep venous thrombosis (DVT) are reported to have a high frequency of clinically silent pulmonary embolism (PE). Little is known, however, about the natural history of asymptomatic PE. Eighty-seven consecutive patients with venographically proved DVT were followed up for 3 months to determine the occurrence of PE and the effects of anticoagulant (AC) therapy on its resolution rate.

Patients and Methods.—Patients eligible for the study had symptoms of DVT for less than 6 days and a diagnosis confirmed by ascending venography within 24 hours. None had symptoms of PE on perfusion lung scintigraphy at study entry, and none had severe cardiovascular diseases. The mean age of the group was 55 years. All patients were ambulated from the first day of admission, wearing graduated compression stockings. Forty-six were randomly assigned to receive AC therapy and 41 to no AC therapy. Those in the AC group received IV heparin for at least 6 days or until a therapeutic level for oral treatment with phenprocoumon was obtained. Oral AC treatment was continued for 3 months. Each group was evaluated for improvement or the presence of new perfusion defects at 10 and 60 days. Repeat venograms were performed after 30 days to compare the effects of AC with those of non-AC treatment.

Results.—Approximately 65% of patients had possible thrombotic risk factors. The overall incidence of silent PE was 49% (table). Distal vein thrombosis embolized in 33% of patients, and femoral vein thrombosis embolized in 53%. The progression rates after 10 days were 13% for the AC group and 8% for the non-AC group; after 60 days, both groups had

Silent Pulmonary Embolism in 87 Patients With DVT
Verified by Venography

DVT localization	Lung scintigraphy positive	negative	Size (lobus) 1	2	> 2
Distal	5 (33%)	10	4	0	1
Distal popliteal femoral	38 (53%)	34	7	14	17
Total	43 (49%)	44	11	14	18

Abbreviation: DVT, deep venous thrombosis.
(Courtesy of Nielsen HK, Husted SE, Krusell LR, et al: Silent pulmonary embolism in patients with deep venous thrombosis: Incidence and fate in a randomized, controlled trial of anticoagulation versus no anticoagulation. *J Intern Med* 235:457–461, 1994. Reprinted with permission from Blackwell Science, Ltd.)

a progression rate of 3%. Clinical signs of PE developed in 2 patients receiving AC therapy, 1 of whom died, and in 1 patient not receiving AC therapy.

Conclusions.—The prognosis of patients with DVT and silent PE was good. Anticoagulation therapy did not affect the resolution rate of PE or the rate of clinical PE during a 3-month follow-up. Late prognosis usually depends on the presence of an underlying illness.

▶ This and many other studies convincingly show that by the time we diagnose lower extremity DVT, about 50% of patients have already had a PE. Ten-day and 60-day lung scans reveal progressive resolution of thrombus in both randomly assigned groups (no AC vs. AC), which appeared unaffected by AC therapy. These investigators conclude that about 53% of the patients with proximal DVT have PE compared with 33% of patients with DVT below the knee. I continue to be unclear as to the role of calf vein thrombosis in the production of PE. I was taught that major PE almost never arose from isolated calf vein thrombosis. Many people disagree, however, concluding that as many as one third of serious PE are derived exclusively from the calf veins. I shall have to consider this matter further. I am surprised that these investigators could get their institutional review board to approve a randomized trial of AC compared with no AC in patients with newly diagnosed DVT. I eagerly await publication of their companion article on DVT outcome that is currently in press (1).

Reference

1. Nielsen HK, Husted SE, Krusell LR, et al: Anticoagulant therapy in deep venous thrombosis. A randomized controlled study. *Thromb Res* (In press).

Risk Factors Associated With Pulmonary Embolism Despite Routine Prophylaxis: Implications for Improved Protection

Winchell RJ, Hoyt DB, Walsh JC, Simons RK, Eastman AB (Univ of California, San Diego)
J Trauma 37:600–606, 1994   145-96-15–8

Background.—Although uncommon, pulmonary embolism (PE) can cause sudden death in patients with trauma who have otherwise survived their injuries. Even with current methods of prophylaxis and detection of patients at risk, PE is still a major cause of post-traumatic illness and death. The risk factors for PE were assessed in patients with trauma in whom this complication developed despite routine prophylaxis.

Methods.—A total of 9,721 patients with trauma discharged during an 8-year period were studied retrospectively. Of these, 36 had clinically evident PE, for an incidence of 0.4%. These complications occurred despite a policy of routine prophylaxis against deep venous thrombosis, including prophylactic use of inferior vena caval filters. In 29 patients, such filters were placed for prophylaxis against PE. A detailed analysis was performed to identify injury-related risk factors.

Results.—Eight of the 36 patients with documented PE died, for a mortality rate of 22%. In no case did PE develop after an inferior vena caval filter was placed. On analysis of pattern of injury, 4 common combinations of significant risk factors were identified as high-risk patterns: head plus spinal cord injury, head plus long bone fracture, severe pelvis plus long bone fracture, and multiple long bone fracture. The percentages of patients in these groups with PE were 1.5%, 2.3%, 3.8%, and 2.9%, respectively. Compared with the control group, the odds ratios of the high-risk groups for PE developing ranged from 4.5 to 12.0. The results of multivariate logistic regression showed that 3 of the 4 high-risk injury patterns were independent predictors of PE (table); only the pattern of head plus spinal cord injury fell short of statistical significance as an independent predictor of PE.

Conclusions.—Improvement of outcome for patients with trauma relies on consistent application of conventional care and consideration of other measures, such as prophylactic inferior vena caval filters, for patients at

Pattern of Injury Analysis Using Multivariate Logistic Regression: Independent Predictors of Pulmonary Embolism

Injury Pattern	Chi Square	Probability
1. Head + spinal cord injury	3.6	0.06
2. Head + long bone fracture	11.6	0.00*
3. Severe pelvis + long bone fracture	7.03	0.01*
4. Multiple long bone fracture	11.8	0.00*

* $P < 0.05$ compared with control group.
(Courtesy of Winchell RJ, Hoyt DB, Walsh JC, et al: Risk factors associated with pulmonary embolism despite routine prophylaxis: Implications for improved protection. *J Trauma* 37:600–606, 1994.)

highest risk for PE. More research is needed to determine the efficacy and long-term complications of prophylactic filter placement. For now, it is suggested that patients whose estimated risk for PE is greater than 2% to 5% despite prophylaxis should be considered for prophylactic vena caval filter placement.

▶ In a large trauma center, 0.37% of patients were recognized as having PE during an 8-year period. Eight of these 36 patients died, with most dying of PE. The multivariate analysis showed the following to be the primary risk factors for PE: axial spine fracture with neurologic deficit, posterior element pelvic fracture, long-bone fracture, and multiple fractures. Pneumatic compression stockings and subcutaneous heparin were being received by 80% of the patients with PE. On the other hand, these investigators had placed 29 prophylactic vena caval filters during the study, and none of these patients had a recognized pulmonary embolus. See also Abstracts 145-96-14–7 to 145-96-14–9.

Recurrent Pulmonary Embolism in Patients Treated Because of Acute Venous Thromboembolism: A Prospective Study
Monreal M, Lafoz E, Ruiz J, Callejas JMa, Arias A (Universidad Autónoma de Barcelona)
Eur J Vasc Surg 8:584–589, 1994   145-96-15–9

Background.—Previous studies of patients having venous thromboembolism have implicated initial pulmonary embolism (PE), neoplastic disease, and proximal vein thrombosis as predictive of an increased risk for recurrence.

Methods.—Baseline lung scans were performed in a prospective series of 348 patients who had deep venous thrombosis (DVT) in the lower extremity or PE. The chest radiograph and lung scan were repeated after 8 days of heparin therapy.

Results.—Twenty-three patients (7%) had recurrent PE. Age, sex, and the proximity of venous thrombosis were not predictive of recurrences, but patients with scintigraphic evidence of PE were initially more likely to have a recurrence regardless of whether the initial diagnosis was PE or DVT (table). Patients in whom DVT developed in the absence of any recognized risk factors were also more likely to have recurrent PE.

Conclusion.—In patients with acute venous thromboembolism, PE not infrequently develops despite adequate heparinization. Patients who have PE initially and those without known risk factors are most at risk.

▶ About 50% of patients with newly diagnosed DVT also had PE, confirming the results in Abstract 145-96-15–7. All patients had repeat scanning 8 days after the initiation of heparin therapy. The important results are that PE recurrences were found in 12% of patients who had a PE at admission but in only 2% of patients with DVT who did not have a PE at admission. The significant incidence of recurrent PE despite heparin is noteworthy and

Logistic Regression of PE Recurrences for Clinical Variables				
Step	Variables included	Odds ratio	95% C.I.	P value
1	PE on admission	6.0	1.7–21.1	<0.01
2	Idiopathic venous thromboembolism	3.0	1.1–8.2	<0.05
3	Age	1.0	0.9–1.0	N.S.
4	Sex (Males)	0.8	0.3–2.0	N.S.
5	Mean heparin dose	0.4	0.02–7.6	N.S.

(Courtesy of Monreal M, Lafoz E, Ruiz J, et al: Recurrent pulmonary embolism in patients treated because of acute venous thromboembolism: A prospective study. *Eur J Vasc Surg* 8:584–589, 1994.)

compatible with the findings of prior studies. As suggested by the authors of the article abstracted in Abstract 145-96-15–7, perhaps the entire matter of anticoagulation for DVT warrants detailed reconsideration.

Deep Venous Thrombosis Prophylaxis

Low Molecular Weight Heparin Versus Warfarin in the Prevention of Recurrences After Deep Vein Thrombosis
Pini M, Aiello S, Manotti C, Pattacini C, Quintavalla R, Poli T, Tagliaferri A, Dettori AG (Ospedale Maggiore, Parma, Italy)
Thromb Haemost 72:191–197, 1994   145-96-15–10

Background.—Subcutaneously injected low-molecular-weight heparins have a long half-life, which allows once-a-day injections, and do not require frequent laboratory monitoring. The role of low-molecular-weight heparins as an alternative to oral warfarin treatment in preventing recurrent venous thromboembolism was evaluated.

Methods.—One hundred eighty-seven patients with symptomatic deep vein thrombosis received a bolus of 5,000 IU of IV heparin sodium, followed by subcutaneous (SC) calcium heparin for 10 days and were then randomly assigned to 1 of 2 secondary prophylaxis groups. The 93 patients in 1 group received SC enoxaparin, 40 mg given once daily, and the 94 patients in the other group received oral warfarin with the dosage adjusted according to prothrombin time results. Symptomatic deep vein thrombosis was diagnosed by strain-gauge plethysmography plus D-dimer latex assay and was usually confirmed by venography.

Results.—During the 3-month treatment, 6% of the patients in the enoxaparin group and 4% of those in the warfarin group had objectively confirmed symptomatic recurrence of deep-vein thromboembolism ($P = 0.5$). Four patients in the enoxaparin group and 12 patients in the warfarin group had bleeding complications ($P = 0.04$). In the following 9 months, venous thromboembolism recurred in 10 patients from the enoxaparin group but in only 4 patients from the warfarin group. However, of more than one third of the patients in the warfarin group had continued prophylaxis after the 3-month prophylaxis study. Only 1 of the 14 late recurrences occurred in a patient with postoperative deep vein thrombosis. During the entire 1-year study period, documented venous thromboembolism recurred in 17% of the enoxaparin group and 9% of the warfarin group ($P = 0.07$).

Conclusions.—Once-daily SC treatment with low-molecular-weight heparin is a viable alternative to oral warfarin in the prophylaxis of patients at risk for recurrence of venous thromboembolism. A slightly higher dosage than the 40 mg of enoxaparin given once daily should be prospectively studied. Patients with postoperative or post-traumatic deep vein thrombosis may require anticoagulation for only 4 weeks.

▶ This randomized trial examined the role of low-molecular-weight heparin compared with warfarin in preventing recurrent venous thromboembolism during 3 months of therapy. Symptomatically recurrent DVT was identical in both groups, with significance at the 5% level. The results after 3 months are impossible to interpret because so many of the patients receiving warfarin continued to do so for other reasons. Because of once-daily dosing and the absence of mandatory laboratory studies, low-molecular-weight heparin may indeed be preferable to warfarin.

Is the Increasing Use of Prophylactic Percutaneous IVC Filters Justified?
Alexander JJ, Yuhas JP, Piotrowski JJ (Case Western Reserve Univ, Cleveland, Ohio; Cleveland Metropolitan Gen Hosp, Ohio)
Am J Surg 168:102–106, 1994   145-96-15–11

Objective.—The ease of placing inferior vena cava (IVC) filters percutaneously may have altered indications for the procedure. To determine whether this has happened, the records of 150 patients given 156 filters were reviewed. In 39 patients, a Greenfield filter was inserted surgically. The other 111 patients received 117 filters percutaneously (Fig 15–3).

Indications.—Patients in the percutaneous and surgical groups had a similar risk for thromboembolism. Indications for surgical filter placement were about evenly divided among prevention of pulmonary embolism (PE), PE in which anticoagulation was contraindicated, complications of anticoagulant therapy, and lack of a response to such treatment. More than half the percutaneous procedures were intended to prevent PE. About one fourth of the patients had PE and contraindications to anticoagulant therapy.

Results.—Early mortality was 26% in the surgical group and 27% in those given IVC filters percutaneously. Half the deaths in the latter group and 10% of those in the surgical group were associated with insertions done to prevent PE. Nearly one fourth of percutaneous procedures (24%) and 8% of surgical insertions caused illness.

Conclusions.—The broadening use of percutaneously placed IVC filters to prevent PE is accompanied by increasing procedural morbidity. Indications for prophylactic IVC filter placement should be reformulated.

IVC Filter Insertion

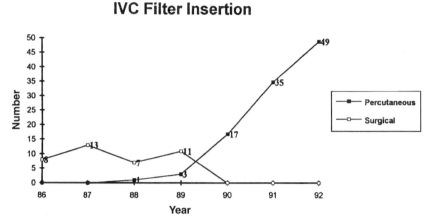

Fig 15–3.—Yearly inferior vena cava (*IVC*) filter insertions. (Courtesy of Alexander JJ, Yuhas JP, Piotrowski JJ: Is the increasing use of prophylactic percutaneous IVC filters justified? *Am J Surg* 168:102–106, 1994. Reprinted with permission from *American Journal of Surgery*.)

▶ When a technique is available that is effective, minimally invasive, and easy to perform and is associated with a low morbidity, it is only natural for clinicians to use it frequently. The seductive nature of percutaneous IVC filter placement threatens to extend the boundaries of indication for PE prophylaxis. Similar to an earlier paper (1), this retrospective study issues a cautionary warning about the inappropriate uses of percutaneous IVC filter insertion. Although the incidences of both DVT and PE were similar on a yearly basis during the study, the marked increase in percutaneous IVC placement for prophylactic reasons is clearly related to more widespread decision making by noncardiovascular physicians. Their unwillingness to use conventional techniques of PE prevention—heparin—and their eagerness to jump to a mechanical IV device may be a natural medical instinct. Outcome data such as those presented in this paper suggest that institutions should develop more uniform policies on patient selection for insertion of this device, which may not always be innocuous.—T. O'Donnell, M.D.

Reference

1. Rohrer MJ, Scheidler MG, Wheeler HB, et al: Extended indications for placement of an inferior vena cava filter. *J Vasc Surg* 10:44–50, 1989.

Miscellaneous

A Strategy of Aggressive Regional Therapy for Acute Iliofemoral Venous Thrombosis With Contemporary Venous Thrombectomy or Catheter-Directed Thrombolysis

Comerota AJ, Aldridge SC, Cohen G, Ball DS, Pliskin M, White JV (Temple Univ Hosp, Philadelphia; Pocono Med Ctr, East Stroudsburg, Pa)
J Vasc Surg 20:244–254, 1994   145-96-15–12

Background.—Patients with deep venous thrombosis of the iliofemoral system are at risk for acute pulmonary embolism and are also likely to have marked post-thrombotic changes. Such patients have not responded well to standard anticoagulant therapy with systemic fibrinolysis. Accordingly, an aggressive approach was taken in caring for 12 consecutive patients who had extensive iliofemoral venous thrombosis, with the goals of eliminating thrombus, providing free venous drainage, and preventing recurrent thrombosis. All but 1 patient had not responded to anticoagulant treatment, and 5 had also received systemic fibrinolysis.

Methods.—Catheter-directed thrombolysis was undertaken by infusing urokinase and, in some cases, recombinant tissue plasminogen activator when no contraindications to lytic treatment were present. When such contraindications were present, patients underwent surgical thrombectomy or venous bypass with a permanent 4-mm arteriovenous fistula.

Results.—Nine of the 12 patients had an excellent or good clinical outcome after an average follow-up of 25 months. Catheter-directed lytic therapy succeeded in 5 of 7 attempts, and 5 of 8 operations were successful. Two of the 3 patients who did not respond to surgery had a residual thrombus in the iliac veins or vena cava after thrombectomy alone. The third patient could not receive anticoagulation and had caval thrombosis develop 2 months after surgery. No patient had symptomatic pulmonary embolism.

Conclusion.—Aggressive treatment, including directed lysis and surgery ensuring unobstructed venous drainage, holds significantly more promise for patients with obliterative iliofemoral venous thrombosis than standard anticoagulant therapy and systemic fibrinolysis.

▶ Twelve consecutive patients with extensive iliofemoral venous thrombosis did not respond to conventional therapy. A variety of treatments were used on these patients, including intraclot infusion of thrombolytic drugs, surgical thrombectomy in 8 patients, vein bypass in 2 patients, and arteriovenous fistula placement in 4. Nine of these patients were considered by the authors to have good or excellent clinical outcome. The inevitable algorithm accompanies this paper, but on balance, I have reservations. We find that large doses of heparin accompanied by exaggerated Trendelenburg position works wonders in these patients. We have not recognized the necessity of the extensive surgical procedures described herein.

Venous Duplex Imaging Follow-Up of Acute Symptomatic Deep Vein Thrombosis of the Leg
Caprini JA, Arcelus JI, Hoffman KN, Size G, Laubach M, Traverso CI, Coats R, Finke N, Reyna JJ (Glenbrook Hosp, Glenview, Ill; Hosp de la Axarquía Vélez-Málaga, Spain)
J Vasc Surg 21:472–476, 1995   145-96-15–13

Background.—Few prospective studies have been done using serial duplex scans to assess the outcome of acute deep vein thrombosis (DVT).

Duplex scanning was used to evaluate the resolution rate of symptomatic DVT 6 months after the initial diagnosis.

Methods.—The study included 73 cases of DVT, all diagnosed by duplex scanning, in 69 patients. These patients received conventional heparin and warfarin therapy. Duplex scanning was repeated 1, 4, 12, and 24 weeks after diagnosis. In addition to defining the rate of resolution, the study sought to determine the proportion of unstable, floating thrombi and the development of chronic damage caused by scarring of the vessel walls.

Results.—By 6 months, 78% of cases of DVT in the common femoral vein, 70% in the superficial femoral vein, 75% in the popliteal vein, and 70% in the calf veins had returned to normal. At the initial duplex scan, 26% of thrombi were deemed unstable. They stabilized within an average of 11 days. Forty-four percent of the patients had vessel wall or valve damage.

Conclusions.—The resolution rate of DVT is similar for the various leg veins studied. Unstable thrombi, which carry an increased risk for embolization, are common. Follow-up duplex scanning for patients with diagnosed DVT provides valuable information on thrombus resolution, propagation, and attachment to the vein wall.

▶ The Seattle group has been interested in evaluating the detailed resolution of venous thrombi. In this study, 73 limbs with DVT underwent duplex scanning 1, 4, 12, and 24 weeks after diagnosis of DVT. About three fourths of the vein segments that initially had a thrombus returned to normal. Damage to the vessel wall or vein was documented in 44% of patients. "Unstable thrombi," whatever that means, were diagnosed in 26% of patients. This information is about what one would expect. On balance, I am not impressed with the concept of "floating thrombus." I suspect the behavior of such thrombi is little different from that of nonfloating thrombi.

Influence of Compression Stockings on Lower-Limb Venous Haemodynamics During Laparoscopic Cholecystectomy
Wilson YG, Allen PE, Skidmore R, Baker AR (Frenchay Hosp, Bristol, England)
Br J Surg 81:841–844, 1994   145-96-15–14

Background.—Laparoscopic techniques are increasingly used to do cholecystectomy and other intra-abdominal procedures. Pneumoperitoneum may produce morbid conditions and significant resistance to venous return in the lower extremities, possibly predisposing patients to thromboembolism.

Methods.—Venous hemodynamics in the lower extremity were examined prospectively in 40 patients having laparoscopic cholecystectomy, half of whom were randomly assigned to wear compression stockings during the procedure. All patients received heparin subcutaneously. Venous capacitance and outflow were estimated noninvasively before and after pneumoperitoneum was established. The intra-abdominal pressure was maintained at 15 mm Hg throughout surgery.

Results.—In most patients in whom compression stockings were not applied, both venous capacitance and outflow decreased during pneumoperitoneum. In those wearing stockings, however, these changes were less marked or were not evident. At the halfway point, the median venous capacitance was 0.9 in control patients and 1.5 in those wearing compression stockings. The respective median outflow ratios were 0.9 and 1.7.

Conclusion.—Establishing pneumoperitoneum produces significant resistance to venous return from the lower extremities, an effect that is countered by the use of compression stockings.

▶ This is an extremely timely paper in view of the logarithmic increase in the number of laparoscopic cholecystectomies being performed. This study shows again that lower extremity venous capacitance and outflow are decreased by pneumoperitoneum used during laparoscopic cholecystectomy. These changes are partially overcome by the wearing of elastic stockings. These results suggest that compressive stockings should be worn to counteract the changes incident to pneumoperitoneum during laparoscopic abdominal procedures. Any disagreement?

16 Chronic Venous and Lymphatic Disease

Chronic Venous Disease

Subfascial Endoscopic Ligation in the Treatment of Incompetent Perforating Veins
Pierik EGJM, Wittens CHA, van Urk H (Sint Franciscus Gasthuis, Rotterdam, The Netherlands; Univ Hosp Rotterdam-Dijkzigt Rotterdam, The Netherlands)
Eur J Vasc Endovasc Surg 9:38–41, 1995   145-96-16–1

Objective.—The efficacy of subfascial endoscopic ligation of incompetent perforating veins was examined prospectively in 38 consecutive patients with prolonged or recurrent venous ulcers in 40 lower extremities.

Technique.—Under spinal anesthesia, a short incision is made at the anteromedial border of the proximal third of the lower leg. After the fascia is horizontally incised, a mediastinoscope 18 cm in length and 12 mm in diameter is inserted to examine the subfascial region (Fig 16–1). All communicating veins are ligated with hemoclips and dissected under direct vision (Fig 16–2). In early cases, a 10-cm fasciotomy is performed after the scope was removed.

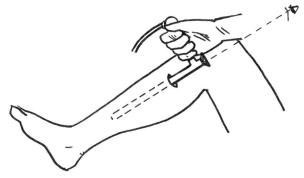

Fig 16–1.—Schematic drawing of a mediastinoscope introduced in subfascial space. (Courtesy of Pierik EGJM, Wittens CHA, van Urk H: Subfascial endoscopic ligation in the treatment of incompetent perforating veins. *Eur J Vasc Endovasc Surg* 9:38–41, 1995.)

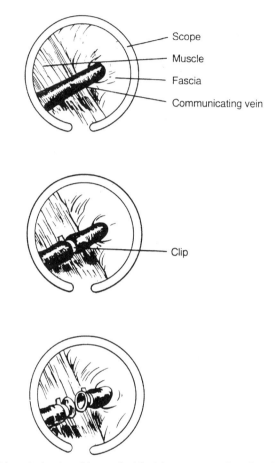

Fig 16–2.—Schematic drawing of image of subfascial space as seen through mediastinoscope. **Top,** communicating vein perforating fascia. **Middle,** clipped perforating vein. **Bottom,** clipped and divided perforating vein. (Courtesy of Pierik EGJM, Wittens CHA, van Urk H: Subfascial endoscopic ligation in the treatment of incompetent perforating veins. *Eur J Vasc Endovasc Surg* 9:38–41, 1995.)

Pathology.—Incompetent perforating veins were clinically evident in all extremities and were confirmed by continuous-wave ultrasonography. Incompetent deep veins were also present in 31 legs. Sixteen patients had active ulcers at the time of surgery.

Results.—Two patients had subfascial infections requiring surgical drainage, and 1 had inflammation at the wound site. All active ulcers healed within 2 months. Only 1 of the 38 patients had recurrent ulceration during an average follow-up of nearly 4 years.

Conclusion.—Subfascial endoscopic ligation using a mediastinoscope is a relatively simple and effective way to treat incompetent perforating veins. The cosmetic results are satisfactory, and ulcers infrequently recur.

▶ Endoscopic subfascial techniques have been developed to avoid traversing the "underprivileged skin and subcutaneous tissue" of the gaiter area, which has been associated with wound slough by the conventional approaches to subfascial ligation of incompetent perforating veins (ICPVs). This report describes the use of a mediastinoscope for visualizing ICPVs in the subfascial space. Although 38 patients underwent interruption of incompetent perforating veins by this method, important pre- and postoperative factors, as well as more detailed technical explanations, are lacking. Preoperative evaluation consisted only of clinical examination and continuouswave ultrasonography. Previous studies have shown this latter technique to be unreliable, with a high false positive rate (1).

Evidently, neither venography nor duplex scanning was used to define both the number and the specific sites of ICPVs. Because the status of the deep venous system plays an important role in venous ulcer recurrence after subfascial ligation, failure to provide the actual incidence of deep venous incompetence makes interpretation of the ulcer recurrence rate difficult. The low ulcer recurrence rate in this study may be more related to the short median follow-up time than to the efficacy of the technique. No assessment of ICPV recurrence after surgery is described. Obviously, the mediastinoscopic technique fails to deal with the paratibial veins, which are quite frequently incompetent. Finally, with laparoscopic techniques available in most centers, this method appears somewhat clumsy.—T. O'Donnell, M.D.

Reference

1. O'Donnell TF, Burnand KG, Clemenson G, et al: Doppler examination versus clinical and phlebographic detection of the location of incompetent perforating veins. *Arch Surg* 112:31–35, 1977.

Venous Diameter and Compliance After Deep Venous Thrombosis
Meissner MH, Manzo RA, Bergelin RO, Strandness DE Jr (Univ of Washington, Seattle; Harborview Med Ctr, Seattle)
Thromb Haemost 72:372–376, 1994   145-96-16–2

Objective and Methods.—Duplex ultrasonography was used to detect changes in diameter in the common femoral, superficial femoral, and popliteal veins in 56 patients who were followed for 6 months or longer after an episode of acute deep venous thrombosis (DVT). Seventeen normal participants were also studied. In addition, venous distensibility was estimated during the Valsalva maneuver as a measure of venous compliance.

Results.—In patients with unilateral DVT, vein segments with residual disease were 0.07 to 0.28 cm smaller in diameter than corresponding segments on the side without disease. Segments that had completely recanalized did not differ significantly, and these patients had ipsilateral/or contralateral vein diameter ratios similar to those of the controls. Vein distensibility was similar in the patients with DVT and controls, regardless of whether disease had resolved.

Conclusions.—Affected leg veins decrease in caliber after acute DVT but return to normal diameter after recanalization is complete. There is no residual change in venous compliance.

▶ See also the commentary for Abstract 145-96-15–13. The Seattle group herein concludes that venous segments with residual disease are slightly smaller than contralateral disease-free segments, whereas completely recanalized segments do not differ from the contralateral normal side. Compliance appeared equal. Because this is a moderately sized negative study, I can see why these authors elected to have it published in this obscure journal.

Venous Function and Clinical Outcome Following Deep Vein Thrombosis
Milne AA, Stonebridge PA, Bradbury AW, Ruckley CV (The Royal Infirmary, Edinburgh, Scotland)
Br J Surg 81:847–849, 1994   145-96-16–3

Objective.—There is currently no way to predict which patients will have symptoms of chronic venous insufficiency after an episode of deep vein thrombosis (DVT) or how severe the symptoms will be or how long they will take to develop. Chronic venous insufficiency is often assumed to result from the development of deep vein reflux, but there is no consistent relationship between deep venous dysfunction and the severity of post-thrombotic symptoms. Thus, other factors, such as superficial venous incompetence, may play an important role. Associations were sought between the severity of post-thrombotic symptoms and abnormalities of deep and superficial venous function as assessed by foot volumetry and duplex ultrasonography.

Methods.—The participants were 107 patients with post-thrombotic symptoms in 111 limbs. All patients had phlebographically confirmed DVT at a median of 8 years before assessment. Superficial and deep venous function was evaluated by foot volumetry in 90 patients and by duplex sonography in 62. The symptoms were rated as mild in 28% of limbs (group 1); moderate in 37% (group 2); and severe in 35% (group 3).

Results.—Symptom severity was unrelated to the site of DVT or the time since DVT. Half-refilling time was significantly shorter for limbs in group 3 than for those in groups 1 and 2, in the absence of tourniquet occlusion of the superficial veins. A nonsignificant trend in the same direction was observed after tourniquet occlusion. Expelled volumes did not significantly differ among the 3 groups. Just more than half of the limbs in all 3 groups showed deep and superficial venous reflux on duplex scanning. Duplex scanning was completely normal in 8 patients, none of whom had severe symptoms. The results of foot volumetry and duplex sonography were poorly correlated.

Conclusions.—Severe postphlebitic syndrome appears to be strongly related to venous reflux, which can be considered necessary for the development of severe post-thrombotic symptoms. However, symptoms are mild in many patients with severe reflux. The development of severe postphlebitic syndrome must therefore involve other factors, perhaps at the microvascular level.

▶ This study relies on foot volumetry, a technique little used in America. Several interesting findings are revealed by this study, the most important of which is that the severity of reflux symptoms in patients is by no means linearly related to demonstrable valvular reflux. Additional unknown factors must contribute to the development of severe postphlebitic syndrome. Although this observation is intuitively obvious, it is nice to have such excellent scientific correlation.

Venous Reflux in Patients With Previous Deep Venous Thrombosis: Correlation With Ulceration and Other Symptoms
Labropoulos N, Leon M, Nicolaides AN, Sowade O, Volteas N, Ortega F, Chan P (St Mary's Hosp, London; Imperial College of Science Technology and Medicine, London)
J Vasc Surg 20:20–26, 1994   145-96-16–4

Background.—In many patients, deep vein thrombosis (DVT) is followed by chronic symptoms in the affected leg, even when recanalization of the affected veins has occurred. Reflux is the main hemodynamic defect seen in recanalized veins. The incidence and extent of venous reflux were correlated with concurrent symptoms in patients with confirmed DVT.

Methods.—The participants were 183 patients with 217 affected limbs. All limbs had a previous venographic diagnosis of DVT. A meticulous duplex scan of the entire venous system was performed to define the sites and extent of reflux. The limbs were classified according to whether the superficial and/or deep venous system was involved and whether the reflux was found proximal and/or distal to the knee.

Results.—Eighty-one limbs were in chronic venous insufficiency class 1, 92 were in class 2, and 38 were in class 3. The reflux involved only the deep venous system in 39% of the limbs, only the superficial venous system in 14%, and both systems in 47%. Twenty-two percent of the limbs had reflux confined to the proximal veins and 26% to the distal veins, whereas 52% had reflux throughout the limb.

Regardless of the venous system involved, the incidence of swelling was greater in limbs with distal or with proximal and distal reflux. The extent of reflux did not influence the incidence of skin changes in limbs with superficial venous insufficiency (SVI) or deep venous insufficiency (DVI) only. However, in limbs with combined SVI and DVI and with reflux throughout the limb, the incidence of skin changes was increased. When distal reflux was absent, the incidence of skin changes was low, even if the limb had DVI. In limbs with SVI, ulceration increased along with the extent of reflux. Limbs without superficial reflux had a low incidence of ulceration, even if DVI was present (table).

Incidence of Ulceration in Relation to Location and Extent of Reflux

System	Extent of Reflux Proximal	Distal	Proximal + Distal	Total
SVI only	0/5 (0.0%)	2/9 (22.2%)	10/17 (58.8%)	12/31 (38.7%)
DVI only	0/14 (0.0%)	1/21 (4.8%)	2/49 (4.1%)	3/84 (3.6%)
SVI + DVI	1/29 (3.4%)	4/26 (15.4%)	18/47 (38.3%)	23/102 (22.5%)
Total	1/48 (2.1%)	7/56 (12.5%)	30/113 (26.5%)	38/217 (17.5%)

Abbreviations: SVI, superficial venous insufficiency; *DVI*, deep venous insufficiency.
(Courtesy of Labropoulos N, Leon M, Nicolaides AN, et al: Venous reflux in patients with previous deep venous thrombosis: Correlation with ulceration and other symptoms. *J Vasc Surg* 20:20–26, 1994.)

Conclusions.—In limbs with previous DVT, distal reflux and superficial venous reflux are associated with skin changes and ulceration. Distal reflux and superficial reflux are more harmful than reflux confined to the deep veins, even when deep vein reflux is present both proximally and distally. Distal antireflux procedures are a necessary adjunct to restore normal limb hemodynamics.

▶ These authors conclude that venous ulceration is most likely to occur with the combination of distal deep vein reflux and superficial vein reflux. In America we have been relatively slow to recognize the significance of superficial vein reflux, but I must say I am impressed by studies showing that isolated superficial vein reflux may be the cause of as many as 50% of venous ulcers. Although I do not believe this is true in America, it probably is true in Northern Europe and England. On the basis of this and similar studies, I shall pay more attention to superficial vein reflux. I note parenthetically that studies such as this one indirectly indicate that isolated valve surgery done at or around the popliteal valve is not likely to be very effective.

Vein Surgery With or Without Skin Grafting Versus Conservative Treatment for Leg Ulcers: A Randomized Prospective Study
Warburg FE, Danielsen L, Madsen SM, Raaschou HO, Munkvad S, Jensen R, Siersen HE (Bispebjerg Hosp, Copenhagen; Humlebaek and Copenhagen Wound Healing Ctr)
Acta Derm Venereol 74:307–309, 1994   145-96-16-5

Objective.—The effectiveness of operating on perforating veins, with or without concomitant skin grafting, was examined in 47 patients with lipodermatosclerosis and leg ulcers in whom ascending phlebography had shown incompetent perforating veins.

Methods.—Forty patients were evaluable a year after entering the study. Fifteen of them had surgery for incompetent perforating veins. Thirteen patients also had excision of ulcerative lesions, followed by skin grafting. A control group consisted of 12 patients. Baseline features were similar in the 3 groups. All patients were treated by compression bandaging. Systemic antibiotic therapy was given when cellulitis was present. Eczema was treated by applying a steroid ointment.

Results.—A review of initial phlebograms showed post-thrombotic changes in the deep veins in most extremities. No difference was noted in median ulcer size either at the outset or at the time of follow-up. The time required for healing averaged 3 months in patients who had vein surgery only and approximately 5 months in the other groups.

Conclusion.—In patients with leg ulcers, neither surgery on incompetent perforating veins nor skin grafting appears to offer substantial benefit beyond what is achieved by conservative treatment.

▶ In this interesting study, 3 groups of patients with perforator vein incompetence and venous ulcerations were randomly assigned to have surgery for incompetent perforators; surgery for perforators with ulcer excision and grafting; or no surgery, with compression therapy only. At the end of 1 year, no difference was seen in the behavior of any of these 3 groups from the others. This confirms our preference for nonoperative therapy for chronic venous disease (1).

Reference

1. Mayberry JC: *Surgery* 109:575–581, 1991.

Iliac Compression Syndrome Treated With Stent Placement

Berger A, Jaffe JW, York TN (Lehigh Valley Hosp, Allentown, Pa)
J Vasc Surg 21:510–514, 1995   145-96-16–6

Background.—The iliac compression syndrome is usually discovered in the third and fourth decades of life as a sequel of iliofemoral deep venous thrombosis. Catheter-directed thrombolysis reportedly is more effective than systemic treatment. One patient with CT-confirmed iliac compression syndrome was successfully managed by stent placement after lysis and an inadequate response to balloon angioplasty.

Case Report.—Man, 51, presented with a painful and swollen left leg 3 weeks after having received heparin and warfarin elsewhere for a deep iliofemoral venous thrombosis. The extremity had been intermittently swollen for 10 years. Venography showed normal femoropopliteal vessels. The external iliac vein was not seen, but extensive pelvic collaterals were noted. Pelvic CT showed extensive thrombosis in the left iliac venous system and compression of the left iliac vein by the right common iliac artery. The patient was given heparin, and warfarin was reversed. Catheter-directed thrombolysis was done with urokinase, with access through the ipsilateral common femoral vein. A large pelvic collateral vein was shown (Fig 16–3) and, after treatment, repeat venography revealed resolution of the thrombus and the presence of bands, webs, or possible residual thrombus at the level of the stricture (Fig 16–4). The placement of stents in the left common iliac vein was followed by much improved transiliac flow into the inferior vena cava and lack of visualization of the collateral veins. The symptoms improved dramatically. The stented vein remained patent 6 months later, when edema was continuing to resolve.

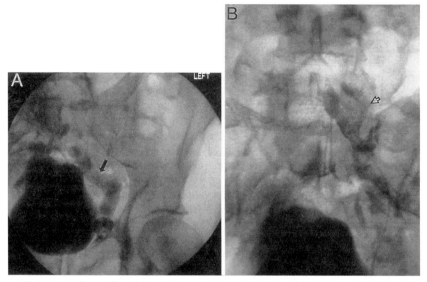

Fig 16–3.—A, large collateral (*arrow*) is seen without visualization of the left iliac vein. **B,** thrombus is seen in left iliac vein (*arrowhead*). (Courtesy of Berger A, Jaffe JW, York TN: Iliac compression syndrome treated with stent placement. *J Vasc Surg* 21:510–514, 1995.)

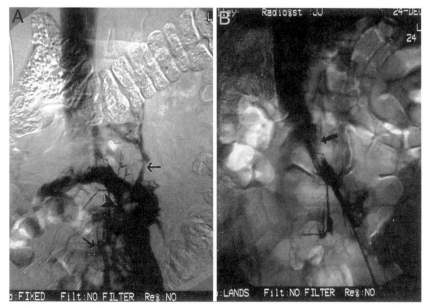

Fig 16–4.—A, extensive collaterals are still seen (*arrows*), along with clot (*arrowhead*) within the common iliac vein. **B,** bands, webs, or residual thrombus are noted within the left common iliac vein (*arrow*). (Courtesy of Berger A, Jaffe JW, York TN: *J Vasc Surg* 21:510–514, 1995.)

▶ Iliac compression syndrome is presumably caused by compression of the first portion of the left common iliac vein behind the right common iliac artery. This condition, although uncommon, is a recognized, albeit infrequent, cause of deep vein thrombosis. Many endovascular and surgical techniques have been described for treatment of this condition, none of which have been particularly successful. This report describes venous balloon dilatation followed by stenting, which does have a certain appeal. If its effectiveness is confirmed by independent reports, this may become the procedure of choice for this uncommon but troublesome condition.

Randomised Trial of Oral Aspirin for Chronic Venous Leg Ulcers
Layton AM, Ibbotson SH, Davies JA, Goodfield MJD (Gen Infirmary at Leeds, England)
Lancet 344:164–165, 1994   145-96-16–7

Background.—The pathogenesis of venous ulcers has not been established. Aspirin treatment may influence thrombocytosis and increase mean platelet volume, both of which are features of gravitational disease. The effect of aspirin on the healing rate of chronic venous ulcers of the leg was therefore studied.

Methods.—Twenty patients with chronic venous leg ulcers were enrolled in the double-blind, placebo-controlled, randomized trial. The patients received 300 mg of enteric-coated aspirin or placebo daily. All received standardized compression bandages.

Findings.—After 4 months of treatment, ulcers healed in 38% of the patients receiving aspirin and in none of those receiving placebo. Ulcer size was significantly decreased in 52% of the patients receiving aspirin and in 26% of those receiving placebo. At 2 and 4 months, aspirin recipients had significantly better ulcer surface area reductions than did placebo recipients. No adverse effects developed.

Conclusions.—Aspirin treatment with standardized compression bandaging improves the healing rates of chronic venous leg ulcers. Aspirin's mechanism of action in such cases, however, is unclear.

▶ Twenty patients with chronic venous ulcers were randomly assigned to receive daily enteric aspirin or placebo along with standard compressive bandaging. A highly significant benefit was noted in favor of the aspirin group. Because thrombocytosis and increased platelet volume are features of chronic venous disease, perhaps aspirin is having a favorable influence on these variables; this, however, is unproven by the study. Although preliminary, I find this information quite interesting. The putative benefits of aspirin continue to accrue.

The Clinical and Hemodynamic Results After Axillary–to–Popliteal Vein Valve Transplantation

Bry JDL, Muto PA, O'Donnell TF, Isaacson LA (New England Med Ctr, Boston; Tufts Univ, Boston)

J Vasc Surg 21:110–119, 1995   145-96-16–8

Introduction.—The rationale for transplantation of the axillary vein to the above-knee popliteal vein position is twofold: (1) to provide a better size match of the transplanted axillary vein segment to the host popliteal vein to avoid late dilatation; and (2) to restore popliteal vein valve function at the critical "gate-keeper" position above the calf muscle venous pump. The clinical, phlebographic, and noninvasive hemodynamic results of axillary vein to popliteal vein valve transplantation were reviewed.

Patients.—Between 1983 and 1992, 15 patients underwent axillary-to-popliteal vein valve transplantation for post-thrombotic destruction of deep venous valves on ascending phlebography and grade III or IV reflux on descending venography. Fourteen patients had moderate-to-severe limb swelling and pain, 13 patients had active ulcers, 1 had intractable symptoms of pain and edema despite aggressive medical management, and 9 had previously undergone surgery including vein stripping or incompetent perforator ligator. Thirteen patients had at least 2 or more ulcer recurrences, and the average duration of stage III disease before surgery was 7.4 years. The mean preoperative venous refill time was abnormal in all patients.

Outcome.—During an average follow-up of 5.3 years, all patients had relief of incapacitating pain, 92% had relief of swelling, and 87% returned to work or household duties. Most patients had improved edema, skin pigmentation, and lipodermatosclerosis. Ulcer recurrence was prevented in 79% of patients, and the probability of remaining free of recurrent ulceration after 5 years was 62%. Only 3 patients (21%) had recurrent ulcers, with an average postoperative ulcer-free interval of 4 years. All 3 patients with recurrent ulcers had a functioning valve on descending phlebography, but 2 patients had recurrent perforating veins and 1 had deep venous thrombosis above a patent and competent valve transplant. Overall, the postoperative mean venous filling index was 6.8 mL/sec and mean valve closure time was 4.9 seconds. Residual volume fraction, which correlates with invasive ambulatory venous pressures, was reduced to a mean of 31%. Late sequential noninvasive values did not further deteriorate.

Conclusion.—Axillary vein to popliteal vein valve transplantation is a durable procedure for preventing recurrent venous ulcers. Deep venous reconstructive surgery should be reserved for highly selected patients in whom conservative management of stage III disease fails. In this series, valve transplantation was restricted to patients with grade III or IV reflux.

▶ Evaluation of this study is difficult because these patients were discharged to receive warfarin, and no comment is made as to whether limb compression was used. One patient had deep venous thrombosis proximal to the valve transplant. Of interest, all patients had a highly abnormal duplex valve closure time. I am not particularly impressed with the apparent improvement shown by air plethysmography because I have significant reservations about the accuracy of the air plethysmographic test in general. In our laboratory, it correlates with nothing. On balance, these investigators achieved a 6-year ulcer-free rate of 62%, less than we would expect with nonoperative therapy. See the commentary for Abstract 145-96-16-5. I would have been much more impressed had the authors randomly assigned these patients and given the nonoperative group appropriate aggressive treatment.

The Development of Valvular Incompetence After Deep Vein Thrombosis: A Follow-Up Study With Duplex Scanning
van Ramshorst B, van Bemmelen PS, Hoeneveld H, Eikelboom BC (St Antonius Hosp, Nieuwegein, The Netherlands)
J Vasc Surg 20:1059–1066, 1994   145-96-16–9

Background.—The long-term clinical outcomes after deep venous thrombosis (DVT) remain unclear. Duplex ultrasound has emerged as a reliable method of diagnosing venous insufficiency in both the deep and superficial veins. Duplex scanning was used to ascertain the physiologic reflux durations in the deep venous system of healthy persons and to show incompetence of the deep vein valves in patients with a history of DVT.

Methods.—Duplex scanning with distal cuff deflation was performed in 21 healthy adults and in 27 patients with phlebographically confirmed DVT. Two hundred fifty-two segments were evaluated in the controls and 160 segments were evaluated in the patients. The patients were studied a mean of 34 months after their episode of DVT.

Results.—The controls had significantly shorter reflux durations in the distal deep vein segments. Almost all reflex durations in this group were less than 0.88 seconds in the common femoral vein, 0.80 seconds in the superficial and deep femoral veins, 0.28 seconds in the popliteal vein, and 0.12 seconds in the posterior tibial vein. In all segments in the superficial

TABLE 1.—Mean Number of Segments With Reflux According to Extent of Thrombosis at Diagnosis

No. of initially affected segments	N	Mean no. of segments with reflux
6	10	2.8
5	3	3.0
4	8	1.9
3	5	0.8
2	—	—
1	1	—

Mann-Whitney, *P* = 0.04.
(Courtesy of van Ramshorst B, van Bemmelen PS, Hoeneveld H, et al: The development of valvular incompetence after deep vein thrombosis: A follow-up study with duplex scanning. *J Vasc Surg* 20:1059–1066, 1994.)

TABLE 2.—Prevalence of Reflux at Different Levels After Thrombosis

Vein segment	No. of segments affected by thrombosis	No. of segments with reflux	Percent
CFV	18	6	30
DFV	12	4	30
SFV	24	17	71
PV	25	17	68
PTVC	21	8	38
PTVA	20	5	25

Note: Both SFV and PV had significantly more reflux than other vein segments; Mann Whitney, $P < 0.01$.
Abbreviations: CFV, common femoral vein; DFV, deep femoral vein; SFV, superficial femoral vein; PV, popliteal vein; PTVC, posterior tibial vein at calf level; PTVA, posterior tibial vein at ankle level.
(Courtesy of van Ramshorst B, van Bemmelen PS, Hoeneveld H, et al: The development of valvular incompetence after deep vein thrombosis: A follow-up study with duplex scanning. J Vasc Surg 20:1059–1066, 1994.)

venous system, the 95th percentile for reflux duration was 0.50 seconds. Reflux peak flow velocity and duration were not significantly correlated.

In the patient group, valve incompetence was detected in 45% of the segments involved in the initial episode of DVT. Of 40 segments that initially showed no thrombus, just 3 exhibited pathologic reflux at follow-up. In the segments with valve incompetence, reflux durations were generally at least twice the normal value. In no patient was valve incompetence detected at all levels of the deep venous system. The extent of initial thrombosis was significantly correlated with the number of refluxing segments (Table 1) but not with the late clinical symptoms. No relationship was seen between the symptoms and the number of incompetent venous segments. Valve incompetence was most common in the superficial femoral and popliteal vein segment (Table 2).

Conclusions.—In patients who have had an episode of DVT, duplex ultrasound scanning permits good discrimination between venous segments with physiologic and abnormal reflux durations. As such, it may play a valuable role in analysis of the post-thrombotic limb. When performed soon after the episode of DVT, duplex scanning may provide important prognostic information. Reflux peak flow velocity is not a useful indicator of the degree of reflux.

▶ This paper compares duplex-measured reflux times induced by the cuff compression techniques in a group of normal persons and those who had a phlebographically documented episode of previous DVT. This study confirms the well-known observation that most segments recanalize rather than remain thrombosed. The authors further extend the previous physiologic observations of van Bemmelen et al. (1) on normal duplex-derived reflux times. Although reflux duration was shorter in distal venous segments (tibials) than in proximal segments, the average was 0.5 seconds. In the post-thrombotic limbs, reflux durations were at least 2 times the duration in normal limbs. One half of the segments with phlebographically documented thrombosis had pathologic reflux at follow-up (mean, 34 months after DVT). Less than 10% of venous segments that were uninvolved by thrombus showed reflux. The extent of initial thrombosis was related to the likelihood of multisegment reflux. The authors also confirm the earlier observation by Browse et al. (2) that no relation was seen between the extent of initial thrombosis and the production of late symptoms.

This study emphasizes the reproducible results for the assessment of valve closure time that can be obtained by the cuff deflation technique. It also challenges several of previous studies indicating (1) that reflux is unlikely to occur in a venous segment previously uninvolved by documented thrombosis (thus supporting the direct damage theory) and (2) a low incidence of calf vein valve reflux. The weakness of this study is the *variability* in the length of time after the initial episode of DVT in which the patients were examined. Studies by the University of Washington group were done at uniformly defined intervals after DVT. In the present study, the superficial femoral and popliteal veins appeared to be particularly susceptible to the development of reflux (34 of 49 [69%]).—T. O'Donnell, M.D.

References

1. van Bemmelen PS, Bedford G, Beach K, et al: Quantitative segmental evaluation of venous valvular reflux with duplex ultrasound scanning. *J Vasc Surg* 10:425–431, 1989.
2. Browse NL, Clemenson G, Lea Thomas M: Is the post-phlebitic leg always post-phlebitic? Relation between phlebographic appearances of deep-vein thrombosis and late sequelae. *BMJ* 281:1167–1170, 1980.

Microangiopathy of the Skin and the Effect of Leg Compression in Patients With Chronic Venous Insufficiency
Abu-Own A, Shami SK, Chittenden SJ, Farrah J, Scurr JH, Smith PDC (Univ College London Med School)
J Vasc Surg 19:1074–1083, 1994   145-96-16–10

Background.—Leg compression is an effective measure in patients with chronic venous insufficiency, but the reasons it is effective remain uncertain. Laser Doppler fluxmetry was used to determine how external compression affects the microcirculation of the skin.

Methods.—Fifteen patients with lipodermatosclerosis secondary to chronic venous insufficiency were examined in the supine and sitting positions. Fifteen control patients of similar age had no venous or arterial disease. A laser Doppler probe incorporated in a polyethylene chamber was applied to the lower leg beneath a pressure cuff, and pressure was increased incrementally to as high as 100 mm Hg. The amount of Doppler-shifted light reflected back from the skin is proportional to the concentration of moving blood cells (CMBCs) in the tissues. The mean frequency shift relates to the average blood cell velocity (BCV). The product of these values constitutes the laser Doppler flux (LDF).

Results.—When patients were supine, compression of 20 mm Hg led to a median increase of 33% in LDF and a 79% increase in BCV. Higher pressures, however, progressively decreased both variables. In the sitting position, a pressure of 20 mm Hg increased median LDF by 84% and BCV by 22%. The CMBC decreased 27% in supine patients with 20 mm Hg of

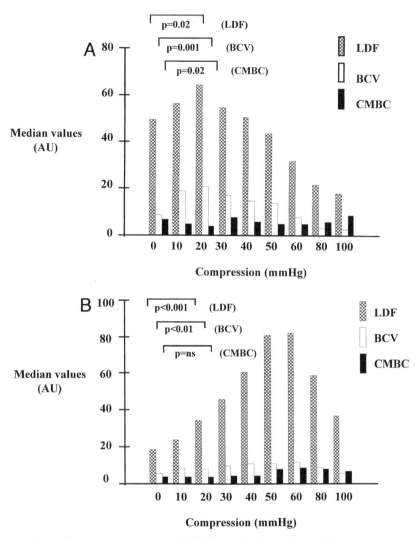

Fig 16–5.—Effect of leg compression on LDF, BCV, and CMBC in patients with lipodermatosclerosis. The medians of LDF, BCV, and CMBC are plotted in AU. *P* is Wilcoxon matched-pairs signed rank test, comparing values at 20 mm Hg compression with basal values at 0 mm Hg. A, horizontal position. B, dependent position. *Abbreviations: LDF*, laser Doppler flux; *BCV*, blood cell velocity; *CMBC*, concentration of moving blood cells; *AU*, arbitrary units; *ns*, not significant. (Courtesy of Abu-Own A, Shami SK, Chittenden SJ, et al: Microangiopathy of the skin and the effect of leg compression in patients with chronic venous insufficiency. *J Vasc Surg* 19:1074–1083, 1994.)

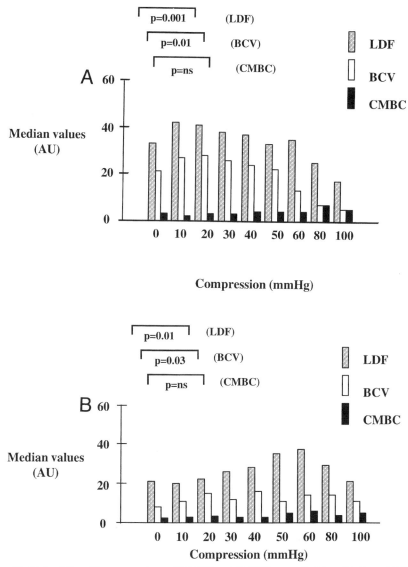

Fig 16–6.—Effect of leg compression on LDF, BCV, and CMBC in control subjects. Medians of LDF, BCV, and CMBC are plotted in AU. *P* is Wilcoxon matched-pairs signed rank test, comparing values at 20 mm Hg compression with basal values at 0 mm Hg. **A**, horizontal position. **B**, dependent position. *Abbreviations: LDF,* laser Doppler flux; *BCV,* blood cell velocity; *CMBC,* concentration of moving blood cells; *AU,* arbitrary units; *ns,* not significant. (Courtesy of Abu-Own A, Shami SK, Chittenden SJ, et al: Microangiopathy of the skin and the effect of leg compression in patients with chronic venous insufficiency. *J Vasc Surg* 19:1074–1083, 1994.)

compression but did not change significantly when the patient was sitting. Similar but less marked changes were seen in the controls (Figs 16–5 and 16–6).

Conclusion.—Part of the clinical effect of compression in patients with chronic venous insufficiency may represent an increase in blood flow velocity in the microcirculation of the leg.

▶ Once again, Doppler fluxmetry rears its ugly head. I refuse to take Doppler fluxmetry seriously until someone convincingly demonstrates what it is measuring. These authors suggest that isolated compression beneath a cuff locally increases Doppler fluxmetry. Remarkably, they conclude that this may be part of the benefit of compressive hosiery in chronic venous disease. Predictably, the senior author attempts to relate this observation to a reduction in leukocyte sludging, a favorite theory of his. Stay tuned. I am sure there will be more to follow.

Saphenous Vein Reflux Without Incompetence at the Saphenofemoral Junction
Abu-Own A, Scurr JH, Smith PDC (Univ College London Med School)
Br J Surg 81:1452–1454, 1994   145-96-16–11

Background.—When duplex ultrasonography is done in patients with primary varicose veins, reflux in the long saphenous vein (LSV) commonly occurs despite a competent saphenofemoral junction (SFJ).

Methods.—Duplex ultrasonography was performed in 167 consecutive patients given a clinical diagnosis of primary varicose veins.

Results.—Reflux of the LSV was identified in 190 extremities, 63 of which lacked findings of an incompetent SFJ. Perforating veins were incompetent in only 5 of these extremities, including perforators in the midthigh in 2 limbs and medial calf perforators in 3 limbs.

Conclusions.—Reflux of the LSV is frequently associated with a competent SFJ. In these cases, saphenofemoral ligation alone is not likely to control varices. Primary varicose veins may develop in an ascending rather than a descending sequence.

▶ A significant number of patients with LSV varicosities do not have incompetence of the SFJ, leading the authors to suggest that in a significant number of patients, LSV varicosities may represent an ascending rather than a descending phenomenon. I wonder.

Iliocaval Complications of Retroperitoneal Fibrosis
Rhee RY, Gloviczki P, Luthra HS, Stanson AW, Bower TC, Cherry KJ Jr (Mayo Clinic and Found, Rochester, Minn)
Am J Surg 168:179–183, 1994   145-96-16–12

Background.—Retroperitoneal fibrosis is known to compress the ureters as well as the nerves and blood vessels in the abdomen, but clinically significant obstruction of large veins has rarely been reported.

Patients.—Seven of 340 patients seen over 17 years with retroperitoneal fibrosis had iliocaval complications. Six of them were seen with features of chronic obstruction, whereas 1 had acute iliocaval thrombosis and underwent immediate venous thrombectomy. Limb edema was a constant feature. Three patients had venous claudication. In all cases, iliocaval occlusion was confirmed by venography, CT, or MRI. The iliocaval tree was involved in 4 cases, the inferior vena cava alone in 2, and the iliac vein alone in 1.

Management and Outcome.—Five patients were treated conservatively by elevation of the legs, compression stockings, and anticoagulation. Two patients were given prednisone. Four of these 5 patients continued to have limb edema. One patient had iliocaval bypass from the external iliac vein to the juxtarenal cava using a ringed polytetrafluoroethylene graft with a femoral arteriovenous fistula (Fig 16–7). Another patient, who had isolated obstruction of the left common iliac vein, underwent a left-to-right femorofemoral saphenous vein bypass (Fig 16–8). Symptoms of venous insufficiency resolved in both these patients. Their grafts remained patent 25 months and 1 year, respectively, after surgery.

Conclusions.—Most patients with iliocaval obstruction complicating retroperitoneal fibrosis may be managed conservatively, but reconstruction

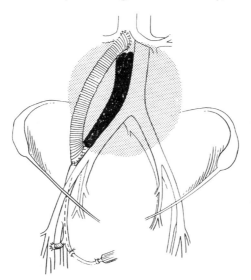

Fig 16–7.—Bypass of the right iliocaval obstruction secondary to retroperitoneal fibrosis with a 14-mm ringed expanded polytetrafluoroethylene (ePTFE) graft. Note the right saphenous vein to femoral artery fistula with an ePTFE sleeve. (Courtesy of Rhee RY, Gloviczki P, Luthra HS, et al: Iliocaval complications of retroperitoneal fibrosis. *Am J Surg* 168:179–183, 1994. Reprinted with permission from *American Journal of Surgery.*)

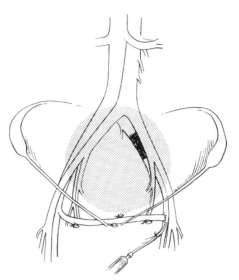

Fig 16–8.—Left to right femorofemoral venous bypass (Palma procedure) for an isolated common iliac vein obstruction secondary to retroperitoneal fibrosis. (Courtesy of Rhee RY, Gloviczki P, Luthra HS, et al: Iliocaval complications of retroperitoneal fibrosis. *Am J Surg* 168:179–183, 1994. Reprinted with permission from *American Journal of Surgery.*)

is feasible for patients who remain symptomatic from chronic venous obstruction. Lifelong anticoagulant therapy should be considered for patients with progressive obstruction.

▶ A remarkable 340 patients with retroperitoneal fibrosis were treated at the Mayo Clinic over 17 years. Seven patients had signs of vena caval compression. Two patients underwent vein bypass, with relief of symptoms at 12 and 25 months. Lifetime anticoagulation is recommended. I continue to be fascinated by the occasional appearance of retroperitoneal fibrosis and its problems of ureteral and vena caval obstruction. I wonder about the relationship between retroperitoneal fibrosis and inflammatory aortic aneurysms. I am sure they are all tied together somewhere, but currently I do not know quite where. I continue to be impressed with Dr. Gloviczki's conservative management of clinical venous problems and his infrequent use of prosthetic venous bypass. I do note, however, that on those occasions when he does use such procedures, they seem to give durable relief. I wish we were all as successful in selecting patients as Dr. Gloviczki obviously has become.

Intramuscular Pressures Beneath Elastic and Inelastic Leggings
Murthy G, Ballard RE, Breit GA, Watenpaugh DE, Hargens AR (NASA Ames Research Ctr, Moffett Field, Calif)
Ann Vasc Surg 8:543–548, 1994   145-96-16–13

TABLE 1.—Intramuscular Pressure Without Leggings (Control Values)

Condition	Soleus (mm Hg)	Tibialis Anterior (mm Hg)
Supine	8 ± 1	11 ± 1
Seated	5 ± 1	9 ± 2
Standing	37 ± 5	35 ± 3
Walking		
Contraction	152 ± 26	84 ± 12
Oscillation	161 ± 29	83 ± 9
Running		
Contraction	226 ± 36	145 ± 19
Oscillation	242 ± 35	153 ± 19

(Courtesy of Murthy G, Ballard RE, Breit GA, et al: Intramuscular pressures beneath elastic and inelastic leggings. *Ann Vasc Surg* 8:543–548, 1994.)

Background.—Devices compressing the leg veins have been widely used by patients with chronic venous insufficiency and, also, by astronauts who experience orthostatic intolerance after space flight. The comparative effects of elastic and inelastic leggings on the calf muscle pump are not clear.

Objective.—Intramuscular pressure (IMP) was recorded in the soleus and tibialis anterior muscles of 11 young adults who were in good general health.

Methods.—Measurements were repeated with elastic and inelastic leggings in place and during recumbency, sitting, standing, walking, and running. Surface compression between the legging and skin was recorded with an air bladder.

Results.—Both types of leggings increased the IMP (Tables 1 and 2). Elastic leggings resulted in significantly greater surface compression than inelastic leggings while the participants recumbent, and IMP values were

TABLE 2.—Intramuscular Pressure and Compression Applied by Level 1 Elastic and Inelastic Leggings

Condition	Elastic legging			Inelastic legging		
	Soleus (mm Hg)	Tibialis Anterior (mm Hg)	External Compression (mm Hg)	Soleus (mm Hg)	Tibialis Anterior (mm Hg)	External Compression (mm Hg)
Supine	21 ± 1*	25 ± 1*	16 ± 1*	14 ± 1	8 ± 1	8 ± 1
Seated	25 ± 1	29 ± 1	16 ± 1	23 ± 1	27 ± 2	14 ± 1
Standing	56 ± 5	48 ± 2	19 ± 1	49 ± 5	45 ± 2	17 ± 1
Walking						
Contraction	162 ± 25	95 ± 11	23 ± 1	156 ± 24	91 ± 10	15 ± 1
Oscillation	153 ± 25	79 ± 10	11 ± 1	154 ± 23	81 ± 8	13 ± 1
Running						
Contraction	254 ± 35	144 ± 19	24 ± 1	241 ± 33	149 ± 17	23 ± 2
Oscillation	263 ± 33	145 ± 21	13 ± 1	247 ± 31	152 ± 17	20 ± 1

* Significantly higher than inelastic legging ($P < 0.05$).
(Courtesy of Murthy G, Ballard RE, Breit GA, et al: Intramuscular pressures beneath elastic and inelastic leggings. *Ann Vasc Surg* 8:543–548, 1994.)

significantly higher at both measurement sites with elastic leggings in place. During sitting, walking, and running, the elastic and inelastic leggings generated similar peak pressures in both muscle compartments.

Implications.—Microcirculatory deficiency and tissue damage may develop if elastic leg compression is applied for a prolonged time in a recumbent patient. Inelastic leggings are safer and may be more effective in promoting venous circulation in patients with chronic venous insufficiency.

▶ We all know external compression devices work, but why? This paper by Murthy et al. attempts to rationalize in physiologic reasons a clinical truism. It is an important physiologic study addressing alternatives in IMPs associated with position as well as with 2 forms of external compression. Intramuscular pressures are important because they relate to the absorption of edema fluid. One weakness of this study is that all participants had normal limbs; therefore, extension of the results to patients with advanced chronic venous insufficiency cannot be direct. The authors confirm the clinical maxim that patients should not wear class I or class II compression bandages to bed because blood flow will certainly be reduced in the supine position. The decreased flow may affect ulcer healing. In addition, despite the higher pressure, the authors found no difference between level I and level II elastic compression garments as to the degree of pressure in mm Hg. Finally, rigid compression devices were no different from elastic stocking compression in the degree of IMP changes. The authors fail to support several investigators' contention that muscle pump function may be improved by elastic compression. In the end, one is left to conclude that it is hard to improve on normal function.—T. O'Donnell, M.D.

▶ I am fascinated that the IMPs under stockings measured in this study were dramatically different from the subcutaneous pressures measured in our laboratory (1). An obvious explanation is that the intracompartmental pressure may be significantly by stockings, whereas the subcutaneous pressure is not. Considerable additional experimental work is needed in this area.—J.M. Porter, M.D

Reference

1. Nehler MR, Moneta GL, Woodard DM, et al: Perimalleolar subcutaneous tissue pressure effects of elastic compression stockings. *J Vasc Surg* 18:783-788, 1993.

Inappropriate Neutrophil Activation in Venous Disease
Whiston RJ, Hallett MB, Davies EV, Harding KG, Lane IF (Univ Hosp of Wales, Cardiff)
Br J Surg 81:695–698, 1994   145-96-16–14

Background.—In chronic venous hypertension, leukocytes accumulate in the dependent extremity and may be in prolonged contact with the vascular endothelium, setting the stage for oxidative damage. Intimal ulcers have healed when treated topically with allopurinol or after oral oxpentifylline. Both these drugs inhibit the production of free oxygen radicals.

Methods.—Production of oxygen radicals by neutrophils was quantified in 18 lower extremities with class 2 or 3 venous disease and in 9 normal extremities. Eleven of the former limbs had active venous ulceration. Neutrophils were isolated from samples of venous blood in the arm and leg, and free radicals were determined by chemiluminescence after stimulation with either the chemotactic peptide formyl-methionyl-leucyl-phenylalanine (FMLP) or the ester phorbol myristate acetate (PMA). Intracellular calcium levels were measured by loading cells with acetoxylmethyl ester.

Results.—The ratio of leg to arm luminescence afer FMLP stimulation was greater in patients with venous disease than in controls. No such difference was found with PMA. Activated neutrophils in blood from the leg had fewer FMLP receptors than those from arm blood. More calcium was released after neutrophils in leg blood were stimulated.

Conclusion.—Neutrophils from an area of chronic venous disease produce an inappropriate amount of oxygen free radicals through an amplified calcium-dependent signal pathway. Activation may result from inflammation in already damaged tissue or may trigger tissue damage in patients with venous hypertension.

▶ The authors believe that neutrophils from patients with chronic venous disease produce more oxygen free radicals than neutrophils from normal patients and that this occurs because of amplification of a calcium-dependent signal pathway. If in some way chronic venous hypertension *does* activate neutrophils and these neutrophils, in turn, damage endothelium, we may have a unifying hypothesis for the production of venous ulcers. I suspect it will not be this simple.

Sclerotherapy

Local Transdermal Glyceryl Trinitrate Has an Antiinflammatory Action on Thrombophlebitis Induced by Sclerosis of Leg Varicose Veins

Berrazueta JR, Fleitas M, Salas E, Amado JA, Poveda JJ, Ochoteco A, Sánchez de Vega MJ, Ruiz de Celis G (Universidad de Cantabria, Santander, Spain)
Angiology 45:347–351, 1994   145-96-16–15

Background.—Recent observations have suggested that transdermal glyceryl trinitrate (GTN) relieves the inflammatory manifestations of infusion-related thrombophlebitis and that it may have an analgesic action.

Methods.—A double-blind, randomized, controlled trial of GTN oint-ment was conducted in 21 patients with mild to moderate varicosities of the legs who underwent bilateral sclerotherapy. Either GTN or placebo ointment was applied along the surface of sclerosed veins at 8-hour inter-vals.

Results.—When assessed 15 minutes after initial treatment, the scle-rosed veins treated with GTN ointment were less than half as intensely inflamed as those treated with placebo ointment. All placebo recipients still had evidence of thrombophlebitis an hour later, but more than one third of those treated with active ointment were free of evident inflammation. All veins in actively treated patients appeared normal within 48 hours, but almost half of those in placebo recipients required longer for signs of inflammation to totally resolve.

Conclusions.—Administered transdermally, GTN speeds the resolution of venous inflammation in patients with sclerotherapy-related throm-bophlebitis. Nitric oxide released from GTN may exert a direct anti-inflammatory action on the inflamed veins and surrounding tissues.

▶ This randomized study examined the effect of topically applied transder-mal GTN compared with that of placebo as an aid in reducing the inflamma-tion and pain associated with cutaneous sclerotherapy. It finds significant benefit with the GTN preparation. It seems like a harmless suggestion, and I suspect those performing sclerotherapy may want to try this.

Hyperosmolar Versus Detergent Sclerosing Agents in Sclerotherapy: Effect on Distal Vessel Obliteration
Sadick NS (New York, NY)
J Dermatol Surg Oncol 20:313–316, 1994   145-96-16–16

Background.—Sclerosing agents are intended to destroy the vascular endothelium locally as far as the adventitia; at the same time, they should not be markedly thrombogenic. They are rapidly inactivated so that dis-tant tissues will not be damaged. Detergent-type sclerosants are suspected of being more likely to cause distal sclerosis than hyperosmolar agents.

Methods.—The ability of a detergent sclerosant, polidocanol (POL), and a hyperosmolar agent, hypertonic saline (HS), to obliterate distal vessels was studied in vivo in 20 women with symmetrical reticular vessels 2–3 mm in diameter in opposite lower extremities. The vessels were injected with 0.5 mL of either 0.5% POL or 23.4% HS, and compression of 20 to 30 mm Hg was maintained for 72 hours. The extent of sclerosis was measured from the inferior patellar tendon at intervals up to 16 weeks after injection.

Results.—Vascular sclerosis extended just over 6 cm from the patellar tendon after injection of each sclerosant. In each case, the treated vessels were no longer clinically seen after 6–6.5 weeks.

Conclusion.—Detergent and hyperosmolar sclerosants have a similar potential for obliterating vessels beyond the injection site.

▶ I have never known the optimal material to use for cutaneous sclerotherapy. The authors note that the only sclerosing agents approved for use by the Food and Drug Administration are sodium morrhuate, ethanolamine oleate, and sodium tetradecyl sulfate. Hypertonic saline is only approved for use as an abortifacient. Polidocanol is currently in a phase III clinical trial in the United States, which it is hoped will lead to a new drug approval. At any rate, this comparative study generally found that HS and POL were similar. Currently, I do not know what the optimal sclerotherapy agent should be. In our clinic we use sodium tetradecyl.

Lymphedema

OK-432 Therapy in 64 Patients With Lymphangioma
Ogita S, Tsuto T, Nakamura K, Deguchi E, Iwai N (Children's Research Hosp, Kyoto Prefectural Univ of Medicine, Japan)
J Pediatr Surg 29:784–785, 1994   145-96-16–17

Background.—OK-432 is a lyophilized preparation of a low-virulence strain of *Streptococcus pyogenes* of human origin. Intralesionally administered OK-432 has been used as an alternative treatment for lymphangioma.
Methods.—Forty-six lymphangiomas were treated primarily by intralesional OK-432. Fourteen other lesions were treated in this way after surgery had failed to remove all of the lesion. In 4 other cases, bleomycin treatment had failed.
Results.—Half of the lesions treated primarily by intralesional injection of OK-432 completely resolved without serious complications. Eight other lesions markedly responded to injection, whereas 12 responded to a slight degree and 3 did not respond at all. All but 2 of 24 cystic lesions responded significantly with treatment, but only 9 of 22 cavernous lesions were improved. Five of the 14 incompletely removed lymphangiomas improved after injection, as did 2 of the 4 previously treated with bleomycin. No recurrences developed during a follow-up interval ranging from 6 months to 7 years. The only side effects were fever and local inflammation; no scars formed.
Conclusion.—Intralesional injection of OK-432 is a safe and effective primary treatment for lymphangioma.

▶ We have seen an increasing interest in the use of drugs for treating lymphangiomas and hemangiomas. Elsewhere in this YEAR BOOK (Abstracts 145-96-1–49 and 145-96-4–18) is reported the use of both interferon-α and antiangiogenesis factor in the treatment of hemangioma. Now we learn that the injection of a lymphangioma with a low-virulence strain of *S. pyogenes* (OK-432) may result in significant improvement in lymphangioma. Total shrinkage was noted in 23 patients, marked shrinkage in 8, slight shrinkage in 12, and no response in only 3. The inflammation did not lead to any scar formation.

Percutaneous Sclerotherapy of Lymphangiomas
Molitch HI, Unger EC, Witte CL, vanSonnenberg E (Univ of Arizona, Tucson; Univ of Texas, Galveston)
Radiology 194:343–347, 1995   145-96-16–18

Objective.—Sclerotherapy was performed using a percutaneous image-guided technique to treat unresectable lymphangiomas in 5 patients. Two patients had lymphangiomas of the pelvis, whereas 1 each had a lesion in the neck, abdomen, and lower extremity.

Methods.—Doxycycline was used as the sclerosant. The volume injected ranged from 5 to 100 mL, depending on the volume of the lymphangiomatous cavity. The procedure was guided by CT, and lymphoscintigraphy, ultrasonography, and MRI were done as needed. The catheter was closed for 6–8 hours after sclerosant was injected and was then aspirated and placed on drainage. Two to 3 treatments generally were given at 24-hour intervals.

Results.—All 5 patients achieved some relief of the symptoms of lymphedema and lymphorrhea or a decrease in size of the lymph pools (table). The dramatic response in 1 of the patients with pelvic lymphangiomatosis is shown in Figure 16–9.

Conclusions.—Percutaneous sclerotherapy using doxycycline is a safe palliative approach to unresectable lymphangiomas. Long-term follow-up is necessary to detect signs of recurrent or new lymphangiomatosis.

Clinical Data and Response to Percutaneous Sclerotherapy

Patent No./ Age (y)/Sex	Location of Lymphangioma	Initial Symptoms	Response to Therapy	Length of Follow-up (mo)
1/16/F	Pelvis, vulva, groin	Vaginal lymphorrhea, inguinal lymphedema	Resolution of vaginal lymphorrhea	24
2/19/M	Pelvis, lower extremity	Massive lymphedema of extremity, lymphorrhea	Decrease in lymphedema, resolved lymphorrhea	10
3/44/F	Neck, anterior mediastinum, chest	Dyspnea, mass effect, deformity	Resolution of mass	24
4/28/F	Left upper quadrant of abdomen, lung, spleen, kidneys	Left upper quadrant abdominal pain	Decrease in mass, resolution of pain	6
5/3/M	Leg	Mass, swelling	Decrease in mass	5

Note: All patients underwent prior surgical procedures.
(Courtesy of Molitch HA, Unger EC, Witte CL, et al: Percutaneous sclerotherapy of lymphangiomas. *Radiology* 194:343–347, 1995.)

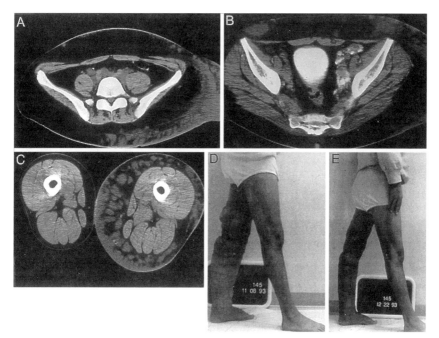

Fig 16–9.—Abdominal and pelvic lymphangiomatosis in a man, 19. **A,** CT scan through the upper pelvis depicts dysplastic deep lymphatic channels, seen as soft-tissue thickening along the iliac vessels, as well as severe left subcutaneous lymphedema. **B,** midpelvic-level CT scan obtained after injection of contrast material into the lymphangioma displays the lymphatic channels along the left iliac vasculature. **C,** massive left leg lymphedema with striking leg asymmetry is seen on this midthigh-level CT scan. **D,** photograph of patient's leg before sclerotherapy. Elephantine lymphedema is shown. **E,** photograph of patient's leg several months after sclerotherapy. Dramatic reduction in lymphedema is apparent. (Photographs courtesy of Marvin Boris, MD, Lymphedema Therapy, Woodbury, NY.) (Courtesy of Molitch HA, Unger EC, Witte CL, et al: Percutaneous sclerotherapy of lymphangiomas. *Radiology* 194:343–347, 1995.)

▶ In 5 patients with unresectable lymphangiomas of the pelvis, intralesional injection with the sclerosant doxycycline appeared to produce significant relief. It is obvious that we should consider both OK-432 and doxycycline sclerosant in the treatment of selected lymphangiomas. See comment after Abstract 145-96-16–17.

17 Portal Hypertension

Three Decades of Experience With Emergency Portacaval Shunt for Acutely Bleeding Esophageal Varices in 400 Unselected Patients With Cirrhosis of the Liver
Orloff MJ, Orloff MS, Orloff SL, Rambotti M, Girard B (Univ of California, San Diego; Univ of Rochester, NY; Univ of California, San Francisco; et al)
J Am Coll Surg 180:257–272, 1995   145-96-17–1

Background.—In patients with portal hypertension and esophagogastric varices, the emergency treatment of acute bleeding is of paramount importance. In 1958, the authors began conducting prospective studies of the various forms of emergency treatment of variceal bleeding, including conventional medical therapy, transesophageal variceal ligation, and especially emergency portacaval shunting (EPCS). The results of EPCS for acutely bleeding esophageal varices in 400 patients with cirrhosis of the liver were reported.

Methods.—The patients were treated from 1963 to 1990. All patients underwent EPCS within 8 hours of initial contact. They were unselected in that EPCS was not denied to any patient with variceal bleeding caused by hepatic disease. A well-defined protocol was followed consistently, and the study data were collected prospectively.

One hundred eighty patients were treated from 1963 to 1978, and 220 were treated from 1978 to 1990. The 1-year follow-up rate of 100% decreased only to 97% at 10 years, and 96% of the patients had EPCS at least 5 years previously. Acute variceal bleeding and cirrhosis were confirmed in every patient; 95% of the patients had alcoholic cirrhosis. Eleven percent of the patients were in Child's risk class A, 65% were in class B, and 24% were in class C. Direct portacaval shunting was performed in all patients, side-to-side in 85% of the cases. This operation decreased the mean portal vein to inferior vena caval pressure gradient from 271 to 21 mm of saline solution.

Results.—Variceal bleeding was controlled immediately and permanently in 99% of the patients. The rate of shunt thrombosis was just 0.5%. For patients in the early group, survival was 58% at 30 days, 40% at 5 years, and 30% at 10 and 15 years. For the recent group, survival improved to 85% at 30 days, 78% at 5 years, 71% at 10 years, and 57% at 15 years (Fig 17–1). Seventy percent of the patients in the recent group abstained from alcohol and had improved liver function values and

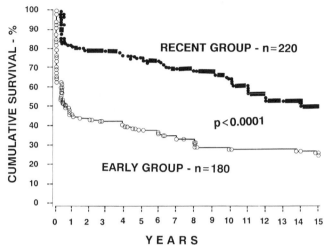

Fig 17–1.—Fifteen-year Kaplan-Meier curves after emergency portocaval shunt in the early group and recent group unadjusted by age and sex for the California population. *Abbreviation: n* number of patients. (Courtesy of Orloff MJ, Orloff MS, Orloff SL, et al: Three decades of experience with emergency portocaval shunt for acutely bleeding esophageal varices in 400 unselected patients with cirrhosis of the liver. *J Am Coll Surg* 180:257–272, 1995. By permission of the *Journal of the American College of Surgeons.*)

Child's class. The rate of recurrent portal-systemic encephalopathy was 9% in the early group and 8% in the recent group.

Conclusions.—For patients with cirrhosis of the liver and bleeding esophageal varices, EPCS yields considerable improvements in survival and quality of life. With prompt diagnosis and surgery, an organized approach to care, and lifelong follow-up emphasizing abstinence from alcohol and control of dietary protein, good results can be reliably achieved. If the patient's bleeding is permanently controlled, liver transplantation will probably not be needed.

► I have been reporting slices of Dr. Orloff's experience in recent YEAR BOOKS (1, 2). We have now come to the mother lode. He reports in this article his experience with 400 emergency portacaval shunts performed over 27 years. His results are absolutely amazing. Ninety-nine percent of the patients had immediate and permanent control of bleeding; shunt thrombosis occurred in only 2 patients; and the survival rate in the recent group was 78%, 71%, and 57% at 5, 10, and 15 years. It is absolutely clear to me that Dr. Orloff's emergency surgery for acutely bleeding varices has produced outstanding results. I have grave reservation as to whether this can be duplicated at other centers. Nonetheless, this does not diminish my admiration for Dr. Orloff's results.

References

1. 1994 YEAR BOOK OF VASCULAR SURGERY, p 455.
2. 1995 YEAR BOOK OF VASCULAR SURGERY, p 37.

Budd-Chiari Syndrome: Successful Treatment by Percutaneous Trans-luminal Angioplasty
Fock KM, Chan CC, Khoo TK (Toa Payoh Hosp, Toa Payoh Rise, Singapore)
Australas Radiol 37:108–110, 1993   145-96-17–2

Background.—The Budd-Chiari syndrome is a rare disorder caused by obstructed hepatic veins. Except in the unusual case in which obstruction is caused by hepatic vein webs or a membranous structure in the inferior vena cava, the prognosis is poor. Such cases are seen more often in Asia and may be managed by percutaneous transluminal angioplasty.

Case Report.—Boy, 17 years, had pain develop in the left hypochondrium, anorexia, nausea, and tea-colored urine. He had an enlarged liver and the classic "spider web" appearance of collateral vessels on wedged hepatic venography. There was no antegrade flow into the inferior cava, and the hepatic segment of this vessel was compressed by the enlarged caudate lobe. Percutaneous angioplasty was done using an 8-mm balloon to obliterate a web, and antegrade flow into the inferior cava was subsequently confirmed. The liver decreased in size and the patient improved clinically.

Indications.—Percutaneous transluminal angioplasty is a useful approach to focal stenosis of the hepatic veins or inferior cava caused by a congenital or postinflammatory web, as well as segmental stenosis or occlusion of the hepatic part of the inferior vena cava.

▶ This is an interesting case report of the Budd-Chiari syndrome success-fully treated in the short-term by balloon venoplasty. Abundant evidence in recent years indicates that the Budd-Chiari syndrome in most patients re-sults from thrombosis of the hepatic veins, with thrombus spilled over into the retrohepatic vena cava. The thrombus then partially lyses and partially thromboses, leaving a fibrotic residual that is the real cause of the long-term Budd-Chiari syndrome. I am not surprised that balloon venoplasty is suc-cessful on occasion. I believe this is the initial treatment of choice in these patients.

Mesocaval Interposition Shunt With Small-Diameter Polytetrafluoro-ethylene Grafts in Sclerotherapy Failure
Paquet K-J, Lazar A, Koussouris P, Hotzel B, Gad HA, Kuhn R, Kalk J-F (Heinz Kalk Hosp, Bad Kissingen, Germany)
Br J Surg 82:199–203, 1995   145-96-17–3

Objective.—The results of mesocaval interposition shunt placement were examined in 57 adult patients with portal hypertension and recurrent bleeding from esophageal varices who had not responded to sclerotherapy.
Patients.—Thirty-one patients (table) had Child-Pugh grade A disease; 26 had grade B disease. Liver volumes ranged from 1,000 to 2,500 mL.

Demographic Features, Etiology, and Severity of Liver Disease in 57
Consecutive Patients Selected for Elective Small-Lumen Mesocaval
Interposition Shunting

Mean (s.d.) age (years)	60(16)
Sex ratio (M:F)	37:20
No. with alcoholic cirrhosis*	46(81)
No. with non-alcoholic cirrhosis*	8(14)
No. with extrahepatic block*	3(5)
Child-Pugh grade*	
A	31(54)
B	26(46)

* Values in parentheses are percentages.
(Courtesy of Paquet K-J, Lazar A, Koussouris P, et al: Mesocaval interposition shunt with
small-diameter polytetrafluoroethylene grafts in sclerotherapy failure. *Br J Surg* 82:199–203, 1995.
Reprinted by permission of Blackwell Science, Ltd.)

Methods.—The patients received an externally supported, ringed polytetrafluoroethylene prosthesis 10 or 12 mm in diameter. Follow-up ranged
from 16 months to 6 years.

Results.—Postoperative mortality was 5%. Two patients had recurrent
variceal bleeding immediately after surgery and 1 in the second year after
surgery. Shunt patency (Fig 17–2) occurred at a cumulative rate of 95%.
Nine percent of patients had encephalopathy that was controlled by protein restriction, lactulose treatment, or both. The overall actuarial survival
at 6 years was 78%; survival was 88% for patients with Child-Pugh grade
A disease and 67% for those with grade B involvement.

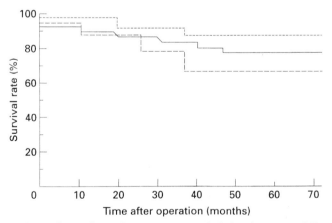

Fig 17–2.—Actuarial survival using the nonparametric method of Kaplan-Meier. *Solid line* indicates all
patients; *short-dashed line*, Child-Pugh grade A (n = 31); *long-dashed line*, Child-Pugh grade B (n = 26).
(Courtesy of Paquet K-J, Lazar A, Koussouris P, et al: Mesocaval interposition shunt with small-diameter
polytetrafluoroethylene grafts in sclerotherapy failure. *Br J Surg* 82:199–203, 1995. Reprinted by permission of Blackwell Science, Ltd.)

Conclusion.—Mesocaval interposition shunting with a small-lumen prosthesis is an effective way to achieve portal decompression while preserving hepatopetal blood flow in patients with recurrent esophageal variceal hemorrhage.

► What makes this group different is the preponderance of patients with Child-Pugh class A and B. Overall, control of bleeding, was good and the incidence of encephalopathy was admirably low at 9%. The actuarial survival of 78% at 6 years is excellent. The small side-to-side shunt preserving hepatic flow does appear to be associated with a desirably low incidence of postoperative encephalopathy. Please see also the comment after Abstract 145-96-17–4, which is next.

Analysis of Nutrient Hepatic Blood Flow After 8-mm Versus 16-mm Portacaval H-Grafts in a Prospective Randomized Trial
Rypins EB, Milne N, Sarfeh IJ (Univ of Illinois, Chicago; Univ of California, Irvine; VA Med Ctrs, Long Beach, Calif)
Am J Surg 169:197–201, 1995   145-96-17–4

Background.—Unrandomized studies have indicated that postoperative portasystemic encephalopathy (PSE) is less frequent after partial portacaval shunting with an 8-mm-diameter H-graft and collateral ablation than after total portacaval shunt surgery. This may be true, because use of an 8-mm graft preserves some nutrient hepatic blood flow.

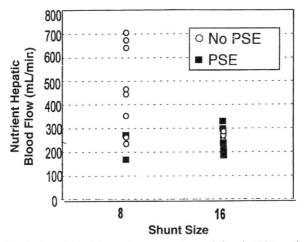

Fig 17–3.—Nutrient hepatic blood flow and portasystemic encephalopathy *(PSE)* are shown separated by shunt size. Patients with total shunts tended to cluster below 350 mL/min, whereas patients with partial shunts had a greater variability in their nutrient hepatic blood flows. (Courtesy of Rypins EB, Milne N, Sarfeh IJ, et al: Analysis of nutrient hepatic blood flow after 8-mm versus 16-mm portacaval H-grafts in a prospective randomized trial. *Am J Surg* 169:197–201, 1995. Reprinted with permission from *American Journal of Surgery.*)

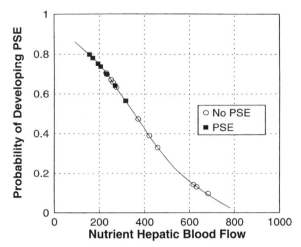

Fig 17–4.—The probability of portasystemic encephalopathy (*PSE*) developing was predicted using logistic regression (all patients are shown). Nutrient flows are plotted on the *line*. Patients with encephalopathy are represented by *filled squares*, and patients without encephalopathy at the time of this report are represented by *open circles*. (Courtesy of Rypins EB, Milne N, Sarfeh IJ, et al: Analysis of nutrient hepatic blood flow after 8-mm versus 16-mm portacaval H-grafts in a prospective randomized trial. *Am J Surg* 169:197–201, 1995. Reprinted with permission from *American Journal of Surgery.*)

Methods.—Nutrient hepatic blood flow was quantified using technetium-99m-Mebrofenin in 10 patients randomly assigned to receive an 8-mm partial portacaval shunt and in 8 others given 16-mm total portacaval H-graft shunts. Blinded observers determined whether PSE was present.

Results.—Encephalopathy developed in 2 of the 10 patients given partial shunts and in 5 of the 8 with total shunts. Nutrient hepatic blood flow was significantly higher in patients with partial shunts than in those with total shunts (Fig 17–3). The average blood flow rates were 403 for the partial-shunt group and 243 mL/min for the total-shunt group. The level of nutrient hepatic flow was the best predictor of PSE, which did not develop in any patient whose nutrient flow exceeded 325 mL/minute (Fig 17–4).

Conclusion.—A partial portacaval shunt preserves some portal blood flow and thereby allows greater nutrient blood flow to the liver than a total shunt. The risk for PSE is therefore minimized.

▶ This is an interesting, albeit small, randomized study comparing side-to-side portacaval shunts of 8-mm compared with 16-mm diameter. The evaluation of the small shunt was complicated by performance of simultaneous portocollateral ligation of the coronary, umbilical, and gastroepiploic veins. Follow-up revealed less encephalopathy in the patients who received partial shunt and increased volume of nutrient blood flow (almost double). Although this series is not large enough to be really convincing, it does add more circumstantial evidence to those favoring the performance of partial shunts. In our area, Dr. Kaj Johansen of the University of Washington has championed this procedure with convincing demonstration of benefit (1). Interestingly, in the superb series described by Orloff et al. in Abstract 145-96-17–1, only 9% of the patients in their recent series have had encephalopathy develop after surgery. They do a side-to-side shunt, but I do not know what size the shunt is.

Reference

1. 1994 YEAR BOOK OF VASCULAR SURGERY, p 456.

Call Mosby Document Express at **1 (800) 55-MOSBY** to obtain copies of the original source documents of articles featured or referenced in the YEAR BOOK series.

Subject Index*

A

Abdomen
angiography of, CT, three-dimensional
spiral, *94:* 91
injury, exsanguinating penetrating,
damage control for improved
survival, *95:* 377
insufflation for laparoscopic
cholecystectomy, venous stasis after,
95: 403
surgery, postoperative thrombosis,
prevention with low molecular
weight heparin, *94:* 416
Abscess
of foot, MRI in, *94:* 137
Acenocoumarol
in proximal vein thrombosis, and
heparin, *94:* 390
Acetazolamide
test, for risk identification of
post-carotid endarterectomy
hyperperfusion syndrome, *95:* 323
Acetylcholine
sweat test, for lumbar sympathectomy
patient selection, *96:* 294
N-Acetylcysteine
in different susceptibility to
nitroglycerine tolerance of
circulation, *94:* 49
Adenoma
aspirin use and risk for, in male health
professionals, *96:* 177
Adenosine
in postischemic spinal cord injury
complete prevention, *95:* 159
Adhesion molecule
1, intercellular
expression, adherence of endothelial
cells to Dacron inducing, *94:* 57
shear stress upregulating expression
of in vascular endothelial cells,
96: 62
Adrenal
hemorrhagic necrosis after aortic
surgery, *96:* 251
Adrenergic
vasoconstriction, α_1- and α_2-, local
temperature modulating, *94:* 48
Adrenoceptors
α_1- and α_2-, and endothelium-derived
relaxing factor, *94:* 48
Age
aortic diameter as function of, *95:* 172
determination of venous thrombi by
ultrasound tissue characterization
(in pig), *94:* 120

in venous physiologic parameters,
95: 408
Aged
aneurysm of, abdominal aortic, aortic
replacement for, *95:* 188
carotid artery disease, extracranial,
echo-Doppler of, *94:* 108
carotid atherosclerotic disease, *94:* 325
endarterectomy for, carotid, *94:* 304
healthy, low dose aspirin adverse effects
in, *95:* 16
myocardial infarction, routine
non-invasive tests do not predict
outcome after, *95:* 146
women
ankle arm blood pressure index
decrease and mortality decrease in,
95: 1
lower extremity arterial disease in,
prevalence and correlates of,
94: 241
AGM-1470
for murine hemangioendothelioma,
96: 60
Air
plethysmography, in chronic venous
insufficiency, *95:* 419
Alcohol
consumption, and carotid
atherosclerosis, Bruneck Study
results, *96:* 1
moderate intake, and myocardial
infarction risk decrease, *95:* 8
Alcoholic
cirrhosis, portacaval shunt for, *95:* 438
Aldosterone
production decrease due to heparin,
94: 6
Allograft
replacement, in situ, of infected
infrarenal aortic prosthetic graft,
94: 345
saphenous vein, cryopreserved, *94:* 366
for below-knee lower extremity
revascularization, *96:* 360
as conduit for limb salvage
procedures, *95:* 344
vein, *95:* 343
bypass, as alternative for
infrapopliteal revascularization,
95: 343
cryopreserved, as alternative coronary
artery bypass conduits, *94:* 365
Allopurinol
to prevent spinal cord injury due to
aortic crossclamping (in animals),
94: 192

---

* All entries refer to the year and page number(s) for data appearing in this and previous
editions of the YEAR BOOK.

Steroids
related complications in giant cell
arteritis, 96: 168
for Vernet's syndrome, ischemic, in
giant cell arteritis, 94: 153
Stockings
compression, in lower extremity venous
hemodynamics during laparoscopic
cholecystectomy, 96: 416
elastic
compression, and venous function
during late pregnancy, 94: 440
compression, perimalleolar
subcutaneous tissue pressure effects
of, 95: 424
in diabetic microangiopathy, 94: 138
Storage
solutions, perioperative, in long-term
vein graft function and
morphology, 95: 43
Strength
training, vs. treadmill exercise for
peripheral arterial disease, 96: 44
Streptokinase
for peripheral thrombolysis, 94: 266
Stress
cold stress testing in Raynaud's
phenomenon, 96: 145
dobutamine stress echocardiography
(see Echocardiography, dobutamine
stress)
shear
fluid, modulating expression of genes
encoding fibroblast growth factor
and platelet derived growth factor
B chain in vascular endothelium,
95: 36
fluid, reversible regulating endothelial
expression of thrombomodulin,
96: 37
in platelet derived growth factor and
fibroblast growth factor release by
arterial smooth muscle cells, 95: 35
upregulating intercellular adhesion
molecule 1 expression in vascular
endothelial cells, 96: 62
testing, cardiac, rupture of abdominal
aneurysm after, 96: 235
thallium heart imaging, and
postoperative heart complications,
96: 193
Stretch
mechanical, increasing protooncogene
expression and phosphoinositide
turnover in vascular smooth muscle
cells, 96: 64
Stroke
associated with nonrheumatic atrial
fibrillation, warfarin to prevent,
94: 13
in cardiopulmonary bypass, 96: 114
carotid endarterectomy after, benefit,
95: 303
carotid endarterectomy and, 94: 333
embolic

aortic atherosclerosis as source of,
94: 144
aortogenic, transesophageal
echocardiography in, 94: 143
European Stroke Prevention Study,
94: 319
hospitalized patients, survival trends
1970 to 1985, 95: 291
hyperhomocyst(e)inemia in, 94: 46
incidence and mortality in Hawaiian
Japanese men, trends, 96: 323
ischemic
acute, deep vein thrombosis in,
prevention with low molecular
weight heparinoid vs.
unfractionated heparin, 94: 418
and anticardiolipin antibodies, 94: 16
and hemorrhagic, in oral
anticoagulants after chronic lower
extremity ischemia reconstruction,
95: 269
recurrence risk factors for, 96: 325
risk, and aortic arch atherosclerosis,
96: 207
in urban population, 95: 285
vitamins A and E and early outcome
after, 94: 53
minor, non-rheumatic atrial fibrillation
after, secondary prevention, 95: 20
mortality, morbidity and risk factors
from 1960 through 1990, 94: 321
nondisabling, carotid artery stenosis
after, early endarterectomy for,
96: 331
prevention
after transient ischemic attacks or
cerebral infarction, 94: 319
late, from carotid stenosis, recurrent,
routine duplex ultrasound not
preventing, 94: 327
late, postendarterectomy duplex
surveillance and, 94: 327
rate
in coronary artery bypass, aortic
ultrasound in, 96: 205
long-term, in carotid endarterectomy,
94: 301
long-term, internal carotid artery
occlusion and contralateral carotid
endarterectomy, 94: 303
risk
after cerebral ischemia in women,
aspirin in, 96: 324
in carotid artery distribution, 96: 345
decrease in women and smoking
cessation, 94: 322
perioperative, in vascular and
coronary surgery, 95: 325
secondary prevention in diabetes,
antiplatelet therapy for, 94: 319
smoking and, in U.S. male physicians,
96: 12
survival, improvement during 1980s,
96: 321

Z

Author Index

A

Abdool-Carrim ATO, 167
Abolafia JM, 22
Abu-Own A, 431, 434
Acar C, 297
Ackerstaff RGA, 334
Adelman M, 188
Adelman MA, 338
Ahn SS, 87
Aho K, 41
Aichner F, 1
Aiello S, 412
Alastrue A, 404
Aldridge SC, 414
Alejo DE, 156
Alexander JJ, 272, 413
Alexander K, 76
Alexander RW, 5
Alexandrova NA, 398
Alfonso F, 137
Alimi Y, 368
Al-Khaffaf H, 341
Al-Kutoubi A, 80
Allan P, 348
Allard L, 128
Allen BT, 239
Allen DR, 240
Allen MK, 390
Allen PE, 416
Allen RC, 312
Almdahl SM, 223
Alpern MB, 125
Alter M, 325
Altomare DF, 294
Amado JA, 439
Amarenco P, 207
Amos AM, 287
Anderson C, 272
Anderson CB, 239
Anderson CM, 110
Anderson KM, 26
Andria G, 48
Anninos E, 347
Aoyama T, 160
Appleberg M, 101, 138
Aprahamian C, 377
Arcelus JI, 415
Arens C, 355
Arias A, 411
Arkoff HM, 185
Arnold T, 394
Ascherio A, 177
Asghar SS, 68
Ashton HA, 240
Atkinson K, 385
Atkinson WJ, 62
Atteberry LR, 380
Auer AI, 402
Austin JK, 326
Aveuarius H-J, 76
Azodo MVU, 96

B

Bachoo P, 242
Bacourt F, 372
Badimon JJ, 34
Badimon L, 34
Baele HR, 272
Baillot R, 222
Baird RN, 134, 284
Baker AR, 416
Baker C, 381
Baker DM, 84
Ball DS, 414
Ballard RE, 436
Bandyk DF, 140
Barie PS, 196
Barkmeier LD, 43
Barnes RW, 301, 335
Barnett HJM, 331, 354
Barone GW, 301, 335
Barone HD, 89
Barratt E, 353
Barrie WW, 270
Barros D'Sa AAB, 295
Barry R, 252
Bartoli J-M, 85
Bartoli S, 215
Baskerville PA, 145
Bassand JP, 401
Bassett FH III, 384
Basson S, 252
Baumann FG, 188
Baumgartner FJ, 391
Bauraind O, 405
Beale PG, 165
Beard JD, 191
Becquemin J-P, 370
Bednarkiewicz M, 384
Belanger AJ, 52
Belcaro G, 351
Bell A, 283
Bell PRF, 75, 111, 280
Bendahan J, 314
Berends F, 38
Bergelin RO, 102, 131, 421
Berger A, 425
Berger KR, 157
Berkman LF, 9
Berkowitz H, 170
Berman PM, 124
Berman SS, 337
Bernhard VM, 337
Bernstein EF, 123
Berrazueta JR, 439
Bertrand B, 207
Besso S, 359
Besson G, 207
Betteridge L, 66
Bevan DH, 35
Bickell WH, 390
Birkmeyer JD, 191
Bjornsson J, 161

Blackbourne LH, 234
Blackburn H, 321
Blackwood JM, 387
Blaisdell FW, 241
Blebea J, 135, 388
Blom HJ, 50
Boccuzzi SJ, 5
Bock DEM, 358
Bode-Böger S, 76
Boerbooms AMT, 68
Boers GHJ, 50
Bojar R, 137
Bolia A, 75
Bond MG, 48
Bongard FS, 391
Bookstein JJ, 94
Bos JD, 68
Bosher LP, 263
Bostom AG, 21, 52
Boswell F, 64
Boulanger B, 398
Bousser M-G, 207
Bower TC, 274, 434
Bowersox JC, 110
Bowles CA, 161
Bradbury AW, 242, 422
Brassard R, 65
Breit GA, 436
Brem H, 60
Brennan FJ, 123
Bressman P, 310
Bridgman AH, 114
Briët E, 406
Brothers TE, 276, 355
Brown CL III, 5
Brown DM, 56
Brown PS Jr, 271
Brown PW, 263
Brown WC, 64
Browning N, 252
Bruno A, 326
Bry JDL, 428
Buchanan SA, 234
Buckmaster MJ, 210
Budd JS, 280
Buehrer JL, 286
Büket S, 155
Bull C, 405
Büller H, 38
Buonocore M, 47
Burgess AM, 268, 275
Burk GL, 107
Burkart DJ, 260
Bush HL Jr, 196
Butt GR, 215
Byrne MP, 133

C

Califf RM, 23, 25, 26, 30
Callejas J Ma, 411